Psychogenic Nonepileptic Seizures

Psychogenic Nonepileptic Seizures
Toward the Integration of Care

Edited By
Barbara A. Dworetzky, MD
Department of Neurology
Chief, Division of Epilepsy
Brigham and Women's Hospital
Harvard Medical School
Boston, MA

Gaston C. Baslet, MD
Department of Psychiatry
Brigham and Women's Hospital
Harvard Medical School
Boston, MA

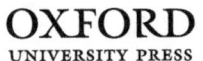

OXFORD
UNIVERSITY PRESS

Oxford University Press is a department of the University of Oxford. It furthers
the University's objective of excellence in research, scholarship, and education
by publishing worldwide. Oxford is a registered trade mark of Oxford University
Press in the UK and certain other countries.

Published in the United States of America by Oxford University Press
198 Madison Avenue, New York, NY 10016, United States of America.

© Oxford University Press 2017

All rights reserved. No part of this publication may be reproduced, stored in
a retrieval system, or transmitted, in any form or by any means, without the
prior permission in writing of Oxford University Press, or as expressly permitted
by law, by license, or under terms agreed with the appropriate reproduction
rights organization. Inquiries concerning reproduction outside the scope of the
above should be sent to the Rights Department, Oxford University Press, at the
address above.

You must not circulate this work in any other form
and you must impose this same condition on any acquirer.

Library of Congress Cataloging-in-Publication Data
Names: Dworetzky, Barbara A., editor. | Baslet, Gaston C., editor.
Title: Psychogenic nonepileptic seizures : toward the integration of care /
edited by Barbara A. Dworetzky, Gaston C. Baslet.
Description: New York, NY : Oxford University Press, [2017] |
Includes bibliographical references and index.
Identifiers: LCCN 2016035148 | ISBN 9780190265045 (alk. paper)
Subjects: | MESH: Seizures—diagnosis | Seizures—physiopathology |
Seizures—therapy | Neurobehavioral Manifestations |
Evidence-Based Practice—methods
Classification: LCC RC372 | NLM WL 340 | DDC 616.85/3—dc23
LC record available at https://lccn.loc.gov/2016035148

This material is not intended to be, and should not be considered, a substitute for medical or
other professional advice. Treatment for the conditions described in this material is highly
dependent on the individual circumstances. And, while this material is designed to offer
accurate information with respect to the subject matter covered and to be current as of the
time it was written, research and knowledge about medical and health issues is constantly
evolving and dose schedules for medications are being revised continually, with new side
effects recognized and accounted for regularly. Readers must therefore always check the
product information and clinical procedures with the most up-to-date published product
information and data sheets provided by the manufacturers and the most recent codes of
conduct and safety regulation. The publisher and the authors make no representations or
warranties to readers, express or implied, as to the accuracy or completeness of this material.
Without limiting the foregoing, the publisher and the authors make no representations or
warranties as to the accuracy or efficacy of the drug dosages mentioned in the material. The
authors and the publisher do not accept, and expressly disclaim, any responsibility for any
liability, loss or risk that may be claimed or incurred as a consequence of the use and/or
application of any of the contents of this material.

3 5 7 9 8 6 4 2
Printed by Sheridan Books, Inc., United States of America

Contents

Preface vii
Contributors List ix

Section I: Clinical Setting
1. Ambulatory Presentations in Adults and Children 3
   Mary Angela O'Neal, MD and Rochelle Caplan, MD

2. Emergency Department and Urgent Care Presentations 14
   Daniel S. Weisholtz, MD and Barbara A. Dworetzky, MD

Section II: Etiological Factors
3. Psychiatric Factors 37
   Kim Bullock, MD and John J. Barry, MD

4. Neurological and Medical Factors 67
   Victoria S. S. Wong, MD and Martin Salinsky, MD

5. Mechanisms of Possible Neurocognitive Dysfunction 86
   Daniel L. Drane, PhD and Dona E. C. Locke, PhD

6. The Neurobiology of PNES and Other Functional Neurological Symptoms 106
   David L. Perez, MD and Valerie Voon, MD, PhD

Section III: Diagnostic Procedures
7. Diagnostic Challenges for the Neurologist 123
   Jigar Rathod, MD and Selim R. Benbadis, MD

8. Diagnostic Challenges for the Mental Health Team and Psychiatrist 139
   Lorna Myers, PhD and John J. Barry, MD

9. Practical and Diagnostic Challenges for the Neuropsychologist 153
   Kim Willment, PhD and David Loring, PhD

Section IV: Principles of Treatment
10. Communicating the Diagnosis 179
    Markus Reuber, MD, PhD

11. Clinicians' Response to the Diagnosis 193
    Sigita Plioplys, MD, Shan Abbas, MD, and Brien Smith, MD

12. Models of Care 202
Tyson Sawchuk, MSc, RPsych, Joan K. Austin, PhD, RN, FAAN, and Debbie Terry, MS CNP

13. Readiness to Start Treatment and Obstacles to Adherence 218
Benjamin Tolchin, MD and Gaston Baslet, MD

Section V: Treatment Interventions

14. Evidence-Based Treatments 235
W. Curt LaFrance Jr., MD, MPH and Laura H. Goldstein, PhD, MPhil

15. The Role of the Neurologist after Diagnosis 253
Adriana Bermeo-Ovalle, MD and Andres M. Kanner, MD, FANA

16. The Roles of the Patient and Family 266
Julia L. Doss, PsyD, LP and Jeffrey Mark Robbins, MSW

Section VI: Long-Term Outcomes and Prognosis

17. Long-Term Outcomes 279
Roderick Duncan, MD, PhD

18. An Integrated Approach to Other Functional Neurological Symptoms and Related Disorders 290
Jon Stone, MB, ChB, FRCP, PhD and Alan Carson, MD

19. Toward the Integration of Care 308
Gaston Baslet, MD and Barbara A. Dworetzky, MD

Index 315

Preface

Psychogenic nonepileptic seizures (PNES), the most common of the functional neurological disorders, affect patients with multiple complex medical and psychiatric comorbidities. Over time, patients see numerous clinicians and specialists and obtain a myriad of diagnostic tests, prescriptions, and other treatments, many of which do not help them become healthier. Patients come away from the diagnostic experience feeling very confused, commonly reporting that they do not understand or accept the diagnosis, feeling blamed for their symptoms as if they should be able to control them. Many may correctly perceive that there is no physician who wants to take the responsibility to follow them. The complexity of their health issues and, in many cases, their difficult lives are mirrored by the response in our divided healthcare system.

Prognosis and outcomes for PNES are poor, which indicates that what we are doing is not effectively working for these patients. These are patients with debilitating and real symptoms who have not been taken seriously by the medical community. Whether PNES is psychological or physiological in origin should not affect whether we as healthcare workers should try to ease the suffering of these patients.

We compiled this book to begin charting a new approach to treating PNES. We have carefully gathered innovative, thoughtful experts from a variety of disciplines who share their compelling arguments for an integrated approach to PNES. The idea of integration of care is not new and has clearly demonstrated improved communication and outcomes in other disciplines where it has been used. It has not yet been applied to PNES, as neurologists and psychiatrists continue to struggle with what to name it, how to distinguish it from epilepsy, and who should take ownership of the follow-up care, rather than how to best help the patient.

Psychogenic Nonepileptic Seizures: Toward the Integration of Care does not claim to contain all the answers to managing this complex disorder. The authors give their own expertise and provide evidence where it exists. Where there is lack of evidence, we encouraged authors to draw from related functional disorders or other complex conditions, such as substance use disorder. Our compilation begins to address how to engage patients in their own recovery and how to deliver care in the most effective way. It is our hope that this book is not a static document but the beginning of a dialogue that will gather enough momentum for functional disorders like PNES to be accepted into the world of modern medicine.

Currently, medicine has become so complex and segmented that we need to take a step back and regain sight of the patient at the helm and the overarching goal of the patient's health, above all other inconveniences. We are encouraged by the power of education in effecting change. We are hopeful that students and teachers will help to forge a new path of acceptance of all patients with functional illness. We believe that change in our approach to the care of these patients is not only possible, but absolutely necessary.

This book is dedicated to the many patients who suffer from psychogenic nonepileptic seizures and deserve better understanding and more compassionate care.

Barbara A. Dworetzky
Gaston Baslet

Contributors List

Shan Abbas, MD
Department of Neurology
Spectrum Health
Grand Rapids, MI

Joan K. Austin, PhD, RN, FAAN
Indiana University School of Nursing
Indianapolis, IN

John J. Barry, MD
Department of Psychiatry and Behavioral
    Sciences
Stanford University Medical Center
Stanford, CA

Gaston Baslet, MD
Department of Psychiatry
Brigham and Women's Hospital
Harvard Medical School
Boston, MA

Selim R. Benbadis, MD
Director, Comprehensive Epilepsy
    Program
Departments of Neurology
    and Neurosurgery
University of South Florida College
    of Medicine
Tampa, FL

Adriana Bermeo-Ovalle, MD
Department of Neurological Sciences
Rush Medical College
Director, EEG Laboratory
Rush University Medical Center
Chicago, IL

Kim Bullock, MD
Department of Psychiatry and
    Behavioral Science
Stanford School of Medicine
Stanford, CA

Rochelle Caplan, MD
Semel Institute for Neuroscience and
    Human Behavior
University of California Los Angeles
Los Angeles, CA

Alan Carson, MD
Department of Clinical Neurosciences
Centre for Clinical Brain Sciences
University of Edinburgh
Western General Hospital
Department of Rehabilitation Medicine
University of Edinburgh
Edinburgh, UK

Julia L. Doss, PsyD, LP
Minnesota Epilepsy Group P.A.
St. Paul, MN

Daniel L. Drane, PhD
Departments of Neurology and Pediatrics
Emory University School of Medicine
Atlanta, GA
Department of Neurology
University of Washington School
    of Medicine
Seattle, WA

Roderick Duncan, PhD
Department of Neurology
Christchurch Hospital
Christchurch, New Zealand

Barbara A. Dworetzky, MD
Chief, Epilepsy
Department of Neurology
Brigham and Women's Hospital
Harvard Medical School
Boston, MA

Laura H. Goldstein, PhD, MPhil
Department of Psychology
Institute of Psychiatry, Psychology
　and Neuroscience
King's College London
London, UK

Andres M. Kanner, MD, FANA
Department of Clinical Neurology
Director, Comprehensive Epilepsy Center
Chief, Epilepsy Section
Miller School of Medicine
University of Miami
Miami, FL

W. Curt LaFrance Jr., MD, MPH
Rhode Island Hospital
Brown University
Providence, RI

Dona E. C. Locke, PhD
Division of Psychology
Mayo Clinic
Scottsdale, AZ

David Loring, PhD
Departments of Neurology and Pediatrics
Director, Neuropsychology
Emory University
Atlanta, GA

Lorna Myers, PhD
Northeast Regional Epilepsy Group
New York, NY

Mary Angela O'Neal, MD
Director of Women's Neurology
Brigham and Women's Hospital
Harvard Medical School
Boston, MA

David L. Perez, MD
Department of Neurology, Cognitive
　Behavioral Neurology Unit
Department of Psychiatry,
　Neuropsychiatry Unit
Massachusetts General Hospital
Harvard Medical School
Boston, MA

Sigita Plioplys, MD
Head, Pediatric Neuropsychiatry Program
Department of Psychiatry and
　Behavioral Sciences
Northwestern University Feinberg
　School of Medicine
Ann & Robert H. Lurie Childrens
　Hospital of Chicago
Chicago, IL

Jigar Rathod, MD
Department of Clinical Neurophysiology
University of South Florida College
　of Medicine
Tampa, FL

Markus Reuber, MD, PhD
Academic Neurology Unit
University of Sheffield
Royal Hallamshire Hospital
Sheffield, UK

Jeffrey Mark Robbins, MSW
Department of Neurology
Brigham and Women's Hospital
Harvard Medical School
Boston, MA

Martin Salinsky, MD
Department of Neurology
Oregon Health & Sciences University
VA Portland Health Care System
Portland, OR

Tyson Sawchuk, MSc, RPsych
Pediatric Neurosciences, Alberta
 Children's Hospital
Brain & Behavior, Alberta Children's
 Hospital Research Institute
Calgary, AB, Canada

Brien Smith, MD
Department of Neurology
Spectrum Health
Grand Rapids, MI

Jon Stone, MB, ChB, FRCP, PhD
Department of Clinical Neurosciences
Centre for Clinical Brain Sciences
University of Edinburgh
Western General Hospital
Edinburgh, UK

Debbie Terry, MS, CNP
Division of Neurology
Nationwide Children's Hospital
Columbus, OH

Benjamin Tolchin, MD
Department of Neurology
Brigham and Women's Hospital
Harvard Medical School
Boston, MA

Valerie Voon, MD, PhD
Department of Psychiatry
Behavioural and Clinical Neurosciences
 Institute
Cambridgeshire and Peterborough NHS
 Foundation Trust
Cambridge University
Cambridge, UK

Daniel S. Weisholtz, MD
Department of Neurology
Brigham and Women's Hospital
Harvard Medical School
Boston, MA

Kim Willment, PhD
Departments of Neurology and Psychiatry
Brigham and Women's Hospital
Harvard Medical School
Boston, MA

Victoria S. S. Wong, MD
Department of Neurology
Oregon Health & Sciences University
VA Portland Health Care System
Portland, OR

Section I
Clinical Setting

1

Ambulatory Presentations in Adults and Children

Mary Angela O'Neal, MD and Rochelle Caplan, MD

1. PREVALENCE

Psychogenic nonepileptic seizures (PNES) represent one of the most common diagnoses of patients referred to tertiary care centers for refractory epilepsy. The prevalence of PNES in the United States has been estimated to be 2 to 33 per 100,000 people.[1] Studies have shown that up to 71% of those afflicted with PNES are women between the ages of 15 and 35. In addition, over 40% of PNES patients have another coexisting neurological condition.[2] These patients have significant long-term disability, which is linked to both their underlying psychiatric morbidity and the length of time to accurate diagnosis.[3,4] They are frequently misdiagnosed as having epilepsy and treated with anticonvulsants.[5]

The prevalence of PNES in children has not been adequately studied and is reported to range from 1% to 46% among youth with epilepsy.[6] Similar to adults with PNES, the differential diagnosis of the first presentation of PNES in children and adolescents can mimic many disorders (Tables 1.1–1.3).[7] As with adults, physicians with different areas of expertise (pediatricians, family doctors, epileptologists, movement disorder neurologists, cardiologists, psychiatrists, and sleep specialists) might evaluate these children and adolescents.

Given the paroxysmal nature of PNES symptoms and of seizures due to epilepsy, seizures do not typically occur in the doctor's office, although this may happen occasionally. Physicians, therefore, have to rely on parents' or significant others' reports, which might appear to be inconsistent owing to the variability of the presenting symptoms. Since pediatric PNES occur more frequently in children with confirmed epilepsy,[6] clinicians often diagnose "break-through" seizures when a child with good seizure control begins to have new paroxysmal symptoms.

The long delay in confirming a diagnosis of PNES in youth—6.5 months to 3 years[8]— and the relationship between poor treatment outcome and long illness duration prior to PNES diagnosis,[8] as well as the cognitive and behavioral/emotional adverse effects of treatment with antiepileptic drugs (AEDs)[9] underscore the importance of early and accurate diagnosis of PNES. Early diagnosis can be achieved by clinicians having information

Table 1.1 Causes of Loss of Consciousness in Adults and Children

Causes of Loss of Consciousness/ Memory	Clinical Characteristics	Risk Factors
Generalized seizure Childhood absence seizures	Postictal confusion, lateral tongue bite, incontinence, cyanosis, minutess in duration, distractibility, no postictal confusion	Genetic, head trauma, structural brain abnormality, metabolic derangements, fever age 5 months to 5 years
Focal dyscognitive seizure	Stereotyped, postictal confusion, automatisms, minutes in duration	Structural brain abnormality
Syncope	Setting—micturition, blood draw, exercise; nausea/vomiting, diaphoresis, tunnel vision, pallor, no post-event confusion	Cardiovascular, older age, vasovagal syncope more common in young women
PNES	Not stereotypic, can occur out of pseudosleep, can occur with triggers, usually no incontinence	**Adults:** PTSD, anxiety, depression **Children:** Anxiety disorders, depression; past medical illnesses; adversities (bullying); learning difficulties; social problems; family dysfunction
Migraine	Prominent headache associated with nausea/vomiting, hormonal triggers, changes in barometric pressure, visual aura (scintillating scotoma or fortification spectra)	Genetic, more common in young women
Obstructive sleep apnea (adults)	Excessive daytime somnolence, snoring	Obesity, thick neck
Parasomnias	Childhood onset, occur during first part of the night, seconds to 1 hour in duration, not stereotyped	Genetic
Encephalopathy	Hours in duration, confusion, visual or tactile hallucinations	Dementia, substance use, medical illness
Transient global amnesia (adults)	Hours in duration, can carry out complex activities, repetitive questions demonstrating poor recent memory	Migraine, can be triggered by cold, sexual activity, exercise
Breath-holding spells	Brief LOC, no post-event confusion, Children age 1.5–3 years	Genetic, triggered when child does not get what he or she wants

FH = Family history; LOC, loss of consciousness; PNES, psychogenic nonepileptic spells; PTSD, post-traumatic stress disorder.

Table 1.2 Shaking Spells in Adults and Children

Spells Associated with Shaking	Clinical Characteristics	Risk Factors
Seizures	Sudden onset, stereotyped, tonic, clonic, tonic-clonic, atonic, myoclonic, aura, 15 seconds to 3 minutes in duration, variable presence of postictal confusion	Head trauma, vascular, neoplastic, degenerative, anoxic, genetic, metabolic derangement, infection
Limb-shaking TIA	Brief, involuntary irregular, wavering movement involving arm-hand alone, or arm-hand and leg together; no amnesia, minutes in duration, sudden onset, often with standing or hypotension	Vascular, older individuals
Movement disorders		
a. RLS/PLM	PLM—repetitive, rhythmic, cramping movements, occurs in sleep often associated with RLS. RLS is present in waking. Sensorimotor disorder is characterized by an overwhelming urge to move the legs.	Iron deficiency, peripheral neuropathy, genetic, alcohol use, ADHD, pregnancy, Parkinson's, ESRD, serotonergic antidepressants; occurs in women more than in men
b. RBD	Complex behaviors during REM sleep, easily awakened, lack of muscle atonia, often disrupts sleep of the bed partner	Older men, occurs with extrapyramidal disorders
c. Paroxysmal movement disorders	Dyskinesia, dystonia, myoclonus, ballismus, tics, tremor, no LOC, improvement in sleep	Genetic, structural brain disease
Encephalopathy	Myoclonus, asterixis, hours to days in duration, LOC, gradual onset	Metabolic derangement, infection, intoxication
Convulsive syncope	Myoclonic, atonic; brief duration, sudden onset, no post-event confusion	See Table 1.1
PNES	Eyelid fluttering, asymmetric limb shaking, side-to-side head movement, pelvic thrusting, can be prolonged, variable LOC, can be triggered	**Adults:** PTSD, depression, anxiety **Children:** Anxiety disorders, depression; past medical illnesses; adversities (bullying); learning difficulties; social issues; family dysfunction

ESRD, end-stage renal disease; LOC, loss of consciousness; PLM, periodic limb movements; PNES, psychogenic nonepileptic seizures; PTSD, post-traumatic stress disorder; RBD, REM behavior disorder; REM, rapid eye movement; RLS, restless leg syndrome; TIA, transient ischemic attack.

Table 1.3 Spells Associated with Falls in Adults and Children

Spells Associated with Falls	Clinical Characteristics	Risk Factors
Seizures	More common with childhood onset; atonic seizures, sudden onset, variable postictal confusion	Often associated with multiple seizure types
Postural orthostatic tachycardia syndrome (POTS)	Orthostatic spells—triggered by changes in posture; typically associated light-headedness without LOC; more common in young women	Pregnancy; autoimmune, mitochondrial, or connective tissue disorders
PNES	Variable LOC, fainting usually without injury	**Adults**: PTSD, depression, anxiety **Children**: Anxiety disorders, depression; past medical illnesses; adversities (bullying); learning difficulties; social problems; family dysfunction
Syncope	Brief LOC (lasting minutes), no post-event confusion, painful trigger for vasovagal syncope	Cardiovascular, older individuals, young women
Breath-holding spells	Brief LOC, no post-event confusion; children age 1.5–3 years; child may be cyanotic or pallid	Genetic; triggered by anger, frustration, fear, or pain
TIA	LOC variable; associated with weakness, vertigo/imbalance, visual symptoms	Vascular
Paroxysmal kinesogenic dyskinesia or dystonia	No LOC, triggered by exercise, sudden movement; childhood and young-adult onset; unilateral or bilateral involuntary movements precipitated by sudden movements, such as standing up from a sitting position, or being startled	Genetic
Cataplexy	Drop attacks, no LOC, sleep related, emotional triggers, hypnagogic hallucinations, sleep paralysis, onset in childhood to young adult	Narcolepsy in relatives
Vestibular disorder	Severe vertigo usually associated with Meniere's disease, no LOC	None

LOC, loss of consciousness; PNES, psychogenic nonepileptic seizures; PTSD, post-traumatic stress disorder; TIA, transient ischemic attack.

This is not a complete list of disorders for children and adolescents. For a detailed list by age group, see Paolicchi JM. The spectrum of nonepileptic events in children. *Epilepsia*. 2002;43(Suppl 3):60–64.

about the risk factors and red flags suggestive of a PNES diagnosis; obtaining a detailed history of the child's symptoms, how they evolved, and the perspective of both the child or adolescent and parents regarding potential stressors; and including PNES in the differential diagnosis of every child with difficult-to-control seizures. Similarly, in adults, a detailed history of the spell characteristics and triggers and the risk factors for development of PNES are important clues for making an early accurate diagnosis.

2. COMMON PRESENTATIONS OF PNES

2.1. Loss of Consciousness

Loss of consciousness (LOC) is a common presentation for many medical and neurological disorders as well as PNES. The patient's history of LOC and its medical context, such as the patient's age, past medical history, and triggers for the event, along with the details of presentation can help guide providers as to the likely etiology. There are multiple causes of LOC and the spells are intermittent, so we rely strongly on historic features, which can be inconsistent. Unresponsiveness without motor features is the most common ictal manifestation of PNES.[10] The ubiquitous presence of phone cameras has been helpful to clinicians for the diagnosis as the spell can be visually documented as it happens. The differential diagnosis is broad. Table 1.1 depicts the most common causes of LOC and their distinguishing clinical features.

Following are two case studies illustrating presentation and diagnosis of adult and adolescent PNES characterized by LOC, along with our comments on each case.

2.1.1. Case 1a–Adult PNES Characterized by LOC

A 24-year-old woman with a history of migraine with aura presented to her internist for evaluation of episodes of twitching associated with LOC. The episodes were described as different each time, some with head movements and others associated with "child-like" speech. She also had episodes of LOC without any motor features. The spells could last hours, and the patient had no memory of the events. Often they would begin with typical migraine symptoms: dots moving throughout her visual field, after which she would develop a throbbing headache, nausea, and vomiting. The spells would improve with sleep and tended to cluster around her menses. They were increasing in frequency and occurred multiple times per month. The family history was remarkable for a maternal aunt with epilepsy.

Her internist was concerned that these events might represent seizures or vasovagal events. The brain magnetic resonance imaging (MRI) was normal. The electroencephalogram (EEG) showed right temporal sharp 4–7 Hz theta slowing without clear epileptiform discharges. The patient was then referred to a neurologist, who was also concerned about seizures with a catamenial exacerbation. An EEG was repeated and was reported as showing right temporal sharp/slow waves. Lamotrigine was started, and the spells initially responded but then recurred with increasing frequency. Given the refractory nature of the episodes, she was switched to valproate and later to carbamazepine. She was then referred for a second neurological opinion and video EEG (vEEG) monitoring was arranged on an inpatient basis. A typical episode was captured and showed no epileptiform discharges during the events.

Comment: The red flags that the episodes represented PNES rather than epilepsy included that they had a painful trigger, were not stereotypic, had a prolonged duration, and did not respond to multiple AEDs. Migraine with aura could be responsible for some of the patient's symptoms. However, the "child-like" speech abnormality, repeated episodes with LOC, and spell-associated movements would be quite atypical. It was appropriate that the internist referred the patient for a neurological evaluation given the uncertain nature of the spells and the abnormal EEG. The EEG abnormality was nondiagnostic and can be seen in many conditions, including migraine. In fact, EEG abnormalities are common in PNES and contribute to the misdiagnosis of epilepsy.[11] In retrospect, owing to the ambiguous EEG test results, poor response to multiple anticonvulsants, as well as the atypical nature of the spells, earlier ambulatory EEG or referral for long-term EEG monitoring to capture the spells would have been useful.

2.1.2. Case 1b—Adolescent PNES Presenting with LOC

This 16-year-old tenth-grade, conscientious student began to faint, mainly on days she had her Advanced Placement (AP) English literature tests. Her pediatrician examined her blood pressure and heart and referred her to a cardiologist. The parents and adolescent became concerned that she might have a genetic heart problem because her first cousin was undergoing assessments for a heart murmur. The episodes of syncope then increased in frequency at school, and she became afraid of going to school because she might faint there. Her parents accessed the school website to make sure she did the homework she missed. She then began to have frequent episodes at home. The cardiologist conducted multiple diagnostic procedures, which were all negative. She missed approximately 20 days of school over a 3-month period. The patient's episodes became more frequent and prolonged with eye rolling and some movements of her limbs. She was then referred to an epileptologist. A vEEG was arranged and demonstrated no epileptiform activity during these episodes. The epileptologist referred the patient to a child psychiatrist to confirm a PNES diagnosis by demonstrating evidence for a conversion disorder.

Comment: The pediatrician did not take a detailed history and thus did not realize that the patient was a conscientious student who became anxious around the time of her AP tests. The parents obtained her homework from the website, which suggests that they might have had high academic achievement expectations for their daughter. Neither physician inquired about possible academic stressors. The cardiologist also did not ask about the patient's fears of fainting at school and about the anxiety and fear both the patient and parents experienced from the multiple medical tests he conducted. The patient missing 20 school days along with the negative cardiovascular testing should have been a red flag for the physicians that the diagnosis was PNES. The epileptologist correctly suspected that evolution of the syncope symptoms into seizure-like episodes indicated the need for a vEEG and psychiatric assessment to confirm the diagnosis of PNES.

2.2. Shaking/Motor Spells

The motor abnormalities that are often used to distinguish epileptic movements from PNES include out-of-phase limb movements, pelvic thrusting, and side-to-side head movements. In a study of 120 seizures (36 PNES and 84 epileptic seizures), the signs that were most reliable in predicting PNES were preserved awareness, eye flutter, and episodes affected by bystanders (intensified or alleviated).[12] Additional useful features include events that come out of sleep, are stereotypic, and are associated with injury such as tongue biting. Table 1.2 lists the potential etiologies of shaking.

Following are two case studies illustrating presentation and diagnosis of adult and pediatric PNES associated with shaking, along with our comments on each case.

2.2.1. Case 2a–Adult PNES Associated with Shaking

A 28-year-old right-handed woman presented to a local hospital with an acute confusional episode and a generalized seizure described as rhythmic tonic-clonic movements with urinary incontinence. The head computed tomography (CT) showed a hypodense left parietal mass. Levetiracetam and decadron were started. Subsequent brain MRI showed a left parietal mass that enhanced with gadolinium. She underwent a left parietal craniotomy with tumor resection. Pathology showed an anaplastic glioma, and treatment was initiated. Unfortunately, she had disease progression with the tumor undergoing a transformation to a glioblastoma multiforme.

She presented to her neuro-oncologist for evaluation of shaking episodes different from her prior seizures with back arching, jaw spasms, and eye deviation to the right that would last hours. A 48-hour ambulatory EEG was abnormal. It showed left more than right high-amplitude theta, particularly in the posterior quadrant, consistent with the known tumor and craniotomy. Initially the spells would occur once a month, but they increased to one to two times per week. She was admitted to the hospital to characterize the spells. The in-hospital monitoring demonstrated that these events were not due to epilepsy.

Comment: The fact that the spells were different from her prior seizures appropriately prompted a new evaluation. This case demonstrates that patients with PNES may have both epileptic and nonepileptic spells.[13] The opisthotonic motor characteristics of her new spells raised a red flag for PNES. In addition, the tempo of worsening events despite treatment is another common feature. Serious health care concerns, in particular, having a neurological problem (as illustrated in this case), are a strong risk for PNES.[14]

2.2.2. Case 2b–Pediatric PNES Associated with Shaking

An 11-year-old girl had well-controlled complex partial seizures (blank stare, chewing, clumsy meaningless random movements followed by sleep, tiredness, and confusion) that were treated with carbamazepine. She began to have episodes in which she had tongue clicking, threw things, was unresponsive, and appeared disoriented after an episode. Her mother reported breakthrough seizures to the treating epileptologist by phone, and he increased her carbamazepine dose. The episodes, which initially occurred at school, now occurred at home and increased in frequency and duration lasting up to 1 hour. After multiple emergency department (ED) visits, her epileptologist added levetiracetam to the child's medication regimen. She became tired, would fall asleep at school, and was sent home.

The patient's parents were divorced, and the mother was about to remarry in a month. The mother was working, so the father who was an independent contractor, would come to the mother's house and spend time with the child, who had stopped going to school. The parents finally convinced her to return to school but she had a prolonged "seizure" at school. An ambulance took her to the ED and she was diagnosed with complex partial seizure status. Both parents were at her bedside in the ED. She would open her eyes, see her parents talking, and then go into another prolonged "seizure." These episodes did not abate despite IV phenytoin, and she was put into phenobarbital coma. When she was taken out of the drug-induced coma, vEEG revealed no epileptiform activity during her tongue thrusting, unresponsive episodes, and when she was throwing things.

Comment: Rather than increasing the patient's AED dose via telephone, when breakthrough seizures occur, clinicians should obtain a detailed history of how symptoms start and evolve, as well as potential stressors the child and family might be facing. When seizures occur primarily at school, it is important to rule out learning difficulties. In this particular case, inquiry during a comprehensive psychiatric evaluation about the child's learning difficulties, the parents' divorce, and the mother's planned marriage—all obvious stressors—could have prevented her from being intubated and sedated by phenobarbital. This is a case of nonepileptic psychogenic status (NEPS) in a child. Further discussion on NEPS can be found in Chapter 2.

2.3. Falls

Falls are a common reason for referral to a neurology clinic. A careful history and examination usually help make the correct diagnosis. However, if the history is unreliable and the exam is normal, the correct diagnosis can be challenging. See Table 1.3.

Following are two case studies illustrating presentation and diagnosis of adult and peditric PNES associated with falls, along with our comments on each case.

2.3.1. Case 3a–PNES Associated with Falls

A 25-year-old woman presented to the psychiatry department after a suicide attempt. She experienced periods of depression as well as occasional episodes of elevated mood and high energy. She had a history of traumatic flashbacks related to sexual abuse. She had multiple different spells; some occurred at night when she would shake and become unarousable. They were associated with urinary incontinence and could lead to her falling out of bed. Afterwards, she would become agitated and aggressive. There were also daytime episodes occurring three to five times a week where she lost time and would find herself in strange places without recall of how she had gotten there. These episodes could last 5 minutes or up to several hours. She also had spells where she would fall without loss of consciousness often triggered by emotional stimuli. She presented to a psychiatrist, who made a diagnosis of bipolar illness and post-traumatic stress disorder (PTSD). The multiple spell types and their manifestations were concerning for dissociative events and the nocturnal events for epileptic seizures. A brain MRI and an EEG were normal. She was referred to neurology. The neurologist obtained a history of hallucinations that occurred around sleep onset. The episodes of falling were triggered by laughing or crying which was concerning for cataplexy. A routine EEG was again normal. A multiple sleep onset test was very abnormal due to early onset of rapid eye movement in all 4 naps. A diagnosis of narcolepsy was made. She was started on sodium oxybate. The drop attacks improved, but the other spells continued. She was referred to an epilepsy specialist and admitted for vEEG monitoring to better characterize the spells. The vEEG demonstrated that both the nocturnal as well as the prolonged episodes where she would lose track of time were PNES.

Comment: Patients may have multiple spells, each of which need to be characterized to allow for appropriate diagnosis and treatment. In addition, beware of the pitfall that the presence of psychiatric disease excludes the possibility of other medical causes for the spells.

2.3.2. Case 3b–Pediatric PNES Associated with Falls

This 10-year-old boy developed racing heart and breathlessness followed by several minutes of disorientation, falling, and LOC that lasted about 20 minutes when he arrived at school in the morning. His family doctor did a physical exam, which was normal. He diagnosed panic attacks and referred the boy to a psychiatrist. The psychiatrist saw the child with his parents and learned that the boy was in a special education class for reading difficulties. However, both the boy and his parents denied any learning problems. On the assumption that this was a panic attack, the psychiatrist prescribed sertraline for the child. Three days later during recess at school, the child had an episode of shortness of breath, sweating, heart racing, and fear that he was going to die followed by loss of consciousness and what looked like a generalized tonic-clonic seizure. An ambulance brought him to the ED by which time the episode had subsided, and his parents joined him there. A diagnosis was made of new onset epilepsy and lamotrigine was prescribed in addition to the sertraline. The child did not want to go back to school because he now had both epilepsy and a learning disorder and would be teased. The parents insisted that he return to school the next day. At recess, he had a full-blown generalized convulsion and once again was taken to the ED. The parents contacted the psychiatrist because they were concerned that something was happening at school that was stressing their son. The psychiatrist saw the boy who denied any problems and had what looked like a generalized tonic-clinic seizure in the psychiatrist's office. The psychiatrist referred the child to an epileptologist who ordered a routine EEG, which was normal. The child continued to have seizures at school despite the addition of levetiracetam to his medication regime so vEEG was arranged. The episodes he had during the vEEG occurred while his mother forced him to do his homework. He would begin to cry and sob with hyperventilation as the mother continued to insist that he do the work. He then had a generalized shaking spell during which the vEEG revealed no epileptic activity.

Comment: The psychiatrist did not assess the importance of the parents' unwillingness to accept that their child had learning problems, the academic pressure they put on him, and the fear of being teased, a form of bullying that the child experienced at school. Under these stressful environmental circumstances, the anti-anxiety drug was ineffective in preventing the child's panic attacks. This case demonstrates how stress-induced hyperventilation and the resulting hypocapnia and/or the changes in acid–base balance can trigger a nonepileptic seizure-like event.[15]

3. SUMMARY

The adult and child cases presented here demonstrate involvement of a wide range of physicians for the various presentations of PNES. These cases also emphasize the importance of obtaining a detailed history, including ancillary information from observers about the development of symptoms, their triggers, and risk factors, as well as the need to include PNES in the differential diagnosis of patients presenting with LOC, shaking, and falls. Finally, as many patients with PNES may have other neurological disorders, a high index of suspicion is needed to not attribute all their symptoms to a functional disorder.

- Patients have complex and variable presentations, so they may present to multiple different providers.
- Collaboration between clinicians can help facilitate an earlier diagnosis of PNES.
- Obtaining a detailed history is critical and should include the following:
  - Ancillary information from family members and observers of the events
  - Development of symptoms
  - Triggers of events
  - Risk factors for events
- PNES should be included in the differential of LOC, shaking, and falls.
- A high index of suspicion is needed in order to not attribute all symptoms to a functional disorder.

REFERENCES

1. Benbadis SR, Hauser WA. An estimate of the prevalence of psychogenic non-epileptic seizures. *Seizure.* 2000;9:280–281.
2. Krumholz A, Niedermeyer E. Psychogenic seizures: a clinical study with follow-up data. *Neurology.* 1983;33:498–502.
3. Kanner AM, Parra J, Frey M, Stebbins G, Pierre-Louis S, Iriarte J. Psychiatric and neurologic predictors of psychogenic pseudoseizure outcome. *Neurology.* 1999;53(5):933–938.
4. Irwin K, Edwards M, Robinson R. Psychogenic non-epileptic seizures: management and prognosis. *Arch Dis Child.* 2000;82:474–478.
5. Patidar Y, Gupta M, Khwaja GA, Chowdhury D, et al. Clinical profile of psychogenic non-epileptic seizures in adults: a study of 63 cases. *Ann Indian Acad Neurol.* 2013;16(2):157–162.

6. Reilly C, Menlove L, Fenton V, Das KB. Psychogenic nonepileptic seizures in children: a review. *Epilepsia*. 2013;54:1715–1724. doi:10.1111/epi.12336
7. Wyllie E, Glazer JP, Benbadis S, Kotagal P, Wolgamuth B. Psychiatric features of children and adolescents with pseudoseizures. *Arch Pediatr Adolesc Med*. 1999;153:244–248.
8. Gudmundsson O, Prendergast M, Foreman D, Cowley S. Outcome of pseudoseizures in children and adolescents: a 6-year symptom survival analysis. *Dev Med Child Neurol*. 2001;43:547–551.
9. Caplan R. Psychopathology in pediatric epilepsy: role of antiepileptic drugs. *Front Neurol*. 2012;3:163–169. doi: 10.3389/fneur.2012.00163
10. Leis AA, Ross MA, Summers AK. Psychogenic seizures: ictal characteristics and diagnostic pifalls. *Neurology*. 1992;42:95–99.
11. Benbadis SR, Tatum WO. Overintepretation of EEGs and misdiagnosis of epilepsy. *J Clin Neurophysiol*. 2003;20(1):42–44.
12. Syed TU, Lafrance WC Jr, Kahriman ES, et al. Can semiology predict psychogenic nonepileptic seizures? A prospective study. *Ann Neurol*. 2011;69(6):997–1004.
13. Martin R, Burneo JG, Prasad A, Powell T, et al. Frequency of epilepsy in patients with psychogenic seizures monitored by video-EEG. *Neurology*. 2003;61(12):1791–1792.
14. O'Sullivan SS, Spillane JE, McMahon EM, et al. Clinical characteristics and outcome of patients diagnosed with psychogenic nonepileptic seizures: a 5-year review. *Epilepsy Behav*. 2007;11(1): 77–84.
15. Brodtkorb E. Common imitators of epilepsy. *Acta Neurol Scand*. 2013;127:5–10. doi:10.1111/ane.12043

2

Emergency Department and Urgent Care Presentations

Daniel S. Weisholtz, MD and Barbara A. Dworetzky, MD

1. INTRODUCTION: THE PROBLEM OF EMERGENCY PRESENTATIONS

1.1. Settings

Although patients with psychogenic nonepileptic seizures (PNES) are mostly managed by neurologists, psychiatrists, and emergency department (ED) physicians, they may present in virtually any clinical setting. Because PNES may present suddenly and without warning and can be quite alarming to the patient and observers, they often trigger emergency medical responses. While few clinicians consider this condition to be one of their areas of expertise, many will encounter it—particularly those working in EDs, urgent care centers, and other primary care settings where these patients may initially seek medical care. PNES may also be encountered by surgeons and anesthesiologists when they occur perioperatively, or by obstetrician/gynecologists when they occur peripartum. All practitioners ought to have a working general knowledge of this condition. It is important that these patients be appropriately diagnosed and followed by clinicians who can help guide management.

1.1.1. The Emergency Department

Patients often find themselves in EDs early on in the course of their illness because the attacks come on suddenly and dramatically and are typically initially mistaken for epileptic seizures. Therefore, an initial ED visit may be appropriate. Patients who develop new-onset seizures ought to be evaluated urgently for structural brain lesions, infection, and other toxic or metabolic disturbances. However, once a diagnosis of PNES is made, patients are often discharged from the hospital or ED almost immediately.[1] When this occurs, there is little time to engage patients, to help them understand their condition, and to solidify a follow-up plan that will work. Therefore, they are often lost to follow-up, only to present again later to new providers who may be unaware of the previous diagnosis.[1] Patients may present to numerous hospitals, such that medical records are scattered among different institutions or providers, interfering with the acquisition of accurate and complete clinical information when a patient arrives in the ED. As a result, patients may undergo unnecessary repeat workups and be given antiepileptic drugs (AEDs) inappropriately by providers who are unfamiliar with this condition and not aware of the previous diagnosis of PNES. Some patients are not told of their diagnosis and are instead given vague explanations by doctors, such as "there's nothing wrong with you," or are treated dismissively, leading them to lose confidence in the doctors and seek help elsewhere, perpetuating the cycle. Education on PNES, including training in effective communication of the diagnosis and management strategies, is necessary for all clinicians seeing patients in the ED and urgent care settings. These clinicians must become familiar with the resources available in their region for the evaluation and treatment of these patients.[2]

1.1.2. Periprocedure PNES

PNES that occur on hospital grounds but outside of the units that are accustomed to caring for seizure patients (i.e., EDs, intensive care units [ICUs], and neurology wards) pose a special problem. Reports of PNES following procedures are scattered in the literature.[3] Medical procedures are stressful and may serve as triggers for patients who are already susceptible to PNES. There have been several reports in the obstetrics and anesthesiology literature of conversion disorder following various procedures.[4-7] This highlights a risk of invasive procedures that is often not considered. Invasive procedures may serve as a PNES trigger in susceptible patients because of the stress the process can engender. Disturbing sensations and dissociative symptoms produced by anesthetic medications may unconsciously trigger PNES. PNES may also be rendered more likely as a result of the behavioral disinhibition that can occur with some anesthetic agents, much the way agitation or aggression can be seen as a paradoxical reaction to benzodiazepines in some patients.[8] These attacks may startle and alarm clinicians unaccustomed to dealing with neurological emergencies and may provoke fears of iatrogenic harm and medicolegal liability, stimulating overreaction. Emergency presentations of PNES can lead to unnecessary repeat testing, intubation, and unnecessary ICU admissions, even when the patient has had similar episodes in the past and the diagnosis of PNES has been previously established.

1.1.3. PNES in Children

Although less well studied in children than in adults, 1–9% of children referred for evaluation of suspected epilepsy have PNES.[9] Children diagnosed with PNES and their families are sometimes reluctant to inform school administrators and nurses about the diagnosis because of fear of social stigma. School officials may feel compelled to follow standard procedures for seizures, which may involve calling 911 (68% of 27 school nurses surveyed indicated this was their school policy).[10] As in adults, ED visits may lead to the administration of unnecessary and potentially harmful treatments if the PNES diagnosis is not suspected by the evaluating clinicians. In children, this may lead to missed school days, potentially interfering with educational progress if frequent. In addition, AEDs prescribed to children may interfere with brain development,[11,12] can worsen mood or other psychiatric symptoms, and can impact cognitive functioning and academic performance. While unnecessary ED visits and AED administration should be avoided in all cases, this is of particular importance in children, whose cognitive, emotional, and social development is still underway.

1.2. Morbidity Associated with Emergency Treatments

In emergency settings, patients are often placed on AEDs when they present after multiple seizure-like events, and patients who are already taking AEDs may have their doses increased or new drugs added to their regimens since clinicians are taught to err on the side of treatment. While initial misdiagnosis is understandable, and it may be reasonable to treat with an AED when epilepsy is suspected even if the initial EEG is normal, clinicians should exercise care to avoid prescribing such medications for patients with established PNES who are presenting with their typical episodes, as these medications are not helpful and may perpetuate PNES or be harmful in other ways. Common AED side effects such as drowsiness, gastrointestinal (GI) symptoms, and cognitive and mood problems overlap with the somatic symptoms commonly experienced by PNES patients, complicating the assessment of these problems. Because of their somatic tendencies, patients with PNES are more likely to have difficulty tolerating AEDs and to experience adverse reactions.[13] In addition to the behavioral and cognitive effects just noted, AEDs may provoke allergic reactions and, in some cases, Stevens-Johnson syndrome. In addition, these medications may cause hepatotoxicity, cytopenia, hyponatremia, pancreatitis, and hyperammonemic encephalopathy depending on which drug is used[14] (Table 2.1). Several of the AEDs are strong inducers of the cytochrome P450 system and have important pharmacokinetic interactions with other medications, including oral contraceptive pills, which may in some cases lead to contraceptive failure.[15] Thus, while these medications are generally well tolerated and effective when used appropriately, they should not be considered entirely benign. When they are prescribed for patients with known PNES who do not have epilepsy, their presence on the medication list may erroneously signal to emergency medical providers that the patient has epilepsy.

1.2.1. The Problem of Nonepileptic Psychogenic Status (NEPS)

Patients who present emergently with markedly prolonged PNES are at particularly high risk for iatrogenic harm, as the condition mimics status epilepticus, a medical emergency that requires aggressive treatment. Nonepileptic psychogenic status (NEPS), formerly referred to as "pseudostatus" or "status pseudoepilepticus," has been defined as a psychogenic nonepileptic seizure lasting 30 minutes or longer, or frequent repetitive nonepileptic seizures without a return to baseline mental state in between. There is no evidence for any risk of brain damage with prolonged PNES as there is with epilepsy, and the absence of electroencephalographic (EEG) evidence of hypersynchronous neuronal activity suggests that cytotoxic injury is not a likely consequence of NEPS, as it can be in status epilepticus.[16-18] Patients also do not typically become hypoxic or develop significant metabolic derangements, as seen with epileptic convulsive seizures.[19-21] Thus, prolonged

Table 2.1. Significant Potential Adverse Reactions Associated with Specific Antiepileptic Drugs

Reaction	Associated Drugs
Agranulocytosis	Carbamazepine, phenytoin, phenobarbital, valproate
Thrombocytopenia/platelet dysfunction	Valproate
Aplastic anemia	Carbamazepine, phenytoin, valproate
Stevens-Johnson syndrome	Carbamazepine, lamotrigine, phenobarbital, phenytoin, valproate, zonisamide
Allergic dermatitis	Most antiepileptic drugs
Hepatic failure	Carbamazepine, phenobarbital, phenytoin, valproate
Pancreatitis	Carbamazepine, valproate
Hyponatremia	Carbamazepine, oxcarbazepine, eslicarbazepine
Nephrolithiasis	Topiramate, zonisamide
Appetite/weight changes	Valproate, carbamazepine, gabapentin (weight gain), topiramate and zonisamide (weight loss)
Psychiatric side effects	Levetiracetam, zonisamide, topiramate, vigabatrin

PNES is likely considerably more benign than status epilepticus, and morbidity is most likely to occur as a result of overly aggressive treatment. The onset and termination of each PNES episode is often indistinct and, in general, PNES are likely to be more prolonged than epileptic seizures.[22] Reuber and colleagues[22] compared retrospective reports of 85 patients with PNES and 64 patients with epilepsy and found that 78% of PNES patients reported that they had experienced seizures lasting for more than 30 minutes as compared with only 33% in the epilepsy group. In the same study, 27% of PNES patients reported that they had been sent to the ICU compared with 22% in the epilepsy group, and 39% had a history of recurrent hospital admissions for "status epilepticus," compared with 13% in the epilepsy group. Recurrent hospitalizations for status epilepticus should raise suspicion for PNES, particularly if EEGs have not been diagnostic for epilepsy and other PNES risk factors are present (see Chapter 3). There have been multiple cases and small series reported on NEPS and the iatrogenic dangers involved, including death.[2,23–28] Reuber et al.[2] report a case of a young man with a previously diagnosed factitious disorder who presented to a hospital he had never been to before with episodes of loss of responsiveness, rolling up of the eyes, stiffening, and body jerking lasting 1–2 minutes and recurring every 5–10 minutes with return to consciousness in between. Episodes did not respond to lorazepam or diazepam. Despite being stable metabolically, he was intubated after 6 hours of recurrent seizures and given intravenous propofol, suxmethonium, and atracrurium. Within 30 seconds of injection of atracurium, he developed electromechanical dissociation, had a cardiopulmonary arrest, and could not be resuscitated.

A survey done by the American Epilepsy Society (AES) Non-Epileptic Seizure (NES) Task Force revealed that the majority of neurologist AES members do not track PNES duration. Additionally, events lasting 20 minutes or longer were considered "markedly prolonged," consistent with NEPS.[29] There are relatively few studies exploring whether it is possible to predict who is at risk of NEPS, whether NEPS patients represent a particular subpopulation within PNES subjects, or whether NEPS is simply a severe form of PNES distinguished primarily by the responses it engenders in healthcare providers who mistake it for status epilepticus.[29] Asadi-Pooya et al.[30] compared patients with PNES only to those with NEPS and found no significant differences between the groups in demographics (age at onset, age at referral, gender, education, or marital status) or risk factors predisposing to PNES (history of abuse as a child, sexual abuse, physical abuse, head trauma, academic failure, confirmed epilepsy, family history of epilepsy, or medical comorbidity). However, patients with NEPS may have an increased tendency toward self-harm behaviors.[22] Compared to PNES patients without prolonged attacks, patients with NEPS were more likely to be admitted to the monitoring unit on an urgent basis, reported a higher frequency of attacks, and were diagnosed sooner in the course of their illness.[31] NEPS events themselves are more varied than short PNES and more likely to demonstrate convulsive movements.[32] Because of the apparent distress associated with ongoing prolonged PNES, patients often receive multiple doses of benzodiazepines when this occurs in the hospital, with the potential for behavioral and physical side effects such as respiratory depression, despite uncertain benefit.

Given the lack of data, there are no guidelines for specific treatment of NEPS. The NES task force survey responses regarding follow-up for NEPS revealed a trend favoring emergency psychiatric consultation and short-term follow-up with the referring neurologist. There was no consistency in the practice of continuing EEG monitoring or hospitalization after presentation of the diagnosis or whether to remove all AEDs to disprove concomitant epilepsy.[29] While epilepsy monitoring units (EMUs) are set up to address these diagnostic questions, they typically accommodate elective admissions, and it can be a challenge to accommodate patients who present emergently and unexpectedly.

1.2.2. PNES in Pregnancy

Seizures that occur during pregnancy cause alarm and often prompt aggressive workups and treatment because of the risks that seizures can pose to the health of a pregnancy. Generalized tonic-clonic seizures can cause maternal and fetal hypoxia, acidosis, fetal heart rate decelerations,[15] and fetal intracranial hemorrhage[33] and may raise concern for eclampsia, which, if diagnosed, may prompt urgent induction and delivery.[34] Treatments for epileptic seizures and eclampsia are not helpful for PNES and can be harmful to the pregnancy. AEDs taken during pregnancy can increase the risk for major congenital malformations and minor anomalies and can worsen neurodevelopmental outcomes.[15] NEPS has also been reported in pregnancy in a case in which inappropriate therapy may have contributed to the death of the fetus in the third trimester.[35] Admitting pregnant women into the EMU and removing medication, a process often necessary in order to diagnose PNES and exclude epilepsy, carries the risk of provoking a generalized convulsion, which could be devastating to the fetus and lead to legal ramifications.[36] Furthermore, the small but real risk of unexpected death in the EMU, possibly related to rapid anticonvulsant withdrawal,[37] may be an unacceptable risk to take in a pregnant woman. Thus, whenever possible, it is essential to clarify the diagnosis of PNES prior to conception, when a woman with uncontrolled seizures is contemplating pregnancy, so that if epilepsy is ruled out, AEDs can be withdrawn, and fetal exposure to AEDs can be prevented.

While there is very little written about pregnancy and PNES, there are multiple case reports and several small case series regarding conversion and pregnancy.[38,39] Much of this literature is largely based on observations from the obstetrics and anesthesiology services. There are a few reports on patients with new-onset PNES during pregnancy, and most of them are single case reports,[40-44] with a rare small case series.[45] If seizures present recurrently during pregnancy, PNES should be considered in the differential diagnosis, and if it is considered to be a significant possibility, diagnostic video EEG should be pursued urgently before escalating medications.[46] This may be done without removing AEDs, if this is felt to be too risky. DeToledo et al.[39] reported five cases of PNES that occurred in pregnancy and concluded that PNES may signal serious emotional instability for the patient and thus a potential concern for the unborn fetus. We are familiar with a case in which a pregnant woman with PNES repeatedly fell on her abdomen during her attacks.[1] This highlights the potentially dangerous nature of the attacks themselves and the need for treatment. The two patients in the series by DeToledo et al. who presented with PNES after learning they were pregnant were dealing with unwanted pregnancies and were from religious families that disapproved of abortion. Self-injurious behaviors occurring in the midst of a PNES, particularly those that are potentially harmful to the fetus, may reflect unconscious ambivalence about the pregnancy. In these cases, urgent psychiatric consultation should be pursued. Psychiatric treatment should focus primarily on support during a very difficult emotional period.

1.3. Educating Emergency Department Physicians

When a patient presents to the ED with prolonged convulsions, neurologists often become involved after the patient is already intubated or loaded with intravenous medications.[22] There are published cases of patients making recurrent emergency visits and undergoing intubations even when doctors are well aware of the diagnosis of PNES, likely because of how closely the episodes resemble epileptic seizures. Nguyen et al.[47] reported on a teenage girl who was sent to the ED for intubation and intravenous medications repeatedly despite staff awareness of the diagnosis, emphasizing the need for educating staff about the appropriate management of PNES. Thus it is incumbent on first responders—particularly ED physicians—to be familiar with PNES as an important consideration in patients presenting with seizures, just as they must recognize panic attack as an important consideration in the differential diagnosis for a patient with complaints of chest pain. The diagnosis may be discovered if the records are requested or the patient's neurologist contacted. PNES should be suspected in patients with atypical seizure semiology, particularly when there are full-body motor seizures without loss of consciousness, when the patient has had numerous admissions for seizures or status epilepticus but repeated EEGs have been normal, when there has been no consistent

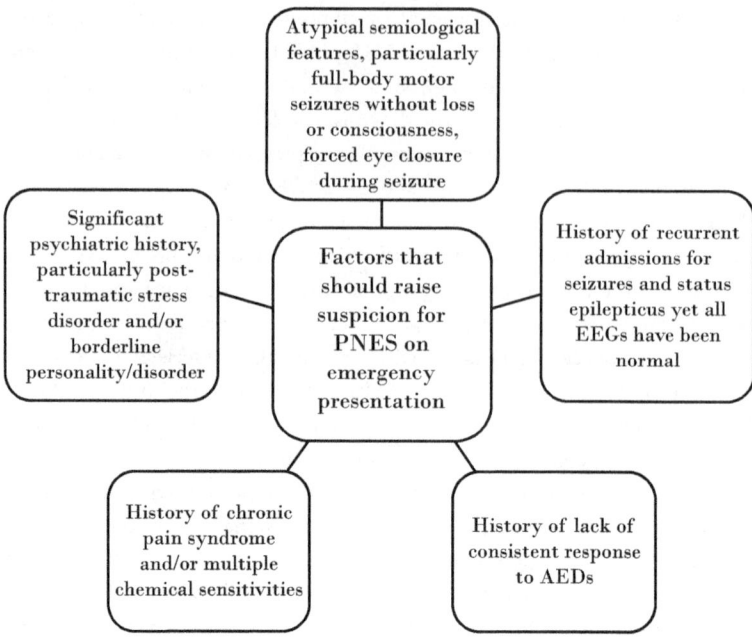

Figure 2.1 Factors that should raise suspicion for psychogenic nonepileptic seizures (PNES) on emergency presentation.
AEDs, antiepileptic drugs.

response to AEDs, when there is a history of recurrent presentations for medically unexplained symptoms, or when there is a substantial psychiatric history (Figure 2.1). Psychiatric risk factors for PNES in adults include a history of depression, anxiety,[9] post-traumatic stress disorder (PTSD), chronic pain,[48-50] substance abuse, borderline personality disorder,[51] and dissociative disorders[52] (see Chapter 3 for more detailed discussion). Risk factors in children include medical, neurological, and psychiatric problems; high utilization of medical services and medications; anxiety sensitivity; solitary emotional coping; and lifetime adversity.[53] A history of sexual or physical abuse is less common in children with PNES than in adults; school difficulties or family discord are more common precipitants for children.[9,54-56]

Overtesting can be an issue in the ED; providers without specialty training in epilepsy may feel understandably wary about diagnosing PNES before excluding other forms of pathology. Unnecessary CT scans of the head are often ordered repeatedly. However, in recent series, there was a relatively low rate of misdiagnosis of conversion disorder.[52] On the other hand, as many as 30% of epilepsy diagnoses may be erroneous,[57,58] mostly as a result of poor histories or over-read EEGs,[58,59] leading to unnecessary prescriptions, procedures, and adverse medication effects. This indicates that there may be a tendency to overdiagnose rather than underdiagnose epilepsy. Excessive reluctance to make a diagnosis of PNES and overtesting may reinforce somatic preoccupation and delay initiation of appropriate treatment. Additionally, overtesting may lead to erroneous diagnoses or further unnecessary tests, since positive test results may be more likely to be false positives than true positives if pretest probability is very low.[60]

Nevertheless, it can be difficult to withhold aggressive treatment for a patient presenting with what appears to be status epilepticus unless a diagnosis of NEPS can be confirmed immediately. In the ED, obtaining an urgent EEG can be very useful when a patient is unresponsive, as a normal result may reduce the need for admission and further testing. The challenge is great for ED physicians dealing with an unfamiliar patient presenting with PNES. ED physicians are often busy with critically ill patients; they need to make rapid diagnoses and the emphasis in treatment is to prevent death or serious morbidity. Additionally, availability of EEG and consultants with expertise in dealing with PNES may be limited in the ED. Thus, it is important to try to prevent patients with chronic PNES from recurrently visiting the ED by providing a satisfactory alternative. These patients are ill and are deserving of empathy and care. Patients presenting to the ED with PNES may be desperate for care but unable to find the appropriate clinical setting in which to receive it. In psychodynamic terms, the transference that these patients project onto the medical system represents their need for care, while at the same time highlights their dissatisfaction and anger toward caring providers. For many, this interpersonal pattern is the center of their psychological conflict. Unfortunately, if patients continue to present only to providers who are either unknowledgeable or uninterested in PNES, the problem can be perpetuated.

If a definitive diagnosis cannot be immediately made in the emergency setting but PNES is suspected, the most important intervention an ED clinician can make is to mention PNES in the differential and to provide a referral to a comprehensive epilepsy center where continuous video EEG (vEEG) monitoring is available. Sending a patient out of the ED without an adequate explanation of the diagnosis or follow-up plan increases the likelihood that the patient will return to the ED or will present to a different ED where the process repeats itself, solidifying this pattern of care-seeking behavior that inevitably leads to disappointment and sometimes anger.

It is important that clinicians working in emergency settings who routinely encounter patients with seizures be familiar with PNES and the procedures or referrals necessary for definitive diagnosis. These clinicians must also recognize that PNES are often a manifestation of significant psychological distress and that the patient may not be aware of this or understand the significance of the psychogenic nature of the attacks and may not know where else to go to seek help. Appropriate follow-up should be arranged prior to discharge from the ED (see Chapter 10).

1.4. Emergency Presentations for Non-Seizure Complaints

Patients with PNES may seek emergency medical care for reasons other than seizure management itself. Patients may present with the sequelae of their events, such as accidents and injuries, or they may present with seemingly unrelated problems that are nevertheless connected to the underlying psychopathology, such as other functional symptoms and suicidal ideation or suicide attempts.

1.4.1. Accidents and Injuries

Accidents and injuries occur in people with epilepsy at four times the rate of the general population and include falls, drowning, and burns.[61] These types of accidents are believed to be uncommon in PNES, as PNES are not believed to impair self-protective reflexes or instincts the way an epileptic seizure may. In fact, one bedside exam maneuver used to identify psychogenic unresponsiveness involves placing the patient's hand over his or her face and dropping it, examining to see if the patient protects the face from the falling hand.[62] However, accidents and injuries do occur during PNES and are reported by patients quite frequently. While most injuries are minor, a significant injury sustained during an attack should not necessarily be considered diagnostic of an epileptic seizure. Peguero et al.[63] contacted 73 of 102 consecutive patients diagnosed with PNES by means of vEEG. Injuries were reported in 40% of cases, with 44% reporting tongue bites and urinary incontinence. The authors did not find a history of burns reported in the PNES patients, only in those with definite epilepsy, although a burn was reported by a PNES patient in another series[64] in which nearly 31% of PNES patients reported injuries. In this study, PNES patients with urinary incontinence were more likely to also report injuries, most commonly minor tongue lacerations, but also more major injuries such as fractures. These statistics are substantial and suggest that the notion that patients are not at risk for injury during PNES is likely erroneous. However, these data must be interpreted with caution. Self-report studies such as these may not reflect actual rates of significant injury, as they are influenced by patient perceptions and recall bias. Patients with functional neurological disorders may have a tendency to grossly overestimate the extent of their symptoms when compared against objective measures.[65] Efforts should be made to obtain objective evidence of injuries. Nevertheless, from the authors' experience, there are definite circumstances where photos and witness reports provide significant evidence that injuries do occur. Falls and injuries have been reported in the EMU during vEEG-proven PNES, particularly when patients were ambulatory,[66] and concerns have been raised about inadequate responses to PNES patients from nursing staff,[66,67] possibly reflecting the misperception among healthcare providers that PNES are not dangerous.

1.4.2. Suicide and Self-Injurious Behavior

PNES are associated with an increased risk of PTSD[50,68] and, in general, antecedent trauma is reported by 75% of patients with PNES, including physical, sexual, and emotional trauma.[69] In addition, anxiety,[50] depressive symptoms,[70] and cluster A and B personality disorders[71] are common in patients with PNES. These psychiatric comorbidities increase a patient's risk of suicidality. Depression, personality disorders,[72] and anxiety disorders[73,74] have all been identified as significant risk factors for suicidality, particularly PTSD.[75] Suicide attempts were reported by 32% of PNES patients in the study by Peguero et al.,[76] Kaufman and Struck[77] reported a case of an attempted suicide in the EMU.

Patients with prolonged PNES, also referred to as NEPS, may have a particularly increased risk of self-harm or suicidal behavior.[22] In addition, patients with PNES who report experiencing injuries or accidents are more likely to report that they had a past suicide attempt,[76] which suggests an association between NEPS and dangerous behavior. Supporting this notion is a series of 18 patients with NEPS, all of whom demonstrated self-destructive behaviors including suicide attempts.[51] This cohort of NEPS patients also had impulse control problems, substance abuse, affective dyscontrol, depression, bulimia, and borderline personality disorder (BPD). Interestingly, although suicide behaviors are relatively common in PNES patients, in one study self-injurious behavior including past suicide attempts was actually a negative predictor of death in patients with PNES who were followed for a mean of 7.9 years after presentation.[78] These patients tended to die of medical illnesses not directly related to seizures or psychiatric illness. Nevertheless, the high rate of psychiatric comorbidity in this patient population and their underlying difficulties with emotion management put these patients at risk for suicidal behaviors.

BPD is highly comorbid in PNES, and may be present in as many as 50% of patients.[79] Individuals with BPD frequently present to EDs in crises, reporting impulsive behaviors including aggression toward others, self-injurious behaviors, or suicidal ideation or attempted suicide. A recent study demonstrated the high cost of healthcare utilization among BPD patients, who tend to use the ED and hospital frequently.[80] Dissociation, which is a major underlying psychopathological mechanism in PNES,[81] is associated in BPD with a high risk of self-injurious behaviors.[82] Thus, one may draw a hypothetical link between self-destructive or suicidal behaviors in BPD, injuries related to PNES, and NEPS. Injuries sustained during PNES, while apparently not intentional, may reflect an underlying self-destructive tendency that manifests during a period of dissociation. Further study is needed to clarify this relationship.

1.4.3. Presentations for Medically Unexplained Symptoms Other Than Seizure

Patients with PNES commonly present to healthcare providers with non-seizure symptoms. These symptoms are typically evaluated by non-neurologist non-psychiatrist clinicians and are considered separately from the seizures. It is quite common that no definitive anatomical or physiological explanation can be found to account for many of these symptoms, and when this occurs recurrently with different symptoms, or when symptoms appear disproportionate to what would be expected based on the patient's medical conditions, somatic symptom disorder[83] should be considered. Medically unexplained symptoms (MUS) other than seizures occur in a large proportion of patients with PNES (57.4% had at least one and 18.5% had multiple MUS in one series[84]), and this association between MUS and PNES likely reflects the role of somatic tendencies in the pathogenesis of PNES (see Chapters 3, 4, and 5).[85,86] Symptoms may include headache, abdominal pain, pelvic pain, chest pain, body pains, fatigue, and medication side effects. Laboratory and imaging workups are usually unrevealing, and patients may be given diagnoses such as migraine headaches, fibromyalgia, chronic fatigue syndrome, atypical or non-cardiac chest pain, or multiple chemical sensitivity. These symptoms are usually predominantly subjective. Other functional neurological symptoms may be seen as well, such as psychogenic tremors, weakness, sensory complaints, or stutter. Non-seizure MUS are not seen in all patients with PNES, and they may reflect certain psychopathological characteristics. When present, they are predictive of a history of prior sexual abuse.[69,87] McKenzie et al.[88] recorded MUS in patients during the 6–12 months following a diagnosis of PNES and found that 23.5% of patients developed new MUS, although most of these had non-seizure MUS prediagnosis as well. Because of the varying nature of these symptoms, a patient may see different medical specialists for each of the symptoms, and MUS contribute to the high healthcare utilization in these patients. While different types of symptoms deserve different types of evaluations and specialist consultations, it is important that these various symptoms not be considered in a vacuum but recognized collectively as part of a syndrome.

2. HANDLING PNES EMERGENCIES
2.1. Acute Management

For patients who have not yet received a definitive diagnosis, plans for diagnostic workup can be instituted at the time of presentation. If a diagnostic workup has been completed, the neurologist may be called upon to provide context and guidance to ED physicians possibly to re-evaluate the patient, particularly if the patient is experiencing a new type of spell. Patients continuing to seize in the ED may require urgent neurological consultation and even repeat vEEG monitoring. The patient may need an urgent psychiatric consultation if significant psychosocial triggers are present or there are immediate safety concerns. A visit to the ED may be a "reachable moment" as the patient's acute stress level is high, and the opportunity to explore psychosocial contributions for the symptoms may be timely. This may be a moment to reinforce the meaning of the diagnosis for patients who have already been given definitive diagnoses of PNES and to solidify the treatment plan. Once the diagnosis of PNES is made, ED physicians may feel uncertain of how to handle a patient who continues to seize in front of them, and the distress of witnessing these episodes may induce providers to administer inappropriate treatments.[47] It is important to note that there is no medication that will acutely stop PNES, short of intubation and general anesthesia, which should be avoided given that the risks are likely greater than the risks of allowing the PNES to continue. Physicians should provide reassurance and support to the patient and the family but must avoid administering doses of sedative medications that can cause a patient to lose the ability to protect his or her airway.

2.2. Understanding PNES Emergencies from the Perspective of Borderline Crises

Patients with PNES may present emergently, apparently desperate for help and looking for answers. In such a state, they may seek urgent care in chaotic and busy EDs where providers may be dealing with acute traumas and critically ill patients. In this setting, health care providers may feel manipulated by these patients once the psychogenic nature of the attacks becomes apparent. Providers are frustrated by how little they have to offer to these patients, and what they can offer—explanations of their diagnosis, mental health referrals, etc.—is often rejected by patients who appear to want what is either unhelpful or not possible: a neurological diagnosis other than PNES and medications that will stop their attacks. The most severe presentations typically lead to short hospitalizations during which referrals are made to neurologists and/or psychiatrists. However, patients often do not follow up or may be seen once or twice in the outpatient setting only to miss subsequent appointments, become lost to follow-up, and then present again in crises to the ED some time later. While there is no easy way to handle this problem, some lessons may be learned from examining the emotional and behavioral crises commonly experienced by patients with BPD and the approaches commonly employed to manage them. As BPD is present in as many as half of patients with PNES, the parallels should not be surprising.

BPD is characterized by affective instability, unstable self-image, and pathological relationships marked by fears of abandonment and transient quasi-psychotic experiences. History of parental abandonment and/or sexual assault at an early age is common among patients with BPD, and many patients exhibit chronic waxing and waning suicidal ideation. BPD patients often present to EDs in crises, exhibiting extreme distress, impulsive aggression, suicidal ideation, or self-destructive or self-injurious behaviors. Underlying these crises is often distress over the uncertainty about the trustworthiness of various relationships, and the patient's maladaptive coping strategy is to challenge those from whom he or she seeks care and support in order to prove or disprove the trustworthiness and dependability of these people. This may take the form of increasing demands, threats, and inappropriate behavior and is ultimately self-defeating, serving only to push caretakers away, rendering judgments about their dependability more uncertain. BPD patients often have difficulty establishing solid therapeutic alliances, leaving providers feeling abused or deceived, and they may refuse to follow well-prepared care plans out of lack of confidence in the provider or low motivation, and then return seeking help primarily during states of crisis. Among patients presenting to psychiatric emergency rooms, patients with personality disorders are the most likely to refuse follow-up care.[89]

Though no evidence-based guidelines exist for managing crises in BPD, efforts are usually made to avoid acute inpatient hospitalization unless the safety risk is felt to be too great. Realistic expectations must be set and a balance struck between ensuring safety and avoiding reinforcing the patient's helplessness and abdication of responsibility. The British Psychological Society and the Royal College of Psychiatrists have published a manual providing guidelines for the treatment of BPD in which management of crises is addressed,[90] emphasizing flexibility, maintaining patient autonomy, and setting limits while maintaining a calm, nonthreatening, and supportive demeanor. These general principles may be applicable to PNES patients in crisis as well (see Table 2.2). Patients presenting to the ED with PNES should be treated with empathy, just as any other patient presenting in crisis. Patients should not be treated dismissively because their understanding of their problem is at odds with the clinicians', but clinicians should not conceal their clinical impressions. Limits may need to be set if the patient demands to be seen immediately by a particular clinician who is not available, but patients should not be discharged without a clear and thoughtful follow-up care plan. Clinicians should be aware of their own feelings of frustration, irritation, and even anger but must not let these feelings interfere with their ability to maintain professionalism throughout the encounter.

3. PREVENTING PNES EMERGENCIES

Once a diagnosis is made, it is important to try to keep patients with chronic PNES from being seen recurrently in the ED. This may require established providers to become more

Table 2.2. Recommendations for Managing PNES Crises*

- *Maintain flexibility so patient autonomy is preserved as much as possible.* Avoid involuntary hospitalizations. If the patient has an established treatment team, the team may be able to help the patient get back into outpatient care. Alternative options should be explored before admitting the patient to the hospital, unless acute hospitalization is necessary for diagnostic clarification (e.g., epilepsy has not been ruled out).
- *Tolerate intense emotions but set necessary limits.* Avoid splitting by presenting a unified front among patient's providers. Consulting neurologists, psychiatrists, and ED physicians should present a single, agreed-upon opinion about the diagnosis management plan.
- *Maintain a calm and unthreatening attitude.* Provide supportive, empathic comments and validating statements. Do not accuse patients of bringing on their seizures voluntarily.
- *Try to understand the crisis from the patient's point of view (i.e., use patient's vocabulary).* Avoid minimizing the patient's stated reasons for crisis or offering solutions before fully clarifying the problem. The patient is likely in a considerable degree of distress if he or she is presenting to the ED with recurrent unexplainable spells.
- *Appropriate follow-up should be offered within an appropriate time frame and with the necessary professionals.*
- *Acute medication use should be limited and short term.* AEDs should be avoided if the patient's spells have already been definitively characterized as PNES.

*Adapted from guidelines for treatment of borderline personality disorder published by the British Psychological Society and the Royal College of Psychiatrists.[90]
AEDs, antiepileptic drugs; ED, emergency department; PNES, psychogenic nonepileptic seizures.

accessible to these patients rather than referring them elsewhere. The patient needs to know that he or she is being heard and not dismissed. Rather than just "ruling out epilepsy" (negative diagnosis), an explanation for the psychogenic origin of the symptoms needs to be offered (positive diagnosis) (see Chapter 10). Explaining PNES as one form of an expression of distress, similar to panic attacks and/or depression, may eventually help patients and professionals to embrace this disorder in a less stigmatizing way. Appropriately explaining the diagnosis may in and of itself reduce ED utilization.[91] However, patients still need somewhere to turn when symptoms continue or recur. A treatment team should be defined for the patient, with specified roles for each member, so that the patient will have alternatives to the ED when crisis is looming.

Following diagnosis, collaboration between various members of the patient's treatment team can be helpful in preventing recurrent ED presentations. Ideally, the treatment team consists of a neurologist, psychiatrist, primary care physician, psychotherapist, and a social worker or care coordinator, all of whom understand the diagnosis and its implications. No one person can assume full responsibility for the patient's PNES management, but it is important that each member of the team have a full understanding of the patient's condition, a sense of his or her own role in the patient's care, and the ability to communicate with other team members when necessary. A unified approach to management should be presented, and each member of the care team must take ownership of his

Table 2.3. Suggested Roles for Members of the Treatment Team

Neurologist	• Uses appropriate procedures to clarify the diagnosis of PNES with a reasonable degree of certainty (usually video EEG confirmation) • Should be called to re-evaluate patients who present to the ED with new types of spells • Should be called to help ED physicians and other medical professionals understand the diagnosis and clarify whether workup is complete or whether further EEG monitoring is indicated
Psychiatrist	• Communicates with neurologist and ED physicians • Screens for psychological stressors that may have precipitated current crisis or predisposed patient to PNES • Screens for psychiatric comorbidities that may necessitate urgent treatment
Psychotherapist	• Must be familiar with the condition and comfortable discussing it with the patient • May serve as the patient's primary contact for handling PNES emergencies, but maintains communication with other members of the patient's treatment team
Case manager	• Helps coordinate care • Helps patient access resources • Provides support and may also serve as psychotherapist
Primary care physician	• May serve as patient's primary contact, particularly if patient has multiple psychosomatic illnesses and is seeing multiple medical subspecialists • Can help address crises in outpatient setting so as to avoid unnecessary ED visits and unnecessary medications and testing

or her particular role (Table 2.3). Knowledge of the patient's PNES and somatic tendencies may help the patient's outpatient providers avoid overtesting and overprescribing while remaining available to the patient to address urgent issues for which the patient may otherwise present to the ED.

3.1. Individualized Treatment Plans

Certain patients who remain high users of emergency services may benefit from individualized treatment plans. These may involve short-duration follow-ups with psychiatry or mental health provider and neurology, combined visits with the neurologist and psychiatrist or other mental health provider, and/or regular telephone contact or visits with a practice nurse or care coordinator. Demonstrating responsiveness in crisis strengthens the doctor–patient alliance, may alleviate the need for actual visits to the ED, and allows the provider to begin to guide the patient toward treatment of underlying psychological issues. Sometimes, merely having a contact person to call in case of emergency may be all that is needed to allay the anxiety over remaining at home. Patients whose events have been clearly characterized as PNES can often be evaluated over the phone when further episodes occur, and reassurance along with a plan for short-term follow-up may be all that is needed to alleviate the need for an ED visit. Patients with PNES who use ED services frequently may need external guidance to contain themselves in times of need. A phone conversation works for some, but in-person contact may be more helpful for others. However, breaking the contingency between a crisis and a medical contact becomes essential to decrease the reinforcing quality of emergency situations. Therefore, such urgent contacts should aim to redirect patients' efforts at developing new skills that will decrease their tendency toward PNES, rather than addressing each emergency individually.

4. CONCLUSIONS

PNES patients may present for urgent or emergent evaluation in a number of settings, but acute treatment is rarely beneficial. Maintaining vigilance to identify patients at risk for accidents or suicide is important, as is preventing iatrogenic harm during an emergency medical encounter. Thus, clinicians dealing with these patients must make it a priority to achieve a definitive diagnosis, communicate the diagnosis effectively to the patient, and establish an outpatient care plan that the patient can accept and will follow up with. Maintaining an empathic demeanor toward the patient and avoiding stigmatizing language are important components of this process (see Chapter 10).

Further research is needed to identify effective strategies for engaging patients in treatment and to identify patients who are at high risk for PNES emergencies. PNES patients who enter the hospital via the ED, are discharged quickly, and do not follow up with outpatient appointments may be at particular risk for future ED visits for PNES-related emergencies. Capturing data on these patients is a major challenge.

5. SUMMARY

- PNES patients frequently present to emergency departments (EDs), where they are initially cared for by providers who are not experts in this condition. Education of emergency physicians is necessary to help patients access appropriate care and avoid inappropriate and at times potentially dangerous treatments intended to treat epileptic seizures.
- When PNES are prolonged (nonepileptic psychogenic status) they may be mistaken for status epilepticus, and patients may inappropriately receive high doses of antiepileptic drugs (AEDs) and sedatives and even be intubated unnecessarily.
- Patients may be injured as a result of PNES itself or medical treatments intended for epilepsy. They may also suffer consequences related to comorbid psychiatric conditions, including self-injurious behavior and suicide attempts. After diagnosis of PNES, patients must be screened and appropriately treated for these conditions.

- PNES is part of a broader psychosomatic illness that commonly involves multiple medical subspecialists. These patients are not best served when they receive a large amount of their care in the ED or from multiple providers who are not in communication with one another. An integrated outpatient treatment team that addresses both the patient's physical symptoms and psychiatric comorbidities may help prevent or limit unnecessary ED visits, reduce health care utilization, and decrease the risk for iatrogenic harm from unnecessary treatments.

REFERENCES

1. Dworetzky BA, Weisholtz DS, Perez DL, Baslet G. A clinically oriented perspective on psychogenic nonepileptic seizure-related emergencies. *Clin EEG Neurosci.* 2015;46(1):26-33.
2. Reuber M, Baker GA, Gill R, Smith DF, Chadwick DW. Failure to recognize psychogenic nonepileptic seizures may cause death. *Neurology.* 2004;62(5):834-835.
3. Parry T, Hirsch N. Psychogenic seizures after general anaesthesia. *Anaesthesia.* 1992;47(6):534.
4. Downs JW, Young PE, Durning SJ. Psychogenic coma following upper endoscopy: a case report and review of the literature. *Mil Med.* 2008;173(5):509-512.
5. Sharma R, Jain A, Singh R, Kumar N. Conversion reaction mimicking a high spinal anesthesia. *J Anesth.* 2012;26(2):316-317.
6. Hirjak D, Thomann PA, Wolf RC, Weidner N, Wilder-Smith EP. Dissociative paraplegia after epidural anesthesia: a case report. *J Med Case Rep.* 2013;7(1):56.
7. Pertek JP, Omar-Amrani M, Artis M, Vignal JP, Chelias A. [Failure to recover after anesthesia attributed to a transient dissociative state]. *Ann Fr Anesth Reanim.* 2000;19(4):257-260.
8. Jones K, Nielsen S, Bruno R, Frei M, Lubman D. Benzodiazepines: their role in aggression and why GPs should prescribe with caution. *Aust Fam Physician.* 2011;40:862-865.
9. Reilly C, Menlove L, Fenton V, Das KB. Psychogenic nonepileptic seizures in children: a review. *Epilepsia.* 2013;54(10):1715-1724.
10. Cole CM, Falcone T, Caplan R, Timmons-Mitchell J, Jares K, Ford PJ. Ethical dilemmas in pediatric and adolescent psychogenic nonepileptic seizures. *Epilepsy Behav.* 2014;37:145-150.
11. Bittigau P, Sifringer M, Genz K, et al. Antiepileptic drugs and apoptotic neurodegeneration in the developing brain. *Proc Natl Acad Sci U S A.* 2002;99(23):15089-15094.
12. Sulzbacher S, Farwell JR, Temkin N, Lu AS, Hirtz DG. Late cognitive effects of early treatment with phenobarbital. *Clin Pediatr.* 1999;38(7):387-394.
13. Robbins NM, Larimer P, Bourgeois JA, Lowenstein DH. Number of patient-reported allergies helps distinguish epilepsy from psychogenic nonepileptic seizures. *Epilepsy Behav.* 2016;55:174-177.
14. Willmore LJ, Fellock JM, Pickens API. Monitoring for adverse effects of antiepileptic drugs. In: Wyllie E, Cascino GD, Gidal BE, eds. *Wyllie's Treatment of Epilepsy: Principles and Practice,* 5th ed. Philadelphia: Wolters Kluwer/Lippincott Williams & Wilkins; 2011:592-600.
15. Pennell PB. Pregnancy, epilepsy, and women's issues. *Continuum (Minneap Minn).* 2013;19(3 Epilepsy):697-714.
16. Chen JW, Naylor DE, Wasterlain CG. Advances in the pathophysiology of status epilepticus. *Acta Neurol Scand.* 2007;115(4 Suppl):7-15.

17. Meldrum BS, Vigouroux RA, Brierley JB. Systemic factors and epileptic brain damage. Prolonged seizures in paralyzed, artificially ventilated baboons. *Arch Neurol.* 1973;29(2):82–87.
18. Sloviter RS. Decreased hippocampal inhibition and a selective loss of interneurons in experimental epilepsy. *Science.* 1987;235(4784):73–76.
19. Hewertson J, Poets CF, Samuels MP, Boyd SG, Neville BG, Southall DP. Epileptic seizure-induced hypoxemia in infants with apparent life-threatening events. *Pediatrics.* 1994;94(2 Pt 1):148–156.
20. Bateman LM, Li CS, Seyal M. Ictal hypoxemia in localization-related epilepsy: analysis of incidence, severity and risk factors. *Brain.* 2008;131(Pt 12):3239–3245.
21. Hirsch LJ, Gaspard N. Status epilepticus. *Continuum (Minneap Minn).* 2013;19(3 Epilepsy):767–794.
22. Reuber M, Pukrop R, Mitchell AJ, Bauer J, Elger CE. Clinical significance of recurrent psychogenic nonepileptic seizure status. *J Neurol.* 2003;250(11):1355–1362.
23. Howell S, Owen L, Chadwick D. Pseudostatus epilepticus. *Q J Med.* 1989;71(266):507–519.
24. Papavasiliou A, Vassilaki N, Paraskevoulakos E, Kotsalis C, Bazigou H, Bardani I. Psychogenic status epilepticus in children. *Epilepsy Behav.* 2004;5(4):539–546.
25. Dobbertin MD, Wigington G, Sharma A, Bestha D. Intubation in a case of psychogenic, non-epileptic status epilepticus. *J Neuropsychiatry Clin Neurosci.* 2012;24(1):E8.
26. Gunatilake SB, De Silva HJ, Ranasinghe G. Twenty-seven venous cutdowns to treat pseudostatus epilepticus. *Seizure.* 1997;6(1):71–72.
27. LaFrance WC Jr, Benbadis SR. Avoiding the costs of unrecognized psychological nonepileptic seizures. *Neurology.* 2006;66(11):1620–1621.
28. Levitan M, Bruni J. Repetitive pseudoseizures incorrectly managed as status epilepticus. *CMAJ.* 1986;134:1029–1031.
29. Dworetzky BA, Bubrick EJ, Szaflarski JP. Nonepileptic psychogenic status: markedly prolonged psychogenic nonepileptic seizures. *Epilepsy Behav.* 2010;19(1):65–68.
30. Asadi-Pooya AA, Emami Y, Emami M, Sperling MR. Prolonged psychogenic nonepileptic seizures or pseudostatus. *Epilepsy Behav.* 2014;31:304–306.
31. Dworetzky BA, Mortati KA, Rossetti AO, Vaccaro B, Nelson A, Bromfield EB. Clinical characteristics of psychogenic nonepileptic seizure status in the long-term monitoring unit. *Epilepsy Behav.* 2006;9(2):335–338.
32. Dworetzky BA, Qureshi N, Weisholtz D, Perez DL, Fantaneanu T, Baslet G. Nonepileptic psychogenic status: longer and more dramatic events. Paper presented at the American Epilepsy Society Annual Meeting, 2014; Seattle, WA.
33. Minkoff H, Schaffer RM, Delke I, Grunebaum AN. Diagnosis of intracranial hemorrhage in utero after a maternal seizure. *Obstetr Gynecol.* 1985;65(3 Suppl):22s–24s.
34. Hart LA, Sibai BM. Seizures in pregnancy: epilepsy, eclampsia, and stroke. *Semin Perinatol.* 2013;37(4):207–224.
35. Peters G, Leach JP, Larner AJ. Pseudostatus epilepticus in pregnancy. *Int J Gynaecol Obstet.* 2007;97(1):47.
36. Weintraub MI. Medicolegal aspects of iatrogenic injuries. *Neurol Clin.* 1998;16(1):217–227.
37. Ryvlin P, Nashef L, Lhatoo SD, et al. Incidence and mechanisms of cardiorespiratory arrests in epilepsy monitoring units (MORTEMUS): a retrospective study. *Lancet Neurol.* 2013;12(10):966–977.
38. Smith PE, Saunders J, Dawson A, Kerr MP. Intractable seizures in pregnancy. *Lancet.* 1999;354(9189):1522.

39. DeToledo JC, Lowe MR, Puig A. Nonepileptic seizures in pregnancy. *Neurology.* 2000;55(1):120–121.
40. Brady WJ, Jr., Huff JS. Pseudotoxemia: new onset psychogenic seizure in third trimester pregnancy. *J Emerg Med.* 1997;15(6):815–820.
41. Carlson RH, Jr., Caplan JP. Pseudolabor born out of psychogenic nonepileptic seizures: a case report of multisymptom conversion disorder. *Psychosomatics.* 2011;52(5):455–458.
42. Tollefson GD, Garvey MJ. Conversion disorder following termination of pregnancy. *J Fam Pract.* 1983;16(1):73–77.
43. Nguyen J, Abola R, Schabel J. Recurrent psychogenic paresis after dural puncture in a parturient. *Int J Obstet Anesth.* 2013;22(2):160–163.
44. Elsharkawy H, Khanna AK, Barsoum S. Caesarean delivery complicated by unintentional subdural block and conversion disorder. *Case Rep Med.* 2013;2013:751648.
45. Munk-Olsen T, Laursen TM, Meltzer-Brody S, Mortensen PB, Jones I. Psychiatric disorders with postpartum onset: possible early manifestations of bipolar affective disorders. *Arch Gen Psychiatry.* 2012;69(4):428–434.
46. Kuruvilla A, Nair M. Pseudoseizures versus epileptic seizures in pregnancy. *Lancet.* 2000;355(9200):318.
47. Nguyen ML, Shapiro MA, Demetree JM, White KA. When non-epileptic seizures fool the experts. *Int J Psychiatry Med.* 2011;42(3):331–338.
48. Dixit R, Popescu A, Bagic A, Ghearing G, Hendrickson R. Medical comorbidities in patients with psychogenic nonepileptic spells (PNES) referred for video-EEG monitoring. *Epilepsy Behav.* 2013;28(2):137–140.
49. Gazzola DM, Carlson C, Rugino A, Hirsch S, Starner K, Devinsky O. Psychogenic non-epileptic seizures and chronic pain: a retrospective case-controlled study. *Epilepsy Behav.* 2012;25(4):662–665.
50. Dworetzky BA, Strahonja-Packard A, Shanahan CW, Paz J, Schauble B, Bromfield EB. Characteristics of male veterans with psychogenic nonepileptic seizures. *Epilepsia.* 2005;46(9):1418–1422.
51. Rechlin T, Loew TH, Joraschky P. Pseudoseizure "status." *J Psychosom Res.* 1997;42(5):495–498.
52. Stone J, Smyth R, Carson A, et al. Systematic review of misdiagnosis of conversion symptoms and "hysteria." *BMJ.* 2005;331(7523):989.
53. Plioplys S, Doss J, Siddarth P, et al. A multisite controlled study of risk factors in pediatric psychogenic nonepileptic seizures. *Epilepsia.* 2014;55(11):1739–1747.
54. Patel H, Scott E, Dunn D, Garg B. Nonepileptic seizures in children. *Epilepsia.* 2007;48(11):2086–2092.
55. Verrotti A, Agostinelli S, Mohn A, et al. Clinical features of psychogenic non-epileptic seizures in prepubertal and pubertal patients with idiopathic epilepsy. *Neurol Sci.* 2009;30(4):319–323.
56. Vincentiis S, Valente KD, Thome-Souza S, Kuczinsky E, Fiore LA, Negrao N. Risk factors for psychogenic nonepileptic seizures in children and adolescents with epilepsy. *Epilepsy Behav.* 2006;8(1):294–298.
57. Chowdhury FA, Nashef L, Elwes RD. Misdiagnosis in epilepsy: a review and recognition of diagnostic uncertainty. *Eur J Neurol.* 2008;15(10):1034–1042.
58. Smith D, Defalla BA, Chadwick DW. The misdiagnosis of epilepsy and the management of refractory epilepsy in a specialist clinic. *QJM.* 1999;92(1):15–23.
59. Benbadis SR. "Just like EKGs!" Should EEGs undergo a confirmatory interpretation by a clinical neurophysiologist? *Neurology.* 2013;80(1 Suppl 1):S47–S51.

60. Mark DB. Decision-making in clinical medicine. In: Kasper DL, Braunwald E, Fauci AS, Hauser SL, Longo DL, Jameson JL, eds. *Harrison's Principles of Internal Medicine*, 16th ed. New York: McGraw-Hill; 2005: 6–13.
61. Beghi E, Cornaggia C. Epilepsy and everyday life risks. A case-referent study: rationale, study design, and preliminary results. Risk in Epilepsy Study Group. *Neuroepidemiology*. 1997;16(4):207–216.
62. Young JL, Rund D. Psychiatric considerations in patients with decreased levels of consciousness. *Emerg Med Clin North Am*. 2010;28(3):595–609.
63. Peguero E, Abou-Khalil B, Fakhoury T, Mathews G. Self-injury and incontinence in psychogenic seizures. *Epilepsia*. 1995;36(6):586–591.
64. Asadi-Pooya AA, Emami M, Emami Y. Ictal injury in psychogenic non-epileptic seizures. *Seizure*. 2014;23(5):363–366.
65. Parees I, Saifee TA, Kassavetis P, et al. Believing is perceiving: mismatch between self-report and actigraphy in psychogenic tremor. *Brain*. 2012;135(Pt 1):117–123.
66. Atkinson M, Shah A, Hari K, Schaefer K, Bhattacharya P. Safety considerations in the epilepsy monitoring unit for psychogenic nonepileptic seizures. *Epilepsy Behav*. 2012;25(2):176–180.
67. Shin HW, Pennell PB, Lee JW, Doucette H, Srinivasan S, Dworetzky BA. Efficacy of safety signals in the epilepsy monitoring unit (EMU): should we worry? *Epilepsy Behav*. 2012;23(4):458–461.
68. D'Alessio L, Giagante B, Oddo S, et al. Psychiatric disorders in patients with psychogenic non-epileptic seizures, with and without comorbid epilepsy. *Seizure*. 2006;15(5):333–339.
69. Duncan R, Oto M. Predictors of antecedent factors in psychogenic nonepileptic attacks: multivariate analysis. *Neurology*. 2008;71(13):1000–1005.
70. Ettinger AB, Devinsky O, Weisbrot DM, Ramakrishna RK, Goyal A. A comprehensive profile of clinical, psychiatric, and psychosocial characteristics of patients with psychogenic nonepileptic seizures. *Epilepsia*. 1999;40(9):1292–1298.
71. Harden CL, Jovine L, Burgut FT, Carey BT, Nikolov BG, Ferrando SJ. A comparison of personality disorder characteristics of patients with nonepileptic psychogenic pseudoseizures with those of patients with epilepsy. *Epilepsy Behav*. 2009;14(3):481–483.
72. Hirschfeld RM, Russell JM. Assessment and treatment of suicidal patients. *N Engl J Med*. 1997;337(13):910–915.
73. Hawton K, Saunders K, Topiwala A, Haw C. Psychiatric disorders in patients presenting to hospital following self-harm: a systematic review. *J Affect Disord*. 2013;151(3):821–830.
74. Kanwar A, Malik S, Prokop LJ, et al. The association between anxiety disorders and suicidal behaviors: a systematic review and meta-analysis. *Depress Anxiety*. 2013;30(10):917–929.
75. Wilcox HC, Storr CL, Breslau N. Posttraumatic stress disorder and suicide attempts in a community sample of urban american young adults. *Arch Gen Psychiatry*. 2009;66(3):305–311.
76. Peguero E, Abou-Khalil B, Fakhoury T, Mathews G. Self-injury and incontinence in psychogenic seizures. *Epilepsia*. 1995;36(6):586–591.
77. Kaufman KR, Struck PJ. Psychogenic nonepileptic seizures and suicidal behavior on a video/EEG telemetry unit: the need for psychiatric assessment and screening for suicide risk. *Epilepsy Behav*. 2010;19(4):656–659.
78. Duncan R, Oto M, Wainman-Lefley J. Mortality in a cohort of patients with psychogenic non-epileptic seizures. *J Neurol Neurosurg Psychiatry*. 2012;83(7):761–762.
79. Bowman ES, Markand ON. Psychodynamics and psychiatric diagnoses of pseudoseizure subjects. *Am J Psychiatry*. 1996;153(1):57–63.

80. Maclean JC, Xu H, French MT, Ettner SL. Mental health and high-cost health care utilization: new evidence from axis II disorders. *Health Serv Res.* 2014;49(2):683–704.
81. Baslet G, Roiko A, Prensky E. Heterogeneity in psychogenic nonepileptic seizures: understanding the role of psychiatric and neurological factors. *Epilepsy Behav.* 2010;17(2):236–241.
82. Brodsky BS, Cloitre M, Dulit RA. Relationship of dissociation to self-mutilation and childhood abuse in borderline personality disorder. *Am J Psychiatry.* 1995;152(12):1788–1792.
83. American Psychiatric Association. *Diagnostic and statistical manual of mental disorders, 5th ed. (DSM-5).* Washington, DC: American Psychiatric Association; 2013.
84. Duncan R, Razvi S, Mulhern S. Newly presenting psychogenic nonepileptic seizures: incidence, population characteristics, and early outcome from a prospective audit of a first seizure clinic. *Epilepsy Behav.* 2011;20(2):308–311.
85. Baslet G. Psychogenic non-epileptic seizures: a model of their pathogenic mechanism. *Seizure.* 2011;20(1):1–13.
86. Reuber M, House AO, Pukrop R, Bauer J, Elger CE. Somatization, dissociation and general psychopathology in patients with psychogenic non-epileptic seizures. *Epilepsy Res.* 2003;57(2-3):159–167.
87. Paras ML, Murad MH, Chen LP, et al. Sexual abuse and lifetime diagnosis of somatic disorders: a systematic review and meta-analysis. *JAMA.* 2009;302(5):550–561.
88. McKenzie PS, Oto M, Graham CD, Duncan R. Do patients whose psychogenic non-epileptic seizures resolve, 'replace' them with other medically unexplained symptoms? Medically unexplained symptoms arising after a diagnosis of psychogenic non-epileptic seizures. *J Neurol Neurosurg Psychiatry.* 2011;82(9):967–969.
89. Bruffaerts R, Sabbe M, Demyttenaere K. Predicting aftercare in psychiatric emergencies. *Soc Psychiatry Psychiatr Epidemiol.* 2005;40(10):829–834.
90. National Collaborating Centre for Mental Health. National Institute for Health and Clinical Excellence: Guidance. *Borderline Personality Disorder: Treatment and Management.* Leicester (UK): British Psychological Society & The Royal College of Psychiatrists; 2009.
91. Jirsch JD, Ahmed SN, Maximova K, Gross DW. Recognition of psychogenic nonepileptic seizures diminishes acute care utilization. *Epilepsy Behav.* 2011;22(2):304–307.

Section II
Etiological Factors

3

Psychiatric Factors

Kim Bullock, MD and John J. Barry, MD

1. INTRODUCTION

Psychogenic nonepileptic seizures (PNES) highlight the challenge of understanding the relationship between mind and body. Reductionistic "root cause" prerogatives of illness are usually ineffective at explaining PNES. Rather, a multifaceted and multifactorial causal model is a more appropriate fit for understanding causality and delivering more precise and personalized care to patients with this condition.

This chapter will review some of the unique psychiatric etiological perspectives of PNES. We will use a "4 P's" (predisposing, precipitating, perpetuating, and prognostic) system of formulation when discussing PNES etiology in this chapter. This sophisticated model can be fused with the traditional multidimensional biopsychosocial (BPS) model to establish a chronology in the development of the disorder and provide an explanatory framework for patients, providers, and families (Figure 3.1).[1,2] This fused "4P-BPS" model may easily be incorporated with other theoretical psychotherapeutic models as well, such as psychodynamic, cognitive-behavioral, interpersonal, and analytical viewpoints. In this way, integration of concepts such as attachment, personality structure, traumatic experiences, behavioral tendencies, defense mechanisms, family and systems can easily be included and adapted creatively by each provider preferences.

In our clinic, we start our psychoeducational approach by reviewing unique predisposing factors and use the analogy that these factors are similar to coenzymes in a chemical reaction. These elements are not completely necessary for a symptom or a disorder to occur but aid in its development. Precipitating factors are explained as similar to the catalysts in a chemical reaction. They are the initial inciting events that are present immediately preceding initial symptom development. From a behavioral viewpoint, they can be seen as the unconditioned stimuli of classical conditioning. Perpetuating factors are those elements that provide reinforcement and create positive feedback loops responsible for keeping PNES symptoms recurring over time. These perpetuating factors are often simply the natural consequences of the symptoms themselves. Often, families are solicited to identify how they may be unintentionally reinforcing symptoms. Prognostic factors describe a patient's strengths, supports, resilience, and liabilities and how these may influence prognosis. Prognostic factors are those that make the chemical reaction more

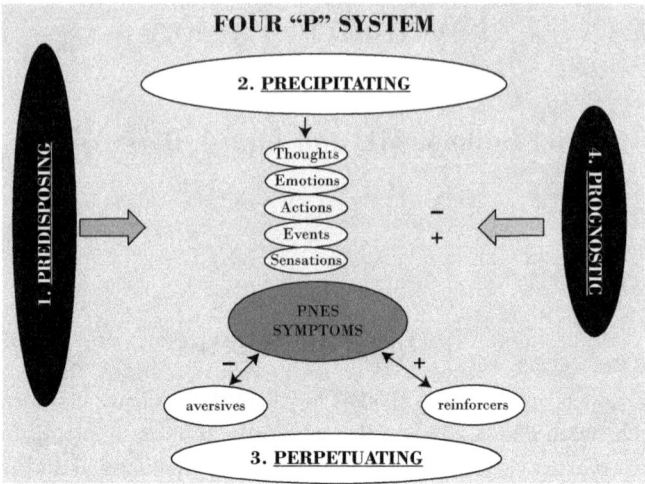

BPS- Biopsychosocial
**PNES- Psychogenic nonepileptic seizures*

Figure 3.1 Causal "4P-BPS" Model of PNES. BPS, biopsychosocial; PNES, psychogenic nonepileptic seizures.

or less likely to occur—environments that metaphorically inactivate or maintain active the enzymes and catalysts or alter homeostasis in either direction. Positive prognostic factors are those elements present in the environment that are non-reinforcing or even aversive or condition PNES symptoms to be less likely. Many of these concepts and factors are not specific to PNES and can be seen in other medical and psychiatric disorders.

The usefulness of the multifactorial model for patients and providers can be profound at the time of diagnosis. Patients often stop pursuing the search for the "golden chalice" cure or a single causal explanation for their symptoms. This is an important function of the model, especially for those patients with comorbid somatic symptom disorder, who tend to demand certainty and a single cause to explain symptoms. We explain the lack of single root cause as "good news" because it offers numerous opportunities for varied treatment modalities. These multifactorial and multidimensional conceptual models allow a more flexible and comprehensive treatment to be prescribed and accepted, which adds resiliency to both patient and caregiving systems. Table 3.1 lists various factors associated with the 4P-BPS model; these are detailed in the discussion below.

2. PREDISPOSING FACTORS

Predisposing factors are biological (including genetic), psychological, or sociocultural features or conditions that render a patient vulnerable to the development of symptoms.

Table 3.1. Fused "4P-BPS" Model of PNES

Factor	Biological	Psychological	Social
Predisposing	Female	Somatic traumatic experiences (i.e. medical, mechanical accident, violence, sexual abuse)	Interpersonal conflict
	Young adulthood	Childhood trauma experiences	Intimate partner violence
	Childhood abuse (verbal, physical, sexual, neglect)	*Psychiatric illness:*	Lifetime adversities
	Fibromyalgia	Depression	Childhood abuse
	Chronic fatigue syndrome, chronic pain syndrome, headaches, irritable bowel syndrome, asthma, GERD	Anxiety disorders	Witnessed seizures in friend/relative
		Somatoform disorders	Exaggerated gender role
		PTSD	Special or favored child status
	Epilepsy	Dissociative disorder	Middle Eastern, Indian, Puerto Rican, Turkish culture
	Lifetime medical and neurological problems	*Personality disorders:*	
	Brain MRI abnormalities	Borderline	
	Mild TBI	Narcissistic	
		Histrionic	
	Neurological developmental and learning disabilities	Antisocial	
		Personality profiles:	
	Medication use	Somatization, hypochondriasis, and hysteria	
	Attentional bias for angry faces	Solitary emotional coping style	
	Lower heart rate variability	Higher hypnotizability	
	Medical service use	Linguistic style: "detailing block" and "focusing resistance"	
	Physical accidents	Fearful attachment style	
	Over age 55: male, health problems	External locus of control beliefs	
		Alexithymia	
		Dissociation	

(*continued*)

Table 3.1. Continued

Factor	Biological	Psychological	Social
Precipitating	Surgical procedures	"Forced choices" or "unspeakable dilemmas"	Bereavement
	Physical accidents	Later onset: traumatic experiences of all types	Interpersonal loss
	Traumatic physical accident, e.g., being hit by a bus or having a fall	*Immediate Triggers:*	Traumatic assault
		Hypnosis	Interpersonal conflict
	Health problems, especially in elderly and males	Being witnessed	Unwanted pregnancy
		Doctor's office	Physical, verbal, or sexual abuse (female: sexual)
	Mild TBI	Emotional stress	Increased job demands
	Epilepsy: especially in early onset	Reminders of past trauma	Litigation
	Immediate Triggers:		Financial problems
	Emergence from general anesthesia		Divorce
	Focal epileptic seizure		Earthquakes
	Sleep		Male: loss of employment or role
	Autonomic arousal		Children: parental discord or divorce, bullying; for boys—academic underachievement
	Transitions out of sympathetic activity		
Perpetuating	Physical health problems	Affective disorders	Family dysfunction
	Antiepileptic drugs (AEDs)	Escape-avoidance behaviors (including avoidance of emotions)	Financial gain
	AED toxicities		Caregiver role
		Bereavement	Isolation
		Health anxiety, hypochondriasis, illness identity	Dependency
		Sexual trauma	Disability status
		Stigmatizing and traumatizing healthcare experiences	Lack of independence, financial problems

			Untreated comorbid psychiatric illness	
Prognostic—Positive	Younger age of onset and time of diagnosis	Acceptance of diagnosis		Greater educational attainment
	Shorter duration of symptoms	Having good relationships with friends as a child		Family structure supporting autonomy
	Female sex	Higher ability to express emotions		Having friends currently
	Semiology: catatonic-like passive behaviors	Less emotional dysregulation		Independent lifestyle
		Lower dissociative scores		
		Seizure induction by suggestion		
Prognostic—Negative	Longer duration of symptoms	Disbelief of PNES diagnosis	Stigma	Lower educational level
	Older age of onset	No formal treatment plan	Transportation difficulties	Social isolation
	Lower IQ	Ongoing stressors	Access to behavioral and mental healthcare	Dependency
	Semiology: dramatic, self-injury, prolonged	Anger	Healthcare system implicit negative bias, untrained healthcare workers	Ongoing litigation
	Comorbid epilepsy	Severe comorbid psychiatric disorder		Ongoing abuse
		Persistent somatization		Unemployment or disability
		Dissociative symptoms		
		Lack of self-disclosure or emotional expression		

GERD, gastroesophageal reflux disease; MRI, magnetic resonance imaging; PNES, psychogenic nonepileptic seizures; PTSD, post-traumatic stress disorder; TBI, traumatic brain injury.

A risk factor (or marker) is difficult to distinguish from a causal variable when examining the few research studies on PNES predisposition. A *risk marker* is defined as being quantitatively associated with a disease indirectly but not directly. A risk marker is not the direct cause but increases the probability of an outcome or disease. Epidemiological studies sometimes identify these risk markers as confounding factors or correlates and control for these when using causal models. For example, being female is correlated with PNES but not all females develop PNES, so it is not considered a direct cause. Predisposing risk factors are important to identify even if they are not directly causal because they can help with screening and with targeting treatments for at-risk populations. Sometimes risk factors that are found to have strong enough associations with a disease can be found to have causal links, as in the case of smoking and lung cancer. This section will review the limited literature on variables presumed to predate seizures, thus possibly representing risk factors for PNES. In most of these studies the precise epidemiological analysis of identifying a risk factor has not been performed and further work in this regard using standardized measures and definitions is needed.[3] Following is a brief review of some of the proposed predisposing factors on PNES.

2.1. Demographics

With the exception of age and gender, other common demographics such as race, years of education, and marital status have not been found to influence the prevalence of PNES,[4] although a recent large retrospective study found that being married was a predictor for PNES more than for epilepsy.[5] While patients of all ages develop PNES, the third decade of life is the most common time for PNES presentation. This may be due to a delay in diagnosis.[4,6-14] Young adulthood appears to be the most common age of symptom onset across cultures.[15-25] In addition, there are data supporting the observation that those with learning disabilities appear to have a younger age of onset.[26] In one study, juvenile-onset PNES patients (below 18 years old), compared to adult-onset patients, showed higher rates of nonsexual and nonphysical abuse (for instance, emotional) and comorbid epilepsy but lower rates of medical comorbidities.[27] Another study showed late-onset PNES (after age 55) to be more likely in males with severe physical health problems, who were less likely to report sexual abuse history.[28]

Female sex is more consistently found in PNES samples and across cultures. PNES studies report a female preponderance ranging from 66% to 99%.[7,8,10,13,29-33] Males appear to predominate in school-aged groups, whereas by adolescence there appears to be a female predominance. One study of 12- to 18-year-old adolescents with PNES reported that 65% were girls and 35% were boys.[34] Although identifying the specific demographic characteristics of PNES patients is not the aim of most studies, no significant demographic sex differences have been reported. There are lower rates of reported physical and sexual abuse, psychiatric illness, and chronic pain in males with PNES.[22]

2.2. Biological

Evidence of pre-existing biological and possibly genetic/epigenetic vulnerabilities in PNES is mounting. Chronic pain, headaches, and fibromyalgia are common among

PNES patients.[35-37] One study showed that patients with PNES were significantly more likely than those with epilepsy to have one or more of the following: fibromyalgia, chronic fatigue syndrome, chronic pain syndrome, headaches, irritable bowel syndrome, asthma, and gastroesophageal reflux disease (GERD).[38] Compared to siblings, PNES patients had significantly more lifetime comorbid medical and neurological problems (including epilepsy) and used more medications and intensive medical services.[39]

2.2.1. Neurological Comorbidities

It is estimated that up to 38% of patients with PNES may show abnormalities on structural brain magnetic resonance imaging (MRI).[8,32,40] Reported MRI abnormalities in PNES without epilepsy include arachnoid cysts, hippocampal sclerosis, venous angiomas, and post-traumatic or gliotic changes, as well as generalized atrophy and white matter lesions.[40] Minor head injury is reported in up to 44% of PNES patients, which is greater than that in epilepsy patients.[13,34,37-43] Mild traumatic brain injury (mTBI) is commonly reported in PNES and is also considered a risk factor.[44] Patients with neurological developmental disabilities have higher rates of PNES than those without, thus intellectual disability (ID) is reported to be a potential risk factor.[13,45,46]

2.2.2. Epilepsy

Comorbid rates of epileptic seizures (ES) vary widely, from 5% to 56%, and are presumed to be due to differences in sampling and non-standardized diagnostic criteria.[13,15,26,32,34,42,47-52] Most often in this circumstance, the epilepsy diagnosis precedes PNES and is presumed to provide some priming of behavioral circuitry, although there are controversies concerning the links between epilepsy and PNES. Some studies define comorbid epilepsy as the presence of interictal spikes, which can be present in some healthy and PNES samples.[3,53,54] It is estimated that 2% to 9% of patients after epilepsy surgery will develop PNES within several months,[55-57] a time when many other postsurgical psychiatric symptoms also manifest. Epilepsy also appears to be more common in juvenile-onset PNES.[27] Further discussion of neurological and medical risk factors can be found in Chapter 4.

2.2.3. Depression

Depression is frequently comorbid with PNES, and the psychobiological aspects of affective illness may also predispose patients to disruptions in hypothalamic, pituitary, neurotransmitter, and brain-derived neurotrophic factor (BDNF) function.[58,59] Potential functional anatomical overlaps between functional neurological symptom disorder (FNSD) and depression can be seen in functional imaging studies (see Chapter 6 for more details).[60-63] In addition, elevation in cortisol, which exists in severe forms of depressive disorders,[64,65] may help explain hippocampal dysfunction in both depression and PNES.

2.2.4. Other

Similar to other populations exposed to traumatic experiences, PNES patients have been reported to display a positive attentional bias for angry faces, which correlates to self-reported sexual trauma and lower heart rate variability (HRV).[66] Autonomic nervous system abnormalities have also been identified.[67] Vulnerability to seizures during the perimenstrual period does not appear to occur in PNES and is more suggestive of ES.[68]

2.3. Traumatic Experiences

Traumatic experiences are a risk factor for PNES. Traumatic experiences can include childhood or adult verbal, physical, or sexual abuse; neglect; intimate partner violence; traumatic medical experiences; or physical accidents.[6,26,32-34,41,69-71] Those with histories of sexual abuse may be at risk of more severe symptoms and may have more self-harm behaviors or medically unexplained symptoms.[26,72] Compared to South America and Asia, there appears to be a stronger association between psychological trauma and PNES in Western countries.[73] Evidence of traumatic experiences as a risk factor rather than a direct cause of PNES comes from studies comparing childhood traumatic experiences in other populations. For example, childhood trauma appears in several studies to be similarly elevated in inpatient epilepsy patients without PNES and may be a risk factor in multiple medical and psychiatric illnesses.[74]

Historically, rates of childhood abuse, specifically sexual abuse, have been assumed to be higher in adult patients with PNES than in people with epilepsy. A review of the adult literature reveals that the evidence to date is mixed (Table 3.2). For example, Alper et al.,[33] Kuyk et al.,[75] Akyuz et al.,[76] and Elliot and Charyton[77] showed that PNES patients had significantly higher rates of childhood sexual trauma than that among individuals with epilepsy. Six other studies, however, reported no significant differences in childhood sexual abuse rates,[41,69,71,74,77-79] and two showed no differences in childhood trauma rates between groups.[69,79] Only one study controlled for gender.[79]

2.4. Psychiatric Illness

Multiple psychiatric conditions are associated with PNES, including depression, anxiety disorders, somatic symptom disorders, post-traumatic stress disorder (PTSD), dissociative disorders, and personality disorders, especially cluster B personality disorders (borderline, narcissistic, histrionic, and antisocial). Often the presence of these disorders is not identified at presentation but is revealed in hindsight during a more in-depth evaluation.[9,32,34,53,80-87] Many of the psychiatric illnesses identified overlap and are also correlated with traumatic experiences. Undifferentiated somatoform disorder (equivalent to somatic symptom disorder in *DSM-5*) is present in up to 30% of patients and includes symptoms such as gastrointestinal complaints, pain, fatigue, and other complaints.[37] Common longstanding personality traits have been found elevated in PNES populations on the basis of personality tests such as the Minnesota Multiphasic Personality Inventory–2 (MMPI-2). The profiles usually elevated in PNES include somatization, hypochondriasis, and

Table 3.2. Studies of Childhood Trauma Comparing PNES and ES Populations

Reference	Screening Tool	PNES (N)	ES (N)	PNES Findings
Alper et al. (1993)[33]	Structured Clinical Interview DSM-III-R	71	140	Higher frequency and severity of sexual abuse and frequency of physical abuse
Kuyk et al. (1999)[75]	The Trauma Questionnaire (TQ)	65	134	Higher sexual abuse on TQ
Rosenberg et al. (2000)[69]	Trauma History Questionnaire (THQ)	8	27	No differences in exposure to childhood traumas
Dikel et al. (2003)[79]	Life Events Checklist, excerpted from the Clinician Administered PTSD Scale used to identify childhood sexual abuse (CSA)	17	34	Controlling for gender (no differences in CSA)
van Merode (2004)[41]	Childhood Trauma Questionnaire (CTQ)	40	138	Higher total CTQ scores
Akyuz et al. (2004)[76]	Childhood Abuse and Neglect Questionnaire (CANQ)	33	30	Higher physical, emotional, and sexual childhood trauma (not neglect or incest)
Koby et al. (2010)[74]	Drossman abuse screen	38	58	Higher frequency of physical abuse, especially in men
Proença et al. (2011)[71]	CTQ	20	20	Higher total CTQ and subscales of emotional neglect and emotional abuse
Kaplan et al. (2013)[78]	CTQ	96	82	Higher total CTQ and subscales of physical abuse and neglect
Elliott & Charyton (2014)[77]	Medical record documentation by clinician	324	281	Higher physical/sexual abuse

DSM-III-R, *Diagnostic and Statistical Manual of Mental Disorders*, Third Edition, Revised; ES, epileptic seizures; PNES, psychogenic nonepileptic seizures; PTSD, post-traumatic stress disorder.

hysteria.[4,32,88–91] Identifying and addressing these premorbid illnesses early may be a preventive measure for PNES and necessary in overall treatment.

One of the most salient psychiatric comorbidities associated with FNSD is depression. In a review by Bowman et al.,[92] of 45 PNES patients, 98% had a past or present history of an affective disorder, and 80% met criteria for major depressive disorder. It is estimated that three out of four patients with depression also present with somatic complaints.[93] The triad of depression, anxiety, and somatization is the most frequent psychiatric complaint seen in primary care.[94] Many patients presenting to a primary care provider (PCP) have somatic symptoms that are considered part of a depressive syndrome.[95] The association between depression and somatization can be understood as involving a psychobiological syndrome consisting of mood complaints, vegetative symptoms, and idiosyncratic cognitive manifestations that influence mood.[95] Patients who somatize usually deny or minimize cognitive and affective complaints and only focus on presumed physical ailments to explain their distress and often embellish the intensity of their affliction. Depression and somatization can be conceptualized as opposite sides of the same coin (one side with primarily affective complaints, the other with somatic ones).

It is also important to understand which psychiatric illnesses are not common in PNES. Comorbid psychotic disorders such as depression with psychosis or schizophrenia are uncommon in PNES.[13] Factitious disorder and malingering have not been associated with or found to be elevated in PNES compared to any other psychiatric disorder. This is important for correcting the stigma that patients face with uninformed providers, often those in emergency settings who may not fully understand the difference between factitious, malingering, and somatic symptoms and related disorders.

2.5. Psychological Characteristics

The rationale for identifying psychological risk factors is to increase understanding of the mechanisms underlying PNES. Specific psychological characteristics have been reported in PNES. In one pediatric study comparing PNES patients to siblings, the PNES patients reported higher anxiety sensitivity, practiced more solitary emotional coping, and experienced more lifetime adversities.[39] Higher hypnotizability scores as well as differences in interactional psycholinguistic style, such as "detailing block" and "focusing resistance," have been reported.[96] *Detailing block* is a term used to describe the paucity of information and incomplete narratives used to describe seizure activity by PNES patients compared to those with epilepsy. *Focusing resistance* refers to the tendency of PNES patients to avoid discussing the topic of seizures except with prompting, as compared to epilepsy patients, who easily volunteer first-person accounts of seizures. These conversational tendencies support avoidant behavioral and cognitive styles. The use of space/place metaphors by PNES patients to describe seizures has also been mentioned and documented.[97] This reveals a semantic preference of PNES patients to metaphorically describe their "seizures" as a place or location they "travel to." In other words, "seizures" are a passive backdrop acted on by the patient. This is in contrast to ES patients, who more often use metaphors of seizures as an active force opposing them or as a volitional opponent. In addition, fearful attachment styles, compared to those with epilepsy, have also been reported.[98] External locus of control, especially with regard to health, have been documented in PNES, alluding to problems with self-efficacy beliefs.[8,99]

2.5.1. Alexithymia

High rates of alexithymia, a personality trait hallmarked by deficits in emotion recognition and processing, is frequently observed in PNES.[100] *Alexithymia* is the term coined by Syphneos in 1973[101] to describe this phenomena. In several studies, this external lack of ability to verbally describe a disturbed internal emotional state has been associated with FNSD.[102,103] In fact, in patients with PNES, alexithymia was found to be an important factor predicting poor quality of life and should be a target for therapeutic intervention.[104] Clinically, it is important for the clinician to pay close attention to somatic complaints and to understand them as a metaphor for distress, especially in the context of alexithymia.

2.5.2. Dissociation

Dissociation is another phenomenon that has been understood as a fundamental defense mechanism commonly present in PNES patients and often conceptualized as essential for the development of FNSD. In the aforementioned study by Bowmen et al.,[92] in 45 patients with PNES, 91% displayed features meeting criteria for a dissociative disorder. The concept that dissociation is necessary for symptom development in PNES has been challenged. The evaluation of dissociation in this population compared to that in epilepsy patients and controls has presented conflicting results. For example, Lawton et al.[105] reviewed the results of seven studies that attempted to clarify these issues and found that only four confirmed a significant difference in dissociation between epilepsy and PNES patients. The authors attributed these findings to the erroneous concept that dissociation is a homogeneous phenomenon and seen in all PNES patients. They tested the hypothesis that dissociation could be bifurcated into two components, detachment (expected to be seen in both groups) and compartmentalization, more characteristic of patients with PNES. The results confirmed the hypothesis, with PNES patients scoring significantly higher on compartmentalization. However, when depression and anxiety were controlled for, this finding disappeared.[105] Other authors have proposed that these differences vary in patient subgroups and that dissociation is not an independent risk factor for all PNES patients.[106,107] Interestingly, patients with both PNES and coexistent epilepsy were found to have significantly elevated levels of dissociation compared to the epilepsy and control groups in a study by Ito et al.[108]

2.5. Culture/Family

Social history and culture may influence and predispose individuals to PNES. PNES patients have often witnessed a seizure of a friend or relative with epilepsy or have been exposed to seizures as a healthcare worker.[32] Few cross-cultural comparison studies have been performed. Prevalence rates of PNES in Turkey, India, and Puerto Rico are estimated at 3% to 4%, which are much greater than prevalence rates for the U.S. general population, estimated to be less than 0.03%. It is unclear which culturally shaped variables are responsible for these prevalence rate differences. Differences in diagnostic procedures, clinical presentation, family and social roles, history of traumatic experiences, comorbidities, and precipitating factors are speculated to be responsible.[109,110] Cultural and role-assignment risk factors may include those reported in Australia and Turkey in which patients with PNES are described as the "special/favorite child," defined by behaviors that include overaccommodation and submissive attitudes.[109,111,112] Areas with rigid gender roles and restrictions on self-expression may have higher incidence rates of PNES, similar to patterns observed in other cultural conceptualizations of emotional distress, such as spirit possession.[113]

Poor communication and interpersonal conflict are reported often in PNES patients and their families.[32,114-116] Maternal rejection and insecure attachment have been reported in PNES patients in Turkey, as is the case in dissociative disorder[117] and somatization.[118] A recent review of childhood traumatic experiences in PNES patients found a significantly stronger association of psychological trauma and PNES in Western countries than in South American or Asian countries.[73]

The elevated overlap between depression and somatization may be best understood when cognitive and sociocultural backgrounds are taken into consideration. The vegetative aspects of depression appear to be universal and cross-cultural.[95] However, cognitive aspects take a variety of forms in different cultures. A somatic focus for depression is the norm in numerous cultures. In many societies, there are no words for depression; somatization provides a more sanctioned way to express grief, emotional upset, or loss in general. It also may function to galvanize family concern and short-circuit interpersonal conflict. For example, in China a symptom called *hsing-ching pu hao* is synonymous with "anxious upset." In Central and South America the term *susto* means "soul loss" and consists of vegetative complaints.[95] Bagayogo et al.[94] have reviewed transcultural aspects of physical symptoms appearing in the context of depressive disorders. The authors note the varied nomenclature from a variety of cultures but with one common aspect: that there is an attempt by the patient to communicate, "I am in some kind of distress but have learned no language other than my body by which to convey this."[119]

2.6. Key Points for Treatment–Predisposing Factors

1. Screen for epilepsy, learning disorders, and childhood abuse (emphasis on juvenile-onset PNES).
2. Address medical illnesses and their traumatic impact (emphasis on late-onset PNES).
3. Sexual trauma is common in females but may not indicate or be an exclusive cause of PNES.
4. Consider screening at-risk patients with standardized measures to identify and treat comorbid psychological illness, especially trauma-related disorders.
5. Engage families and community systems in treatment to improve communication and decrease interpersonal conflict.
6. Teach skills that reinforce internal locus-of-control beliefs.

3. PRECIPITATING FACTORS

The differentiation between predisposing and precipitating factors is often semantic and based on presumed temporal relationships. In reality, precipitating and predisposing events often overlap. Generally, *precipitating factors* are those variables identified as occurring within 1 year of symptom onset and assumed to have a causal link in the development of a disease. These are described as inciting events that are the "last straw" in a series of events or vulnerabilities that finally meet a certain threshold to elicit symptoms consistent with the diagnostic criteria of PNES. This is similar to a quantum event. For example, in the final shovel of dirt that moves a giant boulder, the actual shovel of dirt may not on face value appear that powerful, but in the context of time and previous shoveling it has a huge effect in igniting change. Examining precipitating factors may help identify key causal links to PNES development.

3.1. Symptom Onset

Several studies in the literature point to common precipitants. A study comparing precipitants identified significantly more adverse or traumatic events over the previous year in new-onset PNES than with newly diagnosed epilepsy[120] Psychosocial stressors that have been reported to precipitate the emergence of PNES include unwanted pregnancy, bereavement, physical, verbal, or sexual abuse, increased job demands, litigation, financial problems, divorce or separation, interpersonal conflicts, surgery, earthquakes, medical illness and procedures, and accidents.[3,6,9,32,121] Women more often have precipitants linked to sexual abuse while men report loss of employment or role changes. In older patients, physical illness is the most common precipitant.[122] One study using analysis of 14 video-recorded patient interviews concluded that "forced choices" or unspeakable dilemmas in patients' family and social circumstances were identifiable in 13 of 14 cases.[123] Often these conflicts involve protecting family members at the expense of caring for one's owns needs. For example, a patient may need to move to a community where a past childhood abuser is seen daily in order to better the economic opportunities of his or her children. PNES has often been reported as a sequela from mild traumatic brain injury (TBI).[44] For children, parental discord or divorce may be an inciting event.[11,124] Academic underachievement has been reported as the most prevalent precipitating stressor for young boys.[125] One large study ($N = 288$) of antecedent factors by Duncan and Oto (2008),[26] described all types of traumatic experiences as predicting later age of PNES onset, while bullying and comorbid epilepsy were predictive of earlier onset PNES.

3.2. Immediate Triggers

Another way to define precipitating factors is more immediate and less historical. Precipitating factors can be conceptualized as environment stimuli that currently (i.e., in hours, minutes, or even seconds) trigger symptoms. The term *trigger* is often used when describing precipitants in this way. Triggers in a behavioral paradigm refer to those conditioned and unconditioned stimuli that immediately precede symptoms on an ongoing basis. They are stimuli that are presumed to have been paired to an unconditioned stimulus and then generalized.

Common triggers described in the PNES literature include being "witnessed," for instance, in a doctor's waiting room or during electrode placement during EEG monitoring.[126-128] These triggers may sometimes have predictive and diagnostic value when distinguishing PNES events from epilepsy.[35,129] There is some evidence that patients underreport "stress" triggers, especially emotional stress, and this is better identified by witnesses.[127] Other temporally related triggers include emergence from general anesthesia, from a focal epileptic seizure, or from sleep.[130] More commonly, autonomic arousal caused by a sudden sensory stimulus, either external or interoceptive in nature, or by pain may elicit symptoms. Often, transitions from sympathetic to parasympathetic activities are vulnerable periods, presumably because of a baseline instability in the autonomic nervous system. For example, finally sitting down to rest or watch TV after a stressful day can be a vulnerable period, as it is for migraine headaches. Patients with learning disorders in one study appeared to be more vulnerable to situational triggers.[26]

Often, avoidance of triggers unfortunately strengthens triggers through sensitization. Patients' avoidance and safety behavior patterns develop and increase the chance of autonomic arousal, further increasing the intensity of a trigger or generalizing it to include a new and novel stimulus. This is the same mechanism thought to underlie PTSD. This may explain why some PNES patients are triggered by re-experiencing phenomena related to PTSD and reminders of past traumatic experiences.[98]

3.3. Key Points for Treatment—Precipitating Factors

1. Patients may need others to bring to awareness the initial circumstances that preceded PNES and employ problem-solving strategies if those circumstances still exist.
2. With the help of others, patients should track symptoms to identify triggers, especially emotionally laden ones.
3. As patients become aware of triggers, desensitization can occur through education about avoidance and safety behaviors.
4. Patients should be encouraged to use vagal modulating activities to strengthen autonomic flexibility, such as basic stress management techniques, trauma-focused psychotherapy, yoga, mindfulness, biofeedback, meditation, and exercise. This may be especially important for those with learning disabilities.

4. PERPETUATING FACTORS

Perpetuating factors refer to those elements that keep symptoms present after initial onset and are presumed to be separate from the antecedent causes or precipitants of PNES. These are sometimes the natural consequences or sequelae of symptoms themselves. They can involve the response of the environment or the patient to symptoms and can serve an adaptive value in the short run. These factors may be within a patient's awareness but often are outside of it. Often, perpetuating factors are reinforcing and may have evolutionary value but are hidden from consciousness. They represent the transactional nature of causal factors.

For example, symptoms that create attention from family members may be very embarrassing and humiliating for a patient who is used to being in a caregiving role and for whom independence is a core value. Paradoxically, this same patient may be implicitly rewarded for these PNES behaviors that elicit nurturing or attention that lead to unintended behavioral shaping that is outside volitional control. In this example, the evolutionary value of nurturing and attention overrides the explicit aversive social consequences such as shame or frustration surrounding symptoms. This might be especially true in a patient who normally is in a caregiving role and who rarely allows nurturing or attention to be received directly. In this example, it would be important for this PNES patient in treatment to become aware of nurturing needs and subsequently develop alternate behaviors to obtain these directly and with awareness. Although a literature review may provide some insight into the phenomenon of perpetuation in PNES, its complexity and heterogeneity require reliance on behavioral principals rather than identification of specific factors. Perpetuating factors must be identified and personalized on the basis of intimate knowledge and unique historical and present context of each patient.

Although difficult to measure, some of the literature does shed light on important factors to consider as perpetuating. In a naturalistic study of 59 consecutive cases of functional neurological symptoms seen by one psychotherapist, family dysfunction and affective disorders were identified by the authors as the most common perpetuating factors; other perpetuating factors included bereavement, health anxiety/hypochondriasis, physical health problems, financial gain, illness identity, sexual traumatic experiences, caregiver role, and isolation.[131] A recent review of 14 PNES studies found depressive symptoms to be most strongly associated with quality-of-life indicators. Variables less strongly associated with quality of life included dissociation, somatic symptoms, escape-avoidance behaviors, and family dysfunction. Avoidance of emotions was proposed as a mechanism of perpetuating difficulties with quality of life.[5] The behavioral and emotional avoidance of potential seizure triggers can become a major perpetuating mechanism as patients become more isolated, angry, depressed, and physically deconditioned, increasing the degree of vulnerability. These problems can lead to increasingly more distress, and the "sick role" can then become an entrenched identity and impact the entire family system.[98] Dependency and financial disability often become difficult to reverse.[79,131]

The impact of PNES symptoms on treatment can sometimes also lead to a vicious feed-forward cycle. Often, seizure symptoms lend themselves to lack of independence, financial problems, and transportation difficulties that significantly interfere with consistent healthcare, especially mental health treatment. Another treatment confound occurs when seizure treatment itself may exacerbate symptoms. This is often the case with amplification of PNES with the use of antiepileptic drugs (AEDs) along with their associated toxicities.[98] In addition to the known physiological risks of medical treatment, psychological risks also exist that are linked to medical interventions. Implicit biases and invalidation by providers have been documented [132,133] and may lead to chronic or discrete recurring traumatic experiences. This is especially likely for individuals exposed to traumatic experiences in the past who are sensitized to developing PTSD. The longer the disorder is not accurately diagnosed or treated, the higher the risk of iatrogenic medical and psychological harm.

Although our knowledge of the exact perpetuating factors remains limited,[134] the advantage for patients and providers who identify these factors is powerful. Identifying factors that contribute to these negative feedback loops can ideally lead to commitment to small changes that can eventually lead to impactful gains. One small change in the environment or behavior can start the virtuous cycle of positive feedback and reinforce patients to make further changes. For example, when patients decrease a small amount of their hypervigilance with medications or psychotherapy, there may be an exponential decrease in avoidance patterns, leading to profound symptom improvement. This is also seen in the wider system when family members or providers make a subtle change in their response to a patient and witness the power of this contingency management on the course of the illness.

4.1. Key Points for Treatment—Perpetuating Factors

1. When considering possible perpetuating factors, keep in mind reinforcers that may be outside of the patient's awareness.
2. Treat mood symptoms aggressively, since they are the most strongly reported perpetuating factors that impact quality of life.
3. Minimize and target financial gain from symptoms, family dysfunction, isolation, deconditioning, and comorbid disorders.
4. Teach patients to identify avoidance and safety behaviors and "avoid avoiding."
5. Stop or taper unnecessary antiepileptic drugs as soon as possible.
6. Minimize contact with potentially iatrogenic healthcare settings. Educate providers.
7. Encourage family and provider involvement in making changes.
8. Emphasize and cheerlead small changes that can make impactful differences over time.

5. PROGNOSTIC FACTORS

A *risk factor* is linked to the development of a condition, whereas a *prognostic factor* influences the outcome of a condition. Prognostic factors are sometimes difficult to distinguish from and may overlap with other factors, especially perpetuating ones. Prognostic assessments of PNES report that only 25–38% of patients achieve seizure freedom 6 months to 10 years after diagnosis.[6,8,32,83,135,136] Children have a much better prognosis, with PNES remission rates reaching 70–80%.[137] PNES prognosis will be discussed in more depth in Chapter 17.

It has been argued that event frequency may not be the most ideal measure of clinical outcome. Some studies have instead investigated other variables, most often using quality-of-life measures.[8,135,138,139] State-supported financial benefits at 4 years after diagnosis were reported in 56% in one study sample of 164 PNES patients.[8] A later study showed that 43% of the patients who had reached seizure remission were unproductive and either retired because of ill health or were unemployed a mean of 4.2 years after diagnosis.[135] The unemployed-but-remitted group was significantly older and less educated and had a younger age of onset, longer time to diagnosis, and more severe psychopathology than the remitted employed group. Occupational status and event frequency are often not correlated. This is represented by the fact that despite symptom improvement, social and employment outcomes often remain poor in this group.[79,131] Variables other than event frequency, such as depression and psychosocial issues, are more directly related to disability and quality of life.[80,99,138,139] Some patients may develop new somatic complaints, often pain syndromes and headaches.[36] There is also some evidence pointing to increased mortality among PNES patients.[53] Overall, PNES outcomes are worse than for newly diagnosed epilepsy but similar to those for other somatic symptom disorders.[8]

Table 3.1 lists some of the prognostic variables reported and associated with positive and negative outcomes.[3,7,8,29,36,80,83,84,122,136,140-145] Most of these studies have used event frequency as the outcome measure. In a small retrospective outcome study of 36 PNES patients, Gambini et al.[134] found that the only factor associated with improved long-term outcome was whether the diagnosis was established through induction of PNES symptoms by suggestion. The choice of induction by suggestion in this study was the use of a colored patch imbibed with alcohol on the neck. The use of such suggestion techniques has been questioned by one of the authors (JJB). This may point to the influence of self-efficacy beliefs on the acceptance and outcome of the diagnosis. It is still unclear if factors determining short-term and long-term outcomes are different. Please refer to Chapter 17 for further discussion of long-term outcomes.

5.1. Key Points for Treatment—Prognostic Factors

1. Diagnose and treat PNES aggressively and as early as possible.
2. Spend the time and effort needed to communicate the diagnosis to ensure patient acceptance. Encourage ongoing education on PNES.
3. Diagnose using seizure induction methods when possible, such as hypnosis or other suggestion methods (this can be controversial).
4. Encourage increased socialization.
5. Encourage employment and resolution of litigation quickly.
6. Target aggressive treatment toward dissociative and somatic symptom-related disorders.
7. Encourage and support independence.
8. Target treatment at emotional expression and improved affect regulation.

6. TREATMENT STUDIES AND MECHANISTIC CLUES

Table 3.3 lists randomized control trials (RCTs) performed with PNES subjects. Although the results and details of these studies will be discussed in more detail in Chapter 14, we will briefly explore how these study designs and outcomes might shed light on proposed mechanisms, mediators, and moderators of this illness. The design of an RCT illuminates the hypotheses put forth by experts in the field. Treatments and their targets reveal a researcher's beliefs about the mechanism of PNES, while controlled variables and secondary measures often reveal theories about moderators. In this section we explore some of the assumptions and hypotheses that these studies have about the etiological underpinnings of the disorder.

Table 3.3. Proposed Mechanisms for PNES Suggested by Randomized Controlled Trials

Author/Date	Intervention vs. Control	Authors' Hypothesized Targets
Moene et al. (2002)[145]	Hypnosis + comprehensive inpatient treatment vs. Comprehensive inpatient treatment (with groups, PT) with nonspecific individual therapy	✓ Self-efficacy beliefs/perception of control over symptoms ✓ Dissociation ✓ Hypnotizability ✓ Relaxation/autonomic arousal
Moene et al. (2003)[146]	Outpatient hypnosis vs. Waiting list	✓ Self-efficacy beliefs/perception of control over symptoms ✓ Dissociation ✓ Hypnotizability ✓ Relaxation/autonomic arousal
Ataoglu et al. (2003)[147]	Paradoxical intention (PI), two sessions of imaginal exposure to trauma or attempting to bring on symptoms vs. Diazepam 5–15 mg	✓ Avoidance ✓ Operant conditioning ✓ Secondary gain ✓ Sensitization/desensitization to triggers ✓ Self-efficacy beliefs ✓ Family and environmental response to symptoms
Goldstein et al. (2010)[148]	Cognitive-behavior therapy (CBT) + standard medical care (SMC) vs. SMC CBT nurse delivered	✓ Depression ✓ Anxiety ✓ Avoidance ✓ Response to triggers ✓ Negative thoughts ✓ Illness beliefs ✓ Low self-esteem
LaFrance et al. (2010)[149]	12 weeks of flexible-dose sertraline vs. Placebo	✓ Depression ✓ Anxiety ✓ Impulsivity ✓ Serotonergic activity
Sharpe et al. (2011)[151]	3 months of CBT-based guided self-help (GSH) vs. Usual care (UC)	✓ Somatic awareness ✓ Emotional awareness ✓ Education about illness ✓ Avoidance ✓ Cognitions ✓ Anxiety ✓ Depression

Table 3.3. Continued

Author/Date	Intervention vs. Control	Authors' Hypothesized Targets
Thompson et al. (2013)[152]	Brief semistructured educational intervention by RN using positive reframing while subjects in hospital for video EEG vs. Standard care	✓ Education about illness/treatment ✓ Mental health treatment ✓ Awareness and acceptance of diagnosis
LaFrance et al. (2014)[150]	16 weeks sertraline vs. CBT vs. CBT + sertraline vs. Treatment as usual (TAU)	✓ Serotonergic activity ✓ Depression ✓ Anxiety ✓ Avoidance ✓ Responses to triggers ✓ Negative thoughts ✓ Illness beliefs ✓ Psychoeducation
Chen et al. (2014)[153]	3-monthly psychoeducational group treatment vs. Routine seizure clinic follow-up	✓ Awareness of diagnosis ✓ Education about illness

The first RCTs of this century, by Moene et al.,[145,146] used hypnosis, supporting hypothetical mechanisms such as suggestibility, internal beliefs, and overall sense of control as contributing to symptoms and their improvement. In 2003, Ataoglu et al.[147] used a behavioral approach (paradoxical intention) in an RCT encouraging patients to bring on symptoms or to imagine anxiety-inducing situations or memories in an exposure-based paradigm. This study required patients to actually attempt to elicit symptoms rather than try to cope with or stop symptoms. This design highlighted and its results supported proposed PNES mechanisms of behavioral avoidance patterns, sensitization to cues, "illness identity," and operant reinforcement from the environment.

More standardized studies appeared with the first pilot RCT of cognitive-behavioral therapy (CBT), by Goldstein et al.[148] in 2010. This treatment approach targets comorbidities such as anxiety and depression and encourages the interruption of the behavioral/physiological/cognitive responses to the beginning of a seizure or triggers. Encouragement toward engaging in avoided activities and addressing negative thoughts and illness beliefs, including low self-esteem, was emphasized. Interestingly, this first CBT study found improvement in symptoms but not mood compared to controls. LaFrance et al.,[149,150] in 2010 and 2014, piloted the first pharmacological RCTs of sertraline targeting "Axis I and II serotonergic-mediated symptoms in PNES (i.e., depression, anxiety and impulsivity)". They hypothesized that treating moderating comorbidities in PNES would reduce symptoms. The next RCTs, delivered self-guided CBT in 2011[151] and a multisite individual CBT-informed psychotherapy study in 2014.[150] The design of these studies reiterated hypotheses about the mechanistic targets of PNES such as physical symptoms, emotional states, cognitions, anxiety and depression. "Self-help" can maximize and preserve targeted beliefs and skills related to internal locus of control. The positive results of all of the studies discussed here suggest that their proposed targets may be the mechanisms and moderators involved in PNES.

In more recent RCTs, Thompson[152] and Chen[153] have developed interventions focused on awareness and education about the PNES diagnosis, targeting acceptance of diagnosis and illness, treatment beliefs, and engagement in mental health services. Their results also suggest that these variables are important to recovery and that beliefs about illness may be a salient etiological factor in PNES.

Notably absent targets in the RCT literature include treatments focusing on traumatic experiences and affective regulation. If one returns to the epidemiological evidence of traumatic experiences and autonomic markers in PNES, it appears that correcting the effects of trauma and autonomic dysregulation could also be a useful direction.[154] PNES treatment development in the area of traumatic experiences may consider focusing on prolonged exposure, trauma-sensitive yoga, and mindfulness-based interventions or developing other vagal modulating approaches. Most trauma-related treatments use some form of reshaping of linguistic narratives and episodic memory to enhance locus-of-control beliefs[155] and decrease the negative impact of painful memories. These treatments often use exposure-based techniques to desensitize autonomic arousal and therefore normalize fear habituation abnormalities.

The common sequela of PNES correlates such as traumatic experiences, family and environmental stress, autonomic dysfunction, attachment difficulties, biological sensitivities, and psychiatric and medical illness is often affective dysregulation. Many patients have either alexithymia or lack of accurate interoceptive sensitivity or awareness of emotions. Providing patients with skills to identify and regulate emotions effectively may be the key to regulate sensory, motor, and cognitive dysfunction in PNES. Future treatment approaches will hopefully consider affective dysregulation as an explicit target and common pathway. This would be in alignment with the neurobiological abnormalities found in patients with functional motor disorder, most notably in the area of amygdala habituation that may also underlie PNES.[156]

6.1. Key Points for Treatment–Disease Mechanisms (Based on Treatment Studies)

1. Treatments should target self-efficacy and illness beliefs through psychoeducation and by maximizing the patient's sense of agency with skills acquisition models.
2. Treatment should focus on decreasing avoidance patterns.
3. Use evidence-based treatments that target comorbidities such as depression, anxiety, and trauma-related disorders.

4. Consider targeting trauma-related affective dysregulation in developing and innovating new treatment strategies.
5. Teaching patients skills that aid in identification and regulation of emotion and arousal may be useful in innovating new treatments.

7. SUMMARY

There are numerous perspectives that can explain PNES. PNES exists at the intersection of all the biopsychosocial perspectives of psychiatry. It can be considered a cultural disorder in which shared symbolic meanings of a community bidirectionally influence beliefs and behavior of the individual. It can also be seen as a neuronal and physiological disorder mediated by attachment machinery, autonomic arousal, and limbic dysregulation. Alternatively, it can be regarded as a cognitive and behavioral disorder representing dysfunctional self-efficacy beliefs and maladaptive operant and classical conditioning patterns. PNES can similarly be conceptualized as an interpersonal and traumatic attachment disorder in which symptoms serve to communicate and regulate relationships. More perspectives not mentioned here also exist and reflect the varied narratives, meanings, and distinctions the human language and mind can create to explain PNES complexity and uncertainty.

From the "4P-BPS" model we can conclude that some individuals have neurological substrates that make them vulnerable to PNES via a wide range of possibilities, including genetic and biological predisposition, neurological disability, brain injury, or the neurobiological sequelae of traumatic experiences and depression. These vulnerabilities disturb the normal processing of affective and cognitive regulation. This predisposition in the face of enough environmental stressors or triggers can lead to a dysregulated state which can overflow into voluntary sensory, cognitive, and motor systems causing PNES symptoms. These patterns then can become entrenched over time as the organism adapts through classical and operant conditioning principles, especially via negative reinforcers such as behavioral avoidance. Continuing research and review of PNES data will further elucidate etiologies and their overlapping mechanisms, which will ultimately guide providers in customizing causal formulations specific for each unique patient.

7.1. Key Points for Treatment

- Psychiatric causes of PNES are individual and multifactorial.
- Treatment must address multiple causes or factors using customized formulations.
- Patients and providers need multiple tools and skills for successful outcomes.

REFERENCES

1. Stone J, Carson A. Functional neurologic symptoms: assessment and management. *Neurol Clin.* 2011;29:1–18. doi: 10.1016/j.ncl.2010.10.011
2. Jimenez X, Bautista J, Tesar G. Diagnostic assessment and case formulation in psychogenic nonepileptic seizures: a pilot comparison of approaches. *Epilepsy Behav.* 2015;45:164–168. doi: 10.1016/j.yebeh.2015.02.001

3. Asadi-Pooya A, Sperling M. Epidemiology of psychogenic nonepileptic seizures. *Epilepsy Behav.* 2015;46:60–65. doi:10.1016/j.yebeh.2015.03.015
4. Cragar D, Berry D, Fakhoury T, Cibula JE, Schmitt F. A review of diagnostic techniques in the differential diagnosis of epileptic and nonepileptic seizures. *Neuropsychol Rev.* 2002;12:31–64.
5. Jones B, Reuber M, Norman P. Correlates of health-related quality of life in adults with psychogenic nonepileptic seizures: a systematic review. *Epilepsia.* 2016;57(2):171–181. doi:10.1111/epi.13268.
6. Carton S, Thompson P, Duncan J. Non-epileptic seizures: patients' understanding and reaction to the diagnosis and impact on outcome. *Seizure.* 2003;12:287.
7. Meierkord H, Will B, Fish D, Shorvon S. The clinical features and prognosis of pseudoseizures diagnosed using video-EEG telemetry. *Neurology.* 1991;41(10):1643–1646.
8. Reuber M, Pukrop R, Bauer J, Helmstaedter C, Tessendorf N, Elger CE. Outcome in psychogenic nonepileptic seizures: 1- to 10-year follow-up in 164 patients. *Ann Neurol.* 2003;53(3):305–311.
9. Bowman E. Etiology and clinical course of pseudoseizures. Relationship to trauma, depression, and dissociation. *Psychosomatics* 1993;34(4):333–342.
10. Szaflarski J, Hughes C, Szaflarski M, Ficker D, Cahill W, Li M, Privitera M. Quality of life in psychogenic nonepileptic seizures. *Epilepsia.* 2003;44(2):236–242.
11. Wyllie E, Glazer J, Benbadis S, Kotagal P, Wolgamuth B. Psychiatric features of children and adolescents with pseudoseizures. *Arch Pediatr Adolesc Med.* 1999;153:(3):244–248.
12. McBride A, Shih T, Hirsch L. Video-EEG monitoring in the elderly: a review of 94 patients. *Epilepsia.* 2002;43(2):165–169.
13. Krumholz A, Niedermeyer E. Psychogenic seizures: a clinical study with follow-up data. *Neurology.* 1983;33(4):498–502.
14. Szabó L, Siegler Z, Zubek L, et al. A detailed semiologic analysis of childhood psychogenic nonepileptic seizures. *Epilepsia.* 2012;53(3):565–570. doi:10.1111/j.1528-1167.2012.03404
15. Alessi R, Valente K. Psychogenic non-epileptic seizures at a tertiary care center in Brazil. *Epilepsy Behav.* 2013;26(1):91–95. doi:10.1016/j.yebeh.2012.10.011
16. Scévola L, Teitelbaum J, Oddo S, Loidl C, Kochen S, Centurión E. Psychiatric disorders in patients with psychogenic non-epileptic seizures and drug-resistant epilepsy: a study of an Argentine population. *Epilepsy Behav.* 2013;29(1):155–160. doi:10.1016/j.yebeh.2013.07.012
17. Oto M, Conway P, McGonigal A, Russell A, Duncan R. Gender differences in psychogenic nonepileptic seizures. *Seizure.* 2005;14(1):33–39.
18. Dhiman V, Sinha S, Rawat V, Harish T, Chaturvedi S, Satishchandra P. Semiological characteristics of adults with psychogenic non-epileptic seizures (PNES): an attempt towards a new classification. *Epilepsy Behav.* 2013;27(3):427–432. doi:10.1016/j.yebeh.2013.03.005
19. Cronje G, Pretorius C. The coping styles and health-related quality of life of South African patients with psychogenic non-epileptic seizures. *Epilepsy Behav.* 2013;29(3):581–584.
20. Jones S, O' Brien T, Adams S, et al. Clinical characteristics and outcome in patients with psychogenic non-epileptic seizures. *Psychosom Med.* 2010;72(5):487–497. doi:10.1097/PSY.0b013e3181d96550
21. Abubakr A, Wambacq I. Seizures in the elderly: video/EEG monitoring analysis. *Epilepsy Behav.* 2005;7(3):447–450.
22. Thomas A, Preston J, Scott R, Bujarski K. Diagnosis of probable psychogenic nonepileptic seizures in the outpatient clinic: does gender matter? *Epilepsy Behav.* 2013;29(2):295–297. doi:10.1016/j.yebeh.2013.08.006

23. Noe K, Grade M, Stonnington C, Driver-Dunckley E, Locke D. Confirming psychogenic non-epileptic seizures with video-EEG: sex matters. *Epilepsy Behav.* 2012;23(3):220–223.
24. Asadi-Pooya AA, Emami Y, Emami M. Psychogenic non-epileptic seizures in Iran. *Seizure.* 2014;23(3):175–177. doi:10.1016/j.seizure.2013.11.005
25. Duncan R, Razvi S, Mulhern S. Newly presenting psychogenic nonepileptic seizures: incidence, population characteristics, and early outcome from a prospective audit of a first seizure clinic. *Epilepsy Behav.* 2011;20:308–311. doi:10.1016/j.yebeh.2010.10.022
26. Duncan R, Oto M. Predictors of antecedent factors in psychogenic nonepileptic attacks: multivariate analysis. *Neurology.* 2008;71(13):1000–1005. doi:10.1212/01.wnl.0000326593.50863.21
27. Asadi-Pooya A, Emami M. Juvenile and adult-onset psychogenic non-epileptic seizures. *Clin Neurol Neurosurg.* 2013;115(9):1697–1700. doi:10.1016/j.clineuro.2013.03.009
28. Duncan R, Oto M, Martin E, Pelosi A. Late onset psychogenic non-epileptic attacks. *Neurology.* 2006;66:1644–1647.
29. Reuber M, Elger C. Psychogenic nonepileptic seizures: review and update. *Epilepsy Behav.* 2003;4:205.
30. Metrick M, Ritter F, Gates J, Jacobs M, Skare S, Loewenson R. Nonepileptic events in childhood. *Epilepsia.* 1991;32(3):322–328.
31. Holmes G, Sackellares J, McKiernan J, Ragland M, Dreifuss F. Evaluation of childhood pseudoseizures using EEG telemetry and video tape monitoring. *J Pediatr.* 1980;97(4):554–558.
32. Lancman M, Brotherton T, Asconapé J, Penry J. Psychogenic seizures in adults: a longitudinal analysis. *Seizure.* 1993;2:281–286.
33. Alper K, Devinsky O, Perrine K, Vazquez B, Luciano D. Nonepileptic seizures and childhood sexual and physical abuse. *Neurology.* 1993;43:1950–1953.
34. Say G, Taşdemir H, İnce H. Semiological and psychiatric characteristics of children with psychogenic nonepileptic seizures: gender-related differences. *Seizure.* 2015;31:144–148. doi:10.1016/j.seizure.2015.07.017
35. Benbadis S. A spell in the epilepsy clinic and a history of "chronic pain" or "fibromyalgia" independently predict a diagnosis of psychogenic seizures. *Epilepsy Behav.* 2005;6(2):264–265.
36. Ettinger A, Devinsky O, Weisbrot D, Goyal A, Shashikumar S. Headaches and other pain symptoms among patients with psychogenic non-epileptic seizures. *Seizure.* 1999;8(7):424–426.
37. Mökleby K, Blomhoff S, Malt U, Dahlström A, Tauböll E, Gjerstad L. Psychiatric comorbidity and hostility in patients with psychogenic nonepileptic seizures compared with somatoform disorders and healthy controls. *Epilepsia.* 2002;43(2):193–198.
38. Dixit R, Popescu A, Bagić A, Ghearing G, Hendrickson R. Medical comorbidities in patients with psychogenic nonepileptic spells (PNES) referred for video-EEG monitoring. *Epilepsy Behav.* 2013;28(2):137–140. doi:10.1016/j.yebeh.2013.05.004
39. Plioplys S, Doss J, Siddarth P, et al. A multisite controlled study of risk factors in pediatric psychogenic nonepileptic seizures. *Epilepsia.* 2014;55(11):1739–1747. doi:10.1111/epi.12773
40. Reuber M, Fernández G, Helmstaedter C, Qurishi A, Elger E. Evidence of brain abnormality in patients with psychogenic nonepileptic seizures. *Epilepsy Behav.* 2002;3(3):249–254.
41. van Merode T, Twellaar M, Kotsopoulos I, et al. Psychological characteristics of patients with newly developed psychogenic seizures. *J Neurol Neurosurg Psychiatry.* 2004;75(8):1175–1177.

42. Reuber M, Fernández G, Bauer J, Singh D, Elger C. Interictal EEG abnormalities in patients with psychogenic nonepileptic seizures. *Epilepsia.* 2002;43(9):1013–1020.
43. Barry E, Krumholz A, Bergey GK, Bergey G, Chatha H, Alemayehu S, Grattan L. Nonepileptic posttraumatic seizures. *Epilepsia.* 1998;39(4):427–431.
44. LaFrance W Jr, Deluca M, Machan J, Fava J. Traumatic brain injury and psychogenic nonepileptic seizures yield worse outcomes. *Epilepsia.* 2013;54(4):718–725. doi:10.1111/epi.12053
45. DeToledo J, Lowe M, Haddad H. Behaviors mimicking seizures in institutionalized individuals with multiple disabilities and epilepsy: a video-EEG study. *Epilepsy Behav.* 2002;3(3):242–244.
46. Paolicchi J. The spectrum of nonepileptic events in children. *Epilepsia.* 2002;43(3):60–64.
47. Benbadis S, Agrawal V, Tatum W. How many patients with psychogenic nonepileptic seizures also have epilepsy? *Neurology.* 2001;57(5):915–917.
48. Parra J, Iriarte J, Kanner A. Are we overusing the diagnosis of psychogenic non-epileptic events? *Seizure.* 1999;8(4):223–227.
49. Martin R, Burneo J, Prasad A, et al. Frequency of epilepsy in patients with psychogenic seizures monitored by video-EEG. *Neurology.* 2003;61(12):1791–1792.
50. Lesser R, Lueders H, Dinner D. Evidence for epilepsy is rare in patients with psychogenic seizures. *Neurology.* 1983(4);33:502–504.
51. Marchetti R, Kurcgant D, Gallucci-Neto J, Von Bismark M, Fiore L. Epilepsy in patients with psychogenic non-epileptic seizures. *Arq Neuropsiquiatr.* 2010;68(2):168–173.
52. Hara K, Adachi N, Akanuma N, et al. Dissociative experiences in epilepsy: effects of epilepsy-related factors on pathological dissociation. *Epilepsy Behav.* 2015;44C:185–191.
53. Galimberti C, Ratti M, Murelli R, Marchioni E, Manni R, Tartara A. Patients with psychogenic nonepileptic seizures, alone or epilepsy-associated, share a psychological profile distinct from that of epilepsy patients. *J Neurol.* 2003;250(3):338–346.
54. de Timary P, Fouchet P, Sylin M, Indriets J, de Barsy T, Lefèbvre A, van Rijckevorsel K. Non-epileptic seizures: delayed diagnosis in patients presenting with electroencephalographic (EEG) or clinical signs of epileptic seizures. *Seizure.* 2002;11(3):193–197.
55. Ney GC, Barr WB, Napolitano C, Napolitano C, Decker R, Schaul N. New-onset psychogenic seizures after surgery for epilepsy. *Arch Neurol.* 1998;55(5):726–730.
56. Glosser G, Roberts D, Glosser D. Nonepileptic seizures after resective epilepsy surgery. *Epilepsia.* 1999;40(12):1750–1754.
57. Parra J, Iriarte J, Kanner A, Bergen D. De novo psychogenic nonepileptic seizures after epilepsy surgery. *Epilepsia.* 1998;39(5):474–477.
58. Nemeroff CB. Mood disorders. In: Charney DS, Nestler EJ, eds. *Neurobiology of Mental Illness*, 2nd ed. p357-522 New York: Oxford University Press; 2004.
59. Kanner A, Schachecter S, Barry J, et al. Depression and epilepsy: epidemiologic and neurobiologic perspectives that may explain their high comorbid occurrence. *Epilepsy Behav.* 2012;24(2):156–168. doi:10.1016/j.yebeh.2012.01.007
60. Ye M, Yang T, Qing P, Lei X, Qiu J, Liu G. Changes of functional brain networks in major depressive disorder: a graph theoretical analysis of resting-state fMRI. *PLoS One.* 2015;10(9):1–16. doi:10.1371/journal.pone.0133775
61. Kaiser R, Andrews-Hanna J, Wagner T, Pizzagalli D. Large-scale network dysfunction in major depressive disorder—a meta-analysis of resting-state functional connectivity. *JAMA Psychiatry.* 2015;72(6):603–611.

62. Perez D, Barsky A, Daffner K, Silbersweig D. Motor and somatosensory conversion disorder: a functional unawareness syndrome? *J Neuropsychatry Clin Neurosci.* 2012;24(2):141–151. doi:10.1176/appi.neuropsych.11050110
63. LaFrance W, Leaver K, Stopa E, Papandonatos G, Blum A. Decreased serum BDNF levels in patients with epileptic and psychogenic nonepileptic seizures. *Neurology.* 2010;75(14):1285–1291. doi:10.1212/WNL.0b013e3181f612bb
64. Bijanki K, Hodis B, Brumm M, Harlynn E, McCormick L. Hippocampal and left subcallosal anterior cingulate atrophy in psychotic depression. *PLoS One.* 2014;9(10):1–6. doi:10.1371/journal.pone.0110770
65. Bakvis P, Spinhoven P, Giltay E, Kuyk J, Edelbroek P, Zitman F, Roelofs K. Basal hypercortisolism and trauma in patients with psychogenic nonepileptic seizures. *Epilepsia.* 2010;51(5):752–759. doi:10.1111/j.1528-1167.2009.02394.x
66. Bakvis P, Roelofs K, Kuyk J, Edelbroek P, Swinkels W, Spinhoven P. Trauma, stress, and preconscious threat processing in patients with psychogenic nonepileptic seizures. *Epilepsia.* 2009;50(5):1001–1011. doi:10.1111/j.1528-1167.2008.01862.x
67. Reinsberger C, Sarkis R, Papadelis C, et al. Autonomic changes in psychogenic nonepileptic seizures: toward a potential diagnostic biomarker? *Clin EEG Neurosci.* 2015;46(1):16–25. doi:10.1177/1550059414567739
68. Ettinger A, Weisbrot D, Devinsky O. Patient reporting of seizure exacerbation near the time of menses helps distinguish epileptic from nonepileptic seizures. *J Epilepsy.* 1998;11(6):332–334.
69. Rosenberg H, Rosenberg S, Williamson P, Wolford G. A comparative study of trauma and posttraumatic stress disorder prevalence in epilepsy patients and psychogenic nonepileptic seizure patients. *Epilepsia.* 2000;41(4):447–452.
70. Paras M, Murad M, Chen L, et al. Sexual abuse and lifetime diagnosis of somatic disorders: a systematic review and meta-analysis. *JAMA.* 2009;302(5):550–561. doi:10.1001/jama.2009.109
71. Proença I, Castro L, Jorge C, Marchetti R. Emotional trauma and abuse in patients with psychogenic nonepileptic seizures. *Epilepsy Behav.* 2011:20(2);331–333. doi:10.1016/j.yebeh.2010.11.015
72. Selkirk M, Duncan R, Oto M, Pelosi A. Clinical differences between patients with non-epileptic seizures who report antecedent sexual abuse and those who do not. *Epilepsia.* 2008;49(8):1446–1450. doi:10.1111/j.1528-1167.2008.01611.x
73. Beghi M, Cornaggia I, Magaudda A, Perin C, Peroni F, Cornaggia C. Childhood trauma and psychogenic nonepileptic seizures: a review of findings with speculations on the underlying mechanisms. *Epilepsy Behav.* 2015;52(Pt A):169–173. doi:10.1016/j.yebeh.2015.09.007
74. Koby D, Zirakzadeh A, Staab J, et al. Questioning the role of abuse in behavioral spells and epilepsy. *Epilepsy Behav.* 2010;19(4):584–590. doi:10.1016/j.yebeh.2010.09.014
75. Kuyk J, Spinhoven P, van Emde Boas W, van Dyck R. Dissociation in temporal lobe epilepsy and pseudo-epileptic seizure patients. *J Nerv Ment Dis.* 1999;187(12):713–720.
76. Akyuz G1, Kugu N, Akyuz A, Dogan O. Dissociation and childhood abuse history in epileptic and pseudoseizure patients. *Epileptic Disord.* 2004;6(3):187–192.
77. Elliott J, Charyton C. Biopsychosocial predictors of psychogenic non-epileptic seizures. *Epilepsy Res.* 2014;108(9):1543–1553. doi:10.1016/j.eplepsyres.2014.09.003
78. Kaplan M, Dwivedi A, Privitera M, Isaacs K, Hughes C, Bowman M. Comparisons of childhood trauma, alexithymia, and defensive styles in patients with psychogenicnon-epileptic

seizures vs. epilepsy: implications for the etiology of conversion disorder. *Psychosom Res.* 2013;75(2):142–146. doi:10.1016/j.jpsychores.2013.06.005

79. Dikel T, Fennell E, Gilmore R. Posttraumatic stress disorder, dissociation, and sexual abuse history in epileptic and nonepileptic seizure patients. *Epilepsy Behav.* 2003;4(6):644–650.

80. Ettinger A, Devinsky O, Weisbrot D, Ramakrishna R, Goyal A. A comprehensive profile of clinical, psychiatric, and psychosocial characteristics of patients with psychogenic non-epileptic seizures. *Epilepsia.* 1999;40(9):1292–1298.

81. Westbrook L, Devinsky O, Geocadin R. Nonepileptic seizures after head injury. *Epilepsia.* 1998;39(9):978–982.

82. Reuber M, Pukrop R, Bauer J, Derfuss R, Elger C. Multidimensional assessment of personality in patients with psychogenic non-epileptic seizures. *J Neurol Neurosurg Psychiatry.* 2004;75(5):743–748.

83. Kanner A, Parra J, Frey M, Stebbins G, Pierre-Louis S, Iriarte J. Psychiatric and neurologic predictors of psychogenic pseudoseizure outcome. *Neurology.* 1999;22;53(5):933–938.

84. Bowman E. Nonepileptic seizures: psychiatric framework, treatment, and outcome. *Neurology.* 1999;53(5S2):84.

85. Lacey C, Cook M, Salzberg M. The neurologist, psychogenic nonepileptic seizures, and borderline personality disorder. *Epilepsy Behav.* 2007;11(4):492–498.

86. Harden C, Jovine L, Burgut F, Carey B, Nikolov B, Ferrando S. A comparison of personality disorder characteristics of patients with nonepileptic psychogenic pseudoseizures with those of patients with epilepsy. *Epilepsy Behav.* 2009;14(3):481–483. doi:10.1016/j.yebeh.2008.12.012

87. Testa S, Lesser R, Krauss G, Brandt J. Personality Assessment Inventory among patients with psychogenic seizures and those with epilepsy. *Epilepsia.* 2011;52(8):e84–e88. doi:10.1111/j.1528-1167.2011.03141.x

88. Storzbach D, Binder L, Salinsky M, Campbell B, Mueller R. Improved prediction of nonepileptic seizures with combined MMPI and EEG measures. *Epilepsia.* 2000;41(3):332–337.

89. Dikmen S, Hermann B, Wilensky A, Rainwater G. Validity of the Minnesota Multiphasic Personality Inventory (MMPI) to psychopathology in patients with epilepsy. *J Nerv Ment Dis.* 1983;171(2):114–122.

90. Derry P, McLachlan R. The MMPI-2 as an adjunct to the diagnosis of pseudoseizures. *Seizure.* 1996;5(1):35–40.

91. Schramke C, Valeri A, Valeriano J, Kelly K. Using the Minnesota Multiphasic Inventory 2, EEGs, and clinical data to predict nonepileptic events. *Epilepsy Behav.* 2007;11(3):343–346.

92. Bowman E, Markand O. Psychodynamics and psychiatric diagnoses of pseudoseizure subjects. *Am J Psychiatry.* 1996;153(1):57–63.

93. Kanner A, Schachecter S, Barry J, et al. Depression and epilesy, pain and psychogenic non-epileptic seizures: clinical and therapeutic perspectives. *Epilepsy Behav.* 2012;24(2):169–181. doi:10.1016/j.yebeh.2012.01.008

94. Bagayogo I, Interian A, Escobar J. Transcultural aspects of somatic symptoms in the context of depressive disorders. *Adv Psychosom Med.* 2013;33:64–74. doi:10.1159/000350057

95. Katon W, Kleinman A, Rosen G. Depression and somatization: a review. Part I. *Am J Med.* 1982;72(1):127–135.

96. Plug L1, Sharrack B, Reuber M. Conversation analysis can help to distinguish between epilepsy and non-epileptic seizure disorders: a case comparison. *Seizure.* 2009;18(1):43–50. doi:10.1016/j.seizure.2008.06.002

97. Reuber M1, Monzoni C, Sharrack B, Plug L. Using interactional and linguistic analysis to distinguish between epileptic and psychogenic nonepileptic seizures: a prospective, blinded multirater study. *Epilepsy Behav.* 2009;16(1):139–144. doi:10.1016/j.yebeh.2009.07.018
98. Bowman E, Markand O. The contribution of life events to pseudoseizure occurrence in adults. *Bull Menninger Clin.* 1999;63(1):70–88.
99. Walczak T, Papacostas S, Williams D, Scheuer M, Liebowitz N, Notarfrancesco A. Outcome after diagnosis of psychogenic nonepileptic seizures. *Epilepsia.* 1995;36:1131–1137.
100. Baslet G. Psychogenic non-epileptic seizures: a model of their pathogenic mechanism. *Seizure.* 2011;20(1):1–13.
101. Sifneos P. The prevalence of 'alexithymic' characteristics in psychosomatic patients. *Psychother Psychosom.* 1973;22(2):255–262.
102. Schönenberg M, Jusyte A, Höhnle N, Mayer S, Weber Y, Hautzinger M, Schell C. Theory of mind abilities in patients with psychogenic nonepileptic seizures. *Epilepsy Behav.* 2015;53:20–24. doi:10.1016/j.yebeh.2015.09.036
103. Brown R, Bouska J, Frow A, et al. Emotional dysregulation, alexithymia, and attachment in psychogenic nonepileptic seizures. *Epilepsy Behav.* 2013;29(1):178–183. doi:10.1016/j.yebeh.2013.07.019
104. Wolf L, Hentz J, Ziemba K, et al. Quality of life in psychogenic nonepileptic seizures and epilepsy: the role of somatization and alexithymia. *Epilepsy Behav.* 2015;43:81–88. doi:10.1016/j.yebeh.2014.12.010
105. Lawton G, Baker GA, Brown RJ. Comparison of two types of dissociation in epileptic and non-epileptic seizures. *Epilepsy Behav.* 2008;13(2):333–336. doi:10.1016/j.yebeh.2008.04.015
106. Reuber M, House AO, Pukrop R, Bauer J, Elger CE. Somatization, dissociation and general psychopathology in patients with psychogenic non-epileptic seizures. *Epilepsy Res.* 2003;57(2-3):159–167.
107. Bodde NM, van der Kruijs SJ, Ijff DM, Lazeron RH, Vonck KE, Boon PA, Aldenkamp AP. Subgroup classification in patients with psychogenic non-epileptic seizures. *Epilepsy Behav.* 2013;26(3):279–289. doi:10.1016/j.yebeh.2012.10.012
108. Ito M, Adachi N, Okazaki M, Kato M, Onuma T. Evaluation of dissociative experiences and the clinical utility of the Dissociative Experience Scale in patients with coexisting epilepsy and psychogenic nonepileptic seizures. *Epilepsy Behav.* 2009;16(3):491–494. doi:10.1016/j.yebeh.2009.08.017
109. Martinez-Taboas A, Lewis-Fernandez R, Sar V, Agarwal AL. Cultural aspects of psychogenic nonepileptic seizures. In: Schachter SC, LaFrance CWJr, eds. p121-130 *Gates and Rowan's Nonepileptic Seizures, 3rd* ed. New York: Cambridge University Press; 2010.
110. Benbadis S, Allen Hauser W. An estimate of the prevalence of psychogenic non-epileptic seizures. *Seizure.* 2000;9(4):280–281.
111. Ozturk M, Ozturk O. The intra-family role patterns of children with conversion hysterias. *Med J Soc Psychiatry.* 1981;2:81–87.
112. Kozlowska K. Intergenerational processes, attachment and unexplained medical symptoms. *Aust N Z J Fam Ther.* 2007;28:88–89.
113. Hecker T, Braitmayer L, van Duijl M. Global mental health and trauma exposure: the current evidence for the relationship between traumatic experiences and spirit possession. *Eur J Psychotraumatol.* 2015;6:29126. doi:10.3402/ejpt.v6.29126
114. Krawetz P, Fleisher W, Pillay N, Staley D, Arnett J, Maher J. Family functioning in subjects with pseudoseizures and epilepsy. *J Nerv Ment Dis.* 2001;189(1):38–43.

115. Moore P, Baker G, McDade G, Chadwick D, Brown S. Epilepsy, pseudoseizures and perceived family characteristics: a controlled study. *Epilepsy Res.* 1994;18(1):75–83.
116. Wood B, McDaniel S, Burchfiel K, Erba G. Factors distinguishing families of patients with psychogenic seizures from families of patients with epilepsy. *Epilepsia.* 1998;39:432.
117. Liotti G. Disorganised/disoriented attachment in the aetiology of the dissociative disorders. *Dissociation.* 1992;5:196–204.
118. Waldinger RJ, Schulz MS, Barsky AJ, Ahern DK. Mapping the road from childhood trauma to adult somatization: the role of attachment. *Psychosom Med.* 2006;68(1):129–135.
119. Kreitman N, Swinsbury P, Pearce K, Costain W. Hypochondriasis and depression in outpatients at a general hospital. *Br. J Psychiatry.* 1965;111:607–615.
120. Hudak A, Trivedi K, Harper C, et al. Evaluation of seizure-like episodes in survivors of moderate and severe traumatic brain injury. *J Head Trauma Rehabil.* 2004;19(4):290–295.
121. DeToledo J, Lowe M, Puig A. Nonepileptic seizures in pregnancy. *Neurology.* 2000;55:120.
122. Lesser R. Psychogenic seizures. *Neurology.* 1996;46:1499.
123. Say G, Taşdemir H, İnce H. Semiological and psychiatric characteristics of children with psychogenic nonepileptic seizures: gender-related differences. *Seizure.* 2015;31:144–148. doi:10.1016/j.seizure.2015.07.017
124. Patel H, Scott E, Dunn D, Garg B. Nonepileptic seizures in children. *Epilepsia.* 2007;48:2086.
125. Blumer D, Adamolekun B. Treatment of patients with coexisting epileptic and nonepileptic seizures. *Epilepsy Behav.* 2006;9(3):498–502.
126. Szabó L, Siegler Z, Zubek L, Liptai Z, Körhegyi I, Bánsági B, Fogarasi A. A detailed semiologic analysis of childhood psychogenic nonepileptic seizures. *Epilepsia.* 2012;53(3):565–570. doi:10.1111/j.1528-1167.2012.03404.x
127. Reuber M, Jamnadas-Khoda J, Broadhurst M, et al. Psychogenic nonepileptic seizure manifestations reported by patients and witnesses. *Epilepsia.* 2011;52(11):2028–2035. doi:10.1111/j.1528-1167
128. Woollacott I, Scott C, Fish D, Smith S, Walker M. When do psychogenic nonepileptic seizures occur on a video/EEG telemetry unit? *Epilepsy Behav.* 2010;17(2):228–235. doi:10.1016/j.yebeh.2009.12.002
129. Luther J, McNamara J, Carwile S, Miller P, Hope V. Pseudoepileptic seizures: methods and video analysis to aid diagnosis. *Ann Neurol.* 1982;12(5):458–462.
130. Reuber M. The etiology of psychogenic non-epileptic seizures: toward a biopsychosocial model. *Neurol Clin.* 2009;27(4):909–924. doi:10.1016/j.ncl.2009.06.004
131. Reuber M, Howlett S, Khan A, Grünewald R. Non-epileptic seizures and other functional neurological symptoms: predisposing, precipitating, and perpetuating factors. *Psychosomatics.* 2007;48(3):230–238.
132. Hustvedt S. Philosophy matters in brain matters. *Seizure.* 2013;22(3):169–173. doi:10.1016/j.seizure.2013.01.002
133. Ahern L, Stone J, Sharpe M. Attitudes of neuroscience nurses toward patients with conversion symptoms. *Psychosomatics.* 2009;50(4):336–339. doi:10.1176/appi.psy.50.4.336
134. Gambini O, Demartini B, Chiesa V, Turner K, Barbieri V, Canevini M. Long-term outcome of psychogenic nonepileptic seizures: the role of induction by suggestion. *Epilepsy Behav.* 2014;41:140–143. doi:10.1016/j.yebeh.2014.09.076
135. Reuber M, Mitchell A, Howlett S, Elger C. Measuring outcome in psychogenic nonepileptic seizures: how relevant is seizure remission? *Epilepsia.* 2005;46:1788.

136. McKenzie P, Oto M, Russell A, Pelosi A, Duncan R. Early outcomes and predictors in 260 patients with psychogenic nonepileptic attacks. *Neurology.* 2010;74(1):64-69. doi:10.1212/WNL.0b013e3181c7da6a
137. Wyllie E, Friedman D, Lüders H, Morris H, Rothner D, Turnbull J. Outcome of psychogenic seizures in children and adolescents compared with adults. *Neurology.* 1991;41(5):742-744.
138. Goldstein L, Deale A, Mitchell-O'Malley S, Toone B, Mellers J. An evaluation of cognitive behavioral therapy as a treatment for dissociative seizures: a pilot study. *Cogn Behav Neurol.* 2004;17(1):41-49.
139. Lawton G, Mayor R, Howlett S, Reuber M. Psychogenic nonepileptic seizures and health-related quality of life: the relationship with psychological distress and other physical symptoms. *Epilepsy Behav.* 2009;14(1):167-171. doi:10.1016/j.yebeh.2008.09.029
140. Alsaadi T, Marquez A. Psychogenic nonepileptic seizures. *Am Fam Physician.* 2005;72(5):849-856.
141. Selwa L, Geyer J, Nikakhtar N, Brown M, Schuh L, Drury I. Nonepileptic seizure outcome varies by type of spell and duration of illness. *Epilepsia.* 2000;41(10):1330-1334.
142. Arain A, Hamadani A, Islam S, Abou-Khalil W. Predictors of early seizure remission after diagnosis of psychogenic nonepileptic seizures. *Epilepsy Behav.* 2007;11:409.
143. Ettinger A, Dhoon A, Weisbrot D, Devinsky O. Predictive factors for outcome of nonepileptic seizures after diagnosis. *J Neuropsychiatry Clin Neurosci* 1999;11:458.
144. Lempert T, Schmidt D. Natural history and outcome of psychogenic seizures: a clinical study in 50 patients. *J Neurol.* 1990;237:35.
145. Moene F, Spinhoven P, Hoogduin K, van Dyck R. A randomised controlled clinical trial on the additional effect of hypnosis in a comprehensive treatment programme for in-patients with conversion disorder of the motor type. *Psychother Psychosom.* 2002;71(2):66-76.
146. Moene F, Spinhoven P, Hoogduin K, van Dyck R. A randomized controlled clinical trial of a hypnosis-based treatment for patients with conversion disorder, motor type. *Int J Clin Exp Hypn.* 2003;51(1):29-50.
147. Ataoglu A, Ozcetin A, Icmeli C, Ozbulut O. Paradoxical therapy in conversion reaction. *J Korean Med Sci.* 2003;18(4):581-584.
148. Goldstein L, Chalder T, Chigwedere C, Khondoker M, Moriarty J, Toone B, Mellers J. Cognitive-behavioral therapy for psychogenic nonepileptic seizures: a pilot RCT. *Neurology.* 2010;74(24):1986-1994. doi:10.1212/WNL.0b013e3181e39658
149. LaFrance W, Keitner G, Papandonatos G, Blum A, Machan J, Ryan C, Miller I. Pilot pharmacologic randomized controlled trial for psychogenic nonepileptic seizures. *Neurology.* 2010;28;75(13):1166-1173.
150. LaFrance W, Baird G, Barry J, et al.; NES Treatment Trial (NEST-T) Consortium. Multicenter pilot treatment trial for psychogenic nonepileptic seizures: a randomized clinical trial. *JAMA Psychiatry.* 2014;71(9):997-1005. doi:10.1001/jamapsychiatry.2014.817
151. Sharpe M, Walker J, Williams C, et al. Guided self-help for functional (psychogenic) symptoms: a randomized controlled efficacy trial. *Neurology.* 2011;77(6):564-572. doi:10.1212/WNL.0b013e318228c0c7
152. Thompson N, Connelly L, Peltzer J, Nowack J, Hamera E, Hunter E. Psychogenic nonepileptic seizures: a pilot study of a brief educational intervention. *Perspect Psychiatr Care.* 2013;49(2):78-83.

153. Chen D, Maheshwari A, Franks R, Trolley G, Robinson J, Hrachovy R. Brief group psychoeducation for psychogenic nonepileptic seizures: a neurologist-initiated program in an epilepsy center. *Epilepsia*. 2014;55(1):156–166. doi:10.1111/epi.12481
154. Reinsberger C, Sarkis R, Papadelis C, et al. Autonomic changes in psychogenic nonepileptic seizures: toward apotential diagnostic biomarker? *Clin EEG Neurosci*. 2015;46(1):16–25. doi:10.1177/1550059414567739
155. Stone J, Binzer M, Sharpe M. Illness beliefs and locus of control: a comparison of patients with pseudoseizures and epilepsy. *J Psychosom Res*. 2004;57:541–547. doi:10.1212/WNL.0b013e3181f4d5a9
156. Voon V, Brezing C, Gallea C, et al. Emotional stimuli and motor conversion disorder. *Brain*. 2010;133(Pt 5):1526–1536.

4

Neurological and Medical Factors

Victoria S. S. Wong, MD and Martin Salinsky, MD

This chapter explores neurological and medical comorbidities associated with psychogenic nonepileptic seizures (PNES). These include well-established neurological comorbidities, such as epilepsy and traumatic brain injury (TBI), and subjective complaints, such as pain disorders and other medically unexplained symptoms (MUS). We also review the results of neurodiagnostic tests, including electroencephalography (EEG) and neuroimaging.

1. NEUROLOGICAL AND MEDICAL COMORBIDITY

1.1. Epilepsy and PNES

Epilepsy is usually part of the differential diagnoses when considering a diagnosis of PNES. Due to the possibility of PNES mimicking epileptic seizures (or vice versa), or of comorbid PNES and epilepsy, it is essential to use all available data to reach an accurate diagnosis. If several clinical semiologies are present, effort should be made to characterize each type of episode in order to ensure that epileptic seizures are not missed. Clinical history should be taken into account, including risk factors for PNES or epilepsy, clinical semiology (see Chapter 1), and onset occurring from EEG-confirmed sleep (suggestive of epilepsy).[1] Rates of febrile seizures or a family history of epilepsy have not been found to differ between patients with PNES and patients with epilepsy.[2]

It is well known that some patients have both PNES and epilepsy. The reported percentage of patients with PNES that also have evidence for epilepsy ranges from 5% to 37% (Table 4.1).[3-10] This broad range reflects differences in study definitions and methods. Studies that required unequivocal interictal epileptiform activity (IIEA) or captured epileptic seizures during routine EEG or video-EEG monitoring in order to make the diagnosis of comorbid epilepsy had lower rates, ranging from 5% to 20% (IIEA/ictal epileptiform recording; Table 4.1). Studies that also allowed a diagnosis of epilepsy based on patient history, medical opinion, or prior reports had higher rates. It seems likely that the more conservative estimates, based on direct observation of EEG epileptiform discharges, are more accurate. Indeed, even the most conservative studies in Table 4.1

Table 4.1. Evidence for Coexistent Epilepsy in Patients with PNES

Authors	Year	PNES (N)	Method for Diagnosing Coexistent Epilepsy	IIEA/Ictal Epileptiform Recording	Total Included as Coexistent Epilepsy
Lesser et al.[3]	1983	50	EEG recording	10%	10%
Krumholz & Niedermeyer[4]	1983	41	Records review; medical opinion		37%
Meierkord et al.[5]	1991	110	Clinical evidence, often supported by IIEA		13%
Walczak et al.[6]	1995	51	IIEA recorded, report of IIEA, clinical history	10%	33%
Benbadis et al.[7]	2001	32	Unequivocal IIEA recorded	9%	9%
Martin et al.[8]	2003	514	Unequivocal IIEA recorded	5%	5%
Reuber et al.[9]	2003	329	EEG or "assessment of experienced neurologist"	20%	36%
Jones et al.[10]	2010	221	IIEA recorded, IIEA history, or consensus opinion	8%	14%

IIEA, interictal epileptiform activity. "Total included as coexistent epilepsy" includes patients diagnosed by EEG recording (IIEA/ictal epileptiform) and additional patients diagnosed on the basis of chart review or clinical opinion.

diagnosed comorbid epilepsy primarily on the basis of IIEA alone. As discussed later in the chapter, IIEA is not rare in healthy individuals with no history of epilepsy, and most epileptologists would not make a diagnosis of epilepsy only on the basis of IIEA. So even the "conservative" estimates in Table 4.1 may overestimate the presence of comorbid epilepsy. In summary, comorbid epilepsy is uncommon in patients with PNES but must always be kept in mind.

As compared to studies in adults, there are fewer reports regarding rates of coexistent epilepsy in children with PNES. Studies have reported coexistent epilepsy in 15% to 73% of children with video EEG–documented PNES.[11–16] This broad range again reflects methodological variability (as just discussed), with most studies reporting epilepsy diagnoses based primarily on clinical history. A series of 1,967 patients aged 20 and younger who underwent video EEG monitoring reported 68 patients (4%) with PNES.[16] Within this group, 23 (34%) had documented interictal epileptiform discharges and, ultimately, 26 (38%) total were felt to have coexistent epilepsy. Children under 13 years of age had a higher rate of coexistent epilepsy compared to those aged 13 and older (68% vs. 30%). There are diagnostic challenges unique to the pediatric population. These include subtle risk factors in children with PNES (e.g., school difficulties) and non-motor semiologies as a more common presentation of PNES.[17]

When PNES and epilepsy coexist, the onset of epileptic seizures typically predates the onset of nonepileptic seizures. One study of patients with comorbid PNES and epilepsy found the mean age of onset of epileptic seizures to be 14.5 years and the mean age of onset of PNES to be 27.5 years.[18] Another study noted a mean age of onset for epileptic seizures of 14.3 years and a mean age of onset for PNES of 26.7 years.[9] These observations suggest that living with epilepsy may prime certain patients to experience seizures as a physical manifestation of psychological distress.

Management of patients with comorbid PNES and epilepsy is challenging! After characterization of all seizure types, it is helpful for the patient and caregivers to be educated on the difference between "electrical seizures" (epileptic seizures) and PNES. In some cases, it is helpful for patients and their families to review video recordings of the different episode types, with the epilepsy provider present for explanation. Having the patient or a caregiver keep a seizure log with a description of ongoing events can help with tracking different seizure types so that the epilepsy provider can better manage antiepileptic drug (AED) therapy. Emergence of new seizure types may require further evaluations in the epilepsy monitoring unit (EMU) in order to clarify the diagnosis. This in part explains why patients with both PNES and epilepsy have the highest odds for readmission to the EMU within 30 days of an EMU discharge.[19]

Concurrent treatment for PNES should always be obtained. PNES "treatment as usual" has generally consisted of educating the patient and family regarding PNES (including causes and treatments), discontinuation of AEDs, and mental health referral.[20] When concurrent epileptic seizures are present, discontinuation of AEDs is rarely advisable. Unfortunately, PNES outcomes with "treatment as usual" are generally disappointing, and the presence of concomitant epilepsy does not appear to influence PNES prognosis.[9,21] There have been recent efforts to develop more effective treatment strategies for PNES, with promising results.[22,23]

1.2. Traumatic Brain Injury

TBI is a leading cause of new-onset epilepsy in young adults.[24,25] The risk of developing epilepsy following head trauma is directly related to the severity of the injury.[26,27] Less well known is the strong association between TBI and subsequent development of PNES, now well documented in both civilian studies and studies of U.S. veterans.

Four retrospective series have examined the relationship between an antecedent TBI and the development of PNES in adults (Table 4.2). All were based on EMU diagnoses of PNES. The three civilian studies totaled more than 350 PNES patients, with a range of 24–45% of patients having had one or more TBIs prior to onset of PNES. Motor vehicle accidents were the largest contributor (36–44% of TBIs).[28–30] The somewhat lower TBI rates in the 1998 studies were likely due to the additional requirement that seizures were attributed to the antecedent TBI by the patient or the treating medical team. In all four studies, the diagnosis of TBI was historical; confirmation by review of injury records was not always possible.

A similar review was performed of U.S. veterans with EMU-confirmed PNES.[31,32] A history of antecedent TBI as the proposed cause of seizures was found in 57% of these patients. This rate was significantly higher than the 35% TBI rate found in a comparison group of veterans with epileptic seizures or a comparison group of civilians with PNES (26%), all studied in the same EMU. Half of the TBIs in the Veteran PNES group were military TBIs.

Additional perspective on TBI as the proposed cause for seizures that were ultimately diagnosed as PNES comes from an ongoing multicenter prospective study of seizures in U.S. veterans. This study used a validated patient questionnaire (patient seizure etiology questionnaire [PSEQ]) to assess patient attribution of their seizures to an antecedent TBI or several other common risk factors.[33] Preliminary results are shown in Figure 4.1. TBI was the most common etiology selected by patients as the principal cause of their seizures. TBI was more frequently cited as the probable cause of seizures by patients subsequently diagnosed with PNES than it was by those subsequently diagnosed with epilepsy.

The severity of the TBI was assessed in each of the studies referenced in Table 4.2. Although classification methods differed, the great majority of TBIs reported in patients with PNES would be rated as mild (Table 4.2; loss of consciousness of less than 30 minutes, amnesia of <24 hours, nonpenetrating injury).[26,34] This finding is contrary to the expected predominance of moderate–severe TBI, based on large population-based

Table 4.2. Studies of Association of Prior Traumatic Brain Injury (TBI) and Subsequent Development of PNES

First Author	Year	N	Population	TBI	Mild TBI (% of all TBI)
Barry et al.[29]	1998	157	Civilians	24%	78%
Westbrook et al.[28]	1998	102	Civilians	32%	91%
LaFrance et al.[30]	2013	92	Civilians	45%	73%
Salinsky et al.[32]	2015	67	Veterans	57%	87%

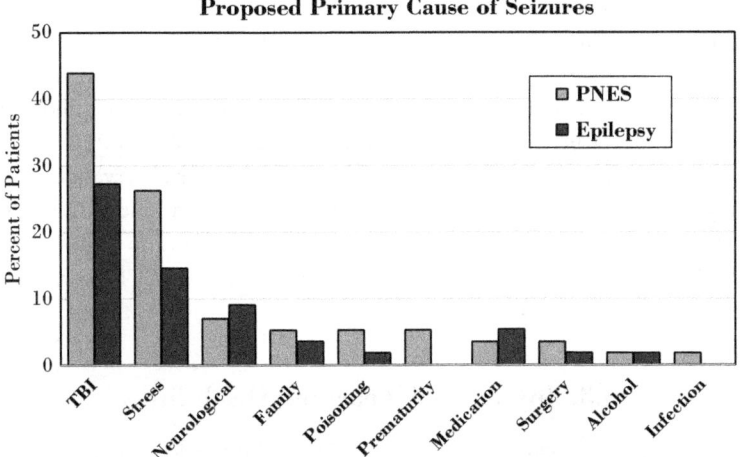

Figure 4.1 Proposed primary cause of seizures from patient questionnaire ($n = 80$; 40 PNES, 40 epilepsy). "Neurological" refers to other neurological disorders. "Family" refers to seizures that run in the family. "Infection" includes meningitis, encephalitis, etc. Twenty-three percent of PNES patients (and 40% of epilepsy patients) did not cite any primary cause. (Totals exceed 100% due to ties.) TBI, traumatic brain injury.

studies of post-traumatic epilepsy. For civilians, Annegers et al. reported a standardized incidence ratio of 17 for severe head injuries but only 1.5 for mild TBI.[26] Similarly, a population-based study of Iraq and Afghanistan veterans showed that post-traumatic seizure risk is directly related to TBI severity, with lowest risk (adjusted odds ratio 1.3) for mild TBI.[27] Consistent with these population-based studies, 63% of veterans with EMU-documented post-traumatic epilepsy had moderate–severe TBI, as compared to only 13% of veterans with post-traumatic PNES ($p < 0.001$).[32] Although most patients with TBI and PNES report mild TBI, PNES can also occur in those with a history of moderate–severe TBI. EMU results for 127 patients with a history of moderate–severe TBI (loss of consciousness greater than 30 minutes) as the presumed cause of seizures were reviewed.[35] Most had documented epilepsy, but even in this select group, 27% had PNES as the only seizure type.

Taken together, these results suggest that patients with poorly controlled seizures ascribed to a mild TBI should be considered at risk for PNES and deserve further investigation to clarify the diagnosis. Early recognition of PNES may redirect therapy away from chronic AED therapy (with associated long-term toxicities) and toward more effective interventions.[22,23]

Reasons for the observed association between PNES and mild TBI are not clear, and there may be multiple factors involved. Mild TBI is relatively common, comprising 61% of all TBIs in the civilian population study of Annegers' and 83% of all U.S. military TBIs over the past 15 years.[26,34] Our experience suggests that patients suffering from unexplained episodes of neurological dysfunction (such as seizures) often associate their symptoms with traumatic events such as a TBI. The well-known association between TBI, particularly military TBI, and the development of epileptic seizures may prime symptom development in patients who are predisposed to conversion symptoms. Also, TBI (particularly mild TBI) is associated with post-traumatic stress disorder (PTSD), and this combination has been strongly associated with PNES in both civilians and veterans.[30,32,36-38] For example, for veterans with documented PNES and mild TBI as the proposed cause of seizures, 67% had previously been diagnosed with PTSD.[32] The association between TBI, PTSD, and PNES is consistent with other observations suggesting that many cognitive and health problems among veterans with mild TBI are mediated by PTSD.[39-41] Issues of compensation/disability may also factor into some cases. In one study, disability rates in PNES patients with a history of preceding TBI were double that of PNES patients without history of TBI.[30]

1.3. Intellectual/Learning Disabilities

Patients with learning disabilities (LD) and patients with intellectual disability (ID) are both overrepresented in series of patients with PNES. The expected population rate of LD is ~5% of children.[42] Among 288 teenage-adult patients with PNES, 9% were diagnosed with a LD through psychiatric interview.[43] Why PNES are overrepresented in patients with LD is unclear. Psychiatric disorders are generally overrepresented in the LD population.[44] Patients with PNES and LD are also more likely to have comorbid epilepsy than patients with PNES without LD (36 vs. 9%).[43] This observation is consistent with the higher rates of epilepsy found among patients with LD as compared to the general population. Epilepsy prevalence rates range from 6% to 50%, commensurate to the severity of LD.[45]

Estimates of ID (IQ less than 75) in patients diagnosed with PNES range from 24% in children to 12–17% in adults, again considerably higher than the expected population rate (~1%).[46,47] Patients with ID and PNES were less likely to have a history of antecedent sexual abuse and were more likely to have immediate situational or emotional triggers for their seizures than patients without ID.[43] A study comparing patients with PNES and epilepsy to patients with epilepsy alone found that 30% in the group with PNES and epilepsy had an IQ below 85, compared to 7% in the group with epilepsy. This again suggests a link between low IQ and a higher rate of PNES.[48]

It is essential that PNES be considered in patients with LD or ID. Within these populations, emerging PNES can easily be misdiagnosed as epileptic seizures, leading to intensification of AED therapy. This may increase the risk of neurotoxicity in patients who already have cognitive limitations. EMU recording or ambulatory EEG can be helpful when new seizure types emerge.

1.4. Prior Brain Surgery

Among patients with PNES, 5% developed nonepileptic seizures after a neurosurgery performed for reasons other than for control of refractory epileptic seizures.[49] Of these, 29% had only nonepileptic seizures while 71% had concurrent epileptic seizures. A preoperative psychiatric diagnosis, particularly depression, conferred a higher risk of postoperative PNES.[50] Risk factors also included female gender. Median time to onset between neurosurgery and first PNES was 1 year. In patients with concurrent epileptic seizures, these developed before the PNES in all cases. De novo PNES after adult epilepsy surgery has also been reported at a frequency of 4%.[50] PNES developed 2 weeks to 10 years following surgery and was independent of seizure outcome.

1.5. Sleep

Few data are available on sleep quality or sleep disorders in patients with PNES. In one study, women with PNES had significantly greater rapid eye movement (REM) sleep than women with epilepsy, but otherwise there were no significant differences in sleep stages, total sleep time, or sleep efficiency.[51] Given the known associations between PNES and PTSD, there are likely commonalities in comorbid sleep disorders such as sleep dysregulation and insomnia.[52] Further studies are needed to elucidate the prevalence of sleep disorders in patients with PNES.

One hallmark of PNES is that the seizures rarely occur between midnight and 6:00 AM (in the EMU) and almost never occur directly out of an EEG-confirmed sleep state.[53] However, on rare occasions it is possible for PNES to arise directly out of EEG-confirmed sleep. In a study of 118 nonepileptic events, eight events in five patients either began during EEG sleep (six episodes) or occurred within 7 seconds after onset of the awake alpha rhythm (two episodes), shortly after stage II or III sleep.[54] It was suggested that recurrent daytime PNES may result in "automatized" episodes that can be triggered in an unconscious or transitional state of consciousness. Recording of events occurring directly out of sleep does not rule out a diagnosis of PNES.

Preictal pseudosleep is defined as "a state that had all the characteristics of normal sleep by behavioral criteria alone, that is, patient supine, motionless, and eyes closed, while EEG shows evidence of wakefulness: alpha rhythm at the same frequency as baseline fully awake, active EMG, rapid eye movements including blinks, and no slow rolling eye movements."[55] Episodes arising out of preictal pseudosleep and lasting at least 1 minute have a sensitivity of 56% and a specificity of 100% for PNES.[55]

1.6. Multiple Sclerosis

Rates of epileptic seizures are increased among patients with multiple sclerosis (MS) as compared to the general population.[56] Whether the prevalence of PNES is likewise increased in MS is unknown. There is a possible association between MS drugs and PNES. On searching for PNES as an adverse drug event in the openFDA database (which contains voluntary reporting of adverse drug events by healthcare professionals and consumers), there were 20 cases reported over the course of 10 years. The most commonly implicated drugs linked to PNES as an adverse drug event included MS disease-modifying drugs (six occurrences: interferon beta [four occurrences], glatiramer, natalizumab), antirheumatic drugs (four occurrences: certolizumab, etanercept, tocilizumab, tofacitinib), anti-seizure drugs (four occurrences: lacosamide, lamotrigine, levetiracetam, oxcarbazepine), and psychiatric drugs (two occurrences: clozapine, sertraline).[57] The association between MS drugs and PNES requires further study.

1.7. Other Medical Comorbidities

There is little information regarding general medical comorbidities in patients with PNES. Psychiatric comorbidities and complaints are discussed in Chapter 3. A recent study of health care utilization (all causes) has shown substantially greater use among patients with PNES as compared to those with epilepsy.[58]

Older patients presenting with PNES may represent a distinct subgroup with greater than expected general medical problems. In patients with onset of PNES after age 55 years, 42% had physical health problems classified as severe (e.g., uncontrolled angina, myocardial infarction, stroke, malignancy), 38% had physical health problems classified as mild–moderate (e.g., controlled hypertension, diabetes, hypercholesterolemia), and 19% had no physical health problems.[59] This is in contrast to 8%, 44%, and 48% having severe, mild–moderate, and no physical health problems, respectively, among patients with PNES onset before age 55. There was no direct comparison to medical rates in older patients with epilepsy or to the general medical population. However, the rates observed in the PNES group were substantially higher than rates previously observed in large population studies.

2. ADDITIONAL NEUROLOGICAL AND MEDICAL COMPLAINTS

2.1. Functional Neurological Symptoms

In the fifth edition of the *Diagnostic and Statistical Manual of Mental Disorders* (*DSM-5*), conversion disorder is also known as *functional neurological symptom disorder*.[60] The term *functional* describes symptoms that "display inconsistency or incongruity with recognized neurological disease."[61] Subtypes of conversion disorder are listed within the following symptom categories: weakness or paralysis, abnormal movement, swallowing symptoms, speech symptoms, attacks or seizures, anesthesia or sensory loss, special sensory symptom (e.g., visual, olfactory, or hearing disturbance), or mixed symptoms. PNES are classified as a conversion disorder with "attacks or seizures."

In an outpatient neurology setting, medically unexplained neurological symptoms are present in 11% to 42% of patients.[62,63] Patients with functional neurological symptoms had a mean of 2.3 unexplained neurological symptoms and a mean symptom duration of 7.7 years.[64] The most common functional neurological symptom was PNES, occurring in 51% of patients. PNES patients had a median of one additional concurrent functional neurological symptom, including weakness, pain, headache, dizziness, numbness, fatigue, memory problems, tremor, visual disturbance, or tinnitus.[64] Another study, based on the Structured Clinical Interview for *DSM-III*, found that among patients with PNES, 42% had evidence of current, and 84% had evidence for lifetime somatoform disorders outside of PNES.[65] These included numbness (58%), weakness (49%), paralysis (42%), fainting (36%), staggering gait (33%), globus hystericus (20%), blindness (18%), muteness (16%), deafness (13%), and visual disturbances (24%).[65] The prognosis of these symptoms is guarded. At 10-year follow-up, more than 40% of patients with functional neurological symptoms (including but not limited to PNES) reported no improvement.[66] This finding is consistent with the generally poor prognosis of PNES with standard medical care.[6,9,21,67,68] Long-term outcomes in PNES are discussed in Chapter 17 of this text.

Similar observations have been made for children with PNES. Among 265 pediatric patients admitted to the EMU, 22 (8%) were diagnosed with PNES (mean age 13.5 years). Psychiatric interview revealed that 11 (50%) of patients with PNES had a secondary conversion or somatic symptom, including headache (most common), abdominal pain, gait abnormality, chest pain, and recurrent hemiparesis.[69]

2.2. Pain Complaints

Pain complaints are overrepresented in patients with PNES: 62% of patients reported a positive pain history, as compared to 31% of a control group with idiopathic generalized epilepsy.[70] In another study, 77% of patients with PNES reported moderate–severe pain. At long-term follow-up of 6 months or greater following diagnosis, 96% of patients with persistent PNES continued to report moderate to severe pain symptoms as compared to 59% of patients whose PNES resolved.[71] Within an epilepsy clinic population, the positive predictive value of a diagnosis of "fibromyalgia" or "chronic pain" for PNES was 75% (sensitivity 9%, specificity 99%).[72] Patients with PNES were more likely to be using one or more pain medications (including opioids) as compared to a control group with epilepsy.[31,70]

Headaches were the most common pain presentation in patients with PNES.[71] Compared to patients with epilepsy, headaches in patients with PNES were reported to be more frequent, more often "migraine" type, longer in duration, and more likely to have nonvisual migraine auras.[73] It has been speculated that patients with PNES may have increased sensory sensitivity, similar to that seen in patients with migraine headaches, although this requires further study.[74,75]

Pain complaints among patients with PNES have a significant impact on health care utilization.[58] Pain complaints (primarily headache, chest pain, and abdominal pain) were the most common reason for presentation to the emergency department and were more common than presentations for seizures (36% vs. 22% of all presentations). The opposite was true for patients with epilepsy, where only 13% of presentations were pain related.

Taken together, these observations underscore the importance of assessing pain complaints in patients with PNES and also highlight the multidimensional nature of medical complaints from patients with conversion disorders. Treatment targeting PNES, without addressing the underlying psychiatric disorder and medical comorbidities, can be expected to have limited impact on overall function.

2.3. Cognitive Complaints

Cognitive complaints are common among patients with PNES. These may complicate the clinical picture by implying the existence of a neurodegenerative or progressive neurological disorder. Cognitive complaints are often difficult to characterize, and the clinician must rely on cognitive testing to separate subjective complaints from objective impairment. The extent and types of cognitive dysfunction seen in PNES are detailed in Chapter 5.

Neuropsychological testing has revealed impaired performance of patients with PNES as compared to that of healthy controls.[76] However, differences between patients with PNES and those with epilepsy were minimal.[76] Patients with both PNES and epilepsy are more impaired than patients with PNES alone.[77] A recent review of the neuropsychological literature reported deficits in attention (particularly executive attention), other executive functions, verbal memory, language performance, and other areas.[78] This is discussed in further detail in Chapters 5 and 9. The causes of poor cognitive performance are less clear. It is important to consider that the PNES population includes an overrepresentation of patients with LD and intellectual dysfunction, as described earlier (see Neurological and Medical Comorbidity: Intellectual/Learning Disabilities). For verbal memory and language, difficulties with higher-order attentional and executive functioning processes may play a role. Anatomical causes such as hippocampal dysfunction have also been associated with chronic stress-related psychiatric disorders such as PTSD.[78–80] Emotional processing can affect cognitive performance of patients with PNES as compared to that of healthy controls.[81,82]

Seizure medications may also contribute to cognitive complaints (and dysfunction). Most PNES patients are on chronic AED therapy at the time of diagnosis.[9,31,67,68,83] Several controlled studies using patients or healthy volunteers have demonstrated significant, and sometimes dramatic, cognitive effects of several commonly used AEDs.[84,85]

Self-perception of cognitive abilities may be altered as well. In a comparison of patients with PNES versus those with severe epilepsy, patients with PNES outperformed patients with epilepsy on objective cognitive tests.[86] Despite this, both groups had similar self-perception of cognitive functioning. There was a significant association between objective and subjective measures of cognitive function in patients with epilepsy, but not in patients with PNES. In the PNES group, a depression scale (MMPI-2) correlated with perceived cognitive dysfunction, and there was no correlation between subjective and objective measurements of cognitive status independent of mood. These results suggest that mood, rather than actual cognitive performance, is the major factor determining self-perception of cognitive function for patients with PNES. Similar observations have been made among patients with epilepsy.[87]

Finally, poor motivation is likely a factor influencing neuropsychological test performance for some patients.[76,88] Patients with PNES were more likely to fail symptom validity testing (SVT; word memory test) than patients with epilepsy.[89] Further, patients with PNES who "failed" SVT performed worse on a battery of cognitive tests than patients who "passed" SVT.[89] These findings are not universal. Using less stringent exclusion criteria, another study found no difference in test effort between patients with epileptic seizures and those with PNES.[90]

2.4. Other Medically Unexplained Symptoms

Patients with PNES often experience non-neurological MUS. *MUS* can be defined as "any current principal somatic complaint reported by patients for which no definite medical diagnosis could be found by physical examination and appropriate investigation."[91] These symptoms can include "bodily distress" symptoms involving numerous organ systems, or they can refer to more specific syndromes, such as irritable bowel syndrome (IBS), chronic fatigue syndrome, and fibromyalgia. A lower degree of somatization has been linked to a better PNES outcome.[9]

One study evaluated patients with PNES and epilepsy for the following conditions: fibromyalgia, chronic fatigue syndrome, chronic pain syndrome, tension headaches, IBS, asthma, migraines, and gastroesophageal reflux disorder (GERD). Sixty-six percent of patients with PNES had at least one of these conditions, versus 27% of patients with epilepsy.[92] A history of at least one of these diagnoses was predictive of PNES over epilepsy, with a sensitivity of 66%, specificity of 73%, and positive predictive value of 76%.[92] As mentioned earlier, fibromyalgia is a predictor of PNES.[72] Six to 12 months after PNES diagnosis, 24% of patients developed new MUS (tension headache, irritable bowel, chronic fatigue, or fibromyalgia).[93] Seventy percent of these patients had evidence for previous MUS.

There is an emerging paradigm of "central sensitization" as a unifying factor for conditions previously labeled using terms such as *functional, somatization disorders*, and *medically unexplained symptoms*.[94] The term describes both the clinical symptomatology and the physiology behind conditions characterized by hypersensitivity (e.g., allodynia, hyperalgesia, pain beyond an area of peripheral nerve supply).[94] Central sensitization is mediated by the central nervous system, thought to be the result of plasticity in pain pathways wherein repeated or sustained noxious stimulation can lead to increased neural responsiveness and thus an exaggerated perception of sensory stimuli.[95] Conditions that fall within this paradigm include fibromyalgia, chronic fatigue syndrome, IBS, myofascial pain syndrome, and multiple chemical sensitivity. Although PNES is not included as a central sensitivity syndrome, it has much in common with listed disorders in regard to risk factors and comorbidities. This issue is discussed further in Chapter 6.

3. ASSOCIATED DIAGNOSTIC TESTS

3.1. EEG Findings in Patients with PNES

3.1.1. Interictal EEG Patterns in PNES

The gold standard for diagnosing PNES is to record typical events on simultaneous video and EEG, with absence of ictal EEG changes before, during, and after the events.[1] Ideally there would be an absence of any pathological pattern on interictal EEG as well, although this is not always the case. Even in healthy adult volunteers without epilepsy, rates of spontaneous IIEA vary from 0% to 6.6%.[96]

Several studies have described EEG dysrhythmias in patients with neuropsychiatric or neurobehavioral disorders, including PNES. These range from benign EEG variants to clearly pathological abnormalities. A comprehensive review defined these patterns as "isolated episodic paroxysmal bursts of slow activity, controversial/anomalous spiky waveforms and/or true non-controversial epileptiform discharges."[97] Within that context, the mean prevalence of interictal EEG dysrhythmias in patients with PNES was 26% (nine studies), with a commonly reported pattern of interictal sharply contoured temporal theta (unilateral or bilateral). The review posited that EEG abnormalities found in patients with PNES and other neuropsychiatric disorders reflect a biological vulnerability to psychiatric disorders.

A blinded, multirater study reviewing EEGs of patients with PNES (excluding those with medical diagnoses or medications that could affect the EEG) revealed that 50% had nonspecific EEG abnormalities (generalized or focal slowing), while 8% had IIEA (spikes, sharp waves).[98] Patients with PNES and IIEA are often classified as having coexistent epilepsy, though this may or may not be true (see earlier section on PNES and epilepsy; Table 4.1). Patients with PNES and no clinically recognizable cause of EEG disturbance were found to have nonspecific EEG abnormalities 1.8 times as often as healthy controls. Some studies have focused on patients with known neurological comorbidities such as ID and/or epilepsy. In these patients, the prevalence of EEG abnormalities ranged from 38% to 80% despite the PNES diagnosis.[98]

3.1.2. EEG as a Neurobiological Marker for PNES

Recent studies suggest that abnormal functional connectivity in specific brain networks is related to the pathophysiology of PNES. One study compared patients with PNES and age- and sex-matched controls, collecting interictal EEG data and using multivariate phase synchronization mapping to create maps of functional connectivity.[99] They did not find a pattern specific to patients with PNES. However, there was an inverse correlation between PNES frequency and synchronicity in frontal and parietal locations. The authors suggested that "reduction or instability in prefrontal EEG synchronization may be a marker of increased susceptibility to PNES."[99] Other EEG studies have identified aberrant patterns of local connectivity in PNES patients as compared to healthy controls.[100,101]

3.2. Neuroimaging in Patients with PNES

3.2.1. MRI

Patients with PNES can have structural abnormalities on brain imaging studies, although the relationship between such lesions and development of PNES is uncertain. In one study, 22 of 311 patients with PNES (7%) *without* concurrent epilepsy had a structural brain imaging abnormality.[102] These included stroke/ischemia/encephalomalacia, cortical dysplasia, TBI, "developmental delay," aneurysm, arteriovenous malformations, cavernous hemangioma, brain tumor (before or after resection), arachnoid cyst, subdural hematoma, and ventriculoperitoneal shunt. In another study, MRI abnormalities were found in 6% of patients with PNES only versus 22% in patients with both PNES and epilepsy.[77] Combined MRI and EEG findings have shown an excess of right hemisphere abnormalities, leading to the theory that functional symptoms are more often mediated by the right cerebral hemisphere.[102] This hypothesis is consistent with observations that lateralized functional symptoms often affect the left side of the body.[102,103]

3.2.2. Functional Imaging

Single-photon emission computed tomography (SPECT) has been used in the evaluation of patients with possible PNES. Although video EEG monitoring is the gold standard for diagnosis of PNES, in complex cases where the ictal semiology or clinical picture is confusing, a negative SPECT study can help support the diagnosis. One report used SISCOM (subtraction SPECT coregistered to MRI) to evaluate patients with video-EEG evidence for PNES and other potentially contradictory findings (seizure semiology consistent with partial epilepsy, abnormal brain MRI, abnormal interictal EEG).[104] SISCOM was negative in 85%, helping to increase the diagnostic certainty of PNES. SISCOM was found to be useful in patients with concurrent epilepsy and PNES, helping to characterize the nature of each seizure type.[105]

Other functional imaging studies including 2-deoxy-2-[fluorine-18]fluoro-d-glucose ((18)FDG-PET)[106] and functional MRI (fMRI)[107–111] have been performed in patients with PNES, primarily to elucidate the pathophysiology of the disorder. These are discussed in Chapter 6.

4. CONCLUSION

This chapter presents considerable evidence that certain neurological and medical factors increase the risk of developing PNES. Epilepsy and TBI are the best-studied examples. The occurrence of previous epileptic seizures may serve as a model or explanation for unexplained new events, and these may be interpreted by patients (or by their providers) as part of their epilepsy. Similarly, the well-known association between TBI and epileptic seizures may prime the development of PNES in patients with a tendency to express psychological distress as physical symptoms, particularly those suffering from PTSD. Patients with learning or intellectual disability also have an increased risk for both epilepsy and PNES, adding to diagnostic confusion when new behaviors emerge. In each case it is important for the clinical care provider to carefully review the circumstances under which the seizures occurred, and the seizure semiology, in order to determine whether further investigation of seizure type is warranted.

Patients with PNES will usually show evidence of other unexplained neurological and medical symptoms. These include various neurological symptoms, pain, cognitive complaints, and general medical complaints such as fibromyalgia and chronic fatigue. In this context, PNES can be considered as one symptom of a more pervasive disorder. These other symptoms, particularly pain, may have a major impact on health care utilization and quality of life and should not be neglected when selecting treatment for PNES. Lastly, results from EEG and MRI have suggested potential biological vulnerabilities that can increase the risk of developing PNES.

5. SUMMARY

- Comorbid epilepsy, as diagnosed by interictal or ictal EEG findings, is present in approximately 5% to 20% of patients with PNES.
- Patients with PNES will often attribute seizures to a TBI. Patients with seizures attributed to mild TBI, particularly those with PTSD, are at increased risk for PNES.
- PNES are overrepresented in patients with learning disorders and intellectual disability.
- Patients with PNES commonly have additional functional neurological symptoms, cognitive complaints, and medically unexplained symptoms.

- A variety of nonspecific abnormalities are seen on interictal EEG and brain MRI in patients with PNES. However, the relationship between these abnormalities and development of PNES is uncertain.

REFERENCES

1. LaFrance WC, Baker GA, Duncan R, Goldstein LH, Reuber M. Minimum requirements for the diagnosis of psychogenic nonepileptic seizures: a staged approach: a report from the International League Against Epilepsy Nonepileptic Seizures Task Force. *Epilepsia.* 2013;54(11):2005–2018.
2. Szaflarski JP, Ficker DM, Cahill WT, Privitera MD. Four-year incidence of psychogenic nonepileptic seizures in adults in Hamilton County, OH. *Neurology.* 2000;55(10):1561–1563.
3. Lesser RP, Lueders H, Dinner DS. Evidence for epilepsy is rare in patients with psychogenic seizures. *Neurology.* 1983;33(4):502–504.
4. Krumholz A, Niedermeyer E. Psychogenic seizures: a clinical study with follow-up data. *Neurology.* 1983;33(4):498–502.
5. Meierkord H, Will B, Fish D, Shorvon S. The clinical features and prognosis of pseudoseizures diagnosed using video-EEG telemetry. *Neurology.* 1991;41(10):1643–1646.
6. Walczak TS, Papacostas S, Williams DT, Scheuer ML, Lebowitz N, Notarfrancesco A. Outcome after diagnosis of psychogenic nonepileptic seizures. *Epilepsia.* 1995;36(11):1131–1137.
7. Benbadis SR, Agrawal V, Tatum WO. How many patients with psychogenic nonepileptic seizures also have epilepsy? *Neurology.* 2001;57(5):915–917.
8. Martin R, Burneo JG, Prasad A, et al. Frequency of epilepsy in patients with psychogenic seizures monitored by video-EEG. *Neurology.* 2003;61(12):1791–1792.
9. Reuber M, Pukrop R, Bauer J, Helmstaedter C, Tessendorf N, Elger CE. Outcome in psychogenic nonepileptic seizures: 1- to 10-year follow-up in 164 patients. *Ann Neurol.* 2003;53(3):305–311.
10. Jones SG, O' Brien TJ, Adams SJ, et al. Clinical characteristics and outcome in patients with psychogenic nonepileptic seizures. *Psychosom Med.* 2010;72:487–497.
11. Szabó L, Siegler Z, Zubek L, et al. A detailed semiologic analysis of childhood psychogenic nonepileptic seizures. *Epilepsia.* 2012;53(3):565–570.
12. Holmes GL, Sackellares JC, McKiernan J, Ragland M, Dreifuss FE. Evaluation of childhood pseudoseizures using EEG telemetry and video tape monitoring. *J Pediatr.* 1980;97(4):554–558.
13. Kramer U, Carmant L, Riviello JJ, et al. Psychogenic seizures: video telemetry observations in 27 patients. *Pediatr Neurol.* 1995;12(1):39–41.
14. Irwin K. Psychogenic non-epileptic seizures: management and prognosis. *Arch Dis Child.* 2000;82(6):474–478.
15. Kotagal P, Costa M, Wyllie E, Wolgamuth B. Paroxysmal nonepileptic events in children and adolescents. *Pediatrics.* 2002;110(4):e46.
16. Patel H, Scott E, Dunn D, Garg B. Nonepileptic seizures in children. *Epilepsia.* 2007;48(11):2086–2092.
17. Dworetzky BA. Psychogenic nonepileptic seizures: children are not miniature adults. *Epilepsy Curr.* 2015;15(4):174–176.
18. Reuber M, Fernandez G, Bauer J, Helmstaedter C, Elger CE. Diagnostic delay in psychogenic nonepileptic seizures. *Neurology.* 2002;58(3):493–495.

19. Caller TA, Chen JJ, Harrington JJ, Bujarski KA, Jobst BC. Predictors for readmissions after video-EEG monitoring. *Neurology.* 2014;83(5):450–455.
20. LaFrance WC, Rusch MD, Machan JT. What is "treatment as usual" for nonepileptic seizures? *Epilepsy Behav.* 2008;12(3):388–394.
21. Kanner AM, Parra J, Frey M, Stebbins G, Pierre-Louis S, Iriarte J. Psychiatric and neurologic predictors of psychogenic pseudoseizure outcome. *Neurology.* 1999;53(5):933–938.
22. Goldstein LH, Chalder T, Chigwedere C, et al. Cognitive-behavioral therapy for psychogenic nonepileptic seizures: a pilot RCT. *Neurology.* 74(24):1986–1994.
23. LaFrance WC, Baird GL, Barry JJ, et al. Multicenter pilot treatment trial for psychogenic nonepileptic seizures: a randomized clinical trial. *JAMA Psychiatry.* 2014;71(9):997–1005.
24. Annegers JF. The epidemiology of epilepsy. In: Wylie E, ed. *The Treatment of Epilepsy: Principles and Practice.* Baltimore, MD; 1996:166–172.
25. Temkin NR, Dikmen SS, Wilensky AJ, Keihm J, Chabal S, Winn HR. A randomized, double-blind study of phenytoin for the prevention of post-traumatic seizures. *N Engl J Med.* 1990;323(8):497–502.
26. Annegers JF, Hauser WA, Coan SP, Rocca WA. A population-based study of seizures after traumatic brain injuries. *N Engl J Med.* 1998;338(1):20–24.
27. Pugh MJ V, Orman JA, Jaramillo CA, et al. The prevalence of epilepsy and association with traumatic brain injury in veterans of the Afghanistan and Iraq wars. *J Head Trauma Rehabil.* 2015;30(1):29–37.
28. Westbrook LE, Devinsky O, Geocadin R. Nonepileptic seizures after head injury. *Epilepsia.* 1998;39(9):978–982.
29. Barry E, Krumholz A, Bergey GK, Chatha H, Alemayehu S, Grattan L. Nonepileptic posttraumatic seizures. *Epilepsia.* 1998;39(4):427–431.
30. LaFrance WC, Deluca M, MacHan JT, Fava JL. Traumatic brain injury and psychogenic nonepileptic seizures yield worse outcomes. *Epilepsia.* 2013;54(4):718–725.
31. Salinsky M, Spencer D, Boudreau E, Ferguson F. Psychogenic nonepileptic seizures in US veterans. *Neurology.* 2011;77(10):945–950.
32. Salinsky M, Storzbach D, Goy E, Evrard C. Traumatic brain injury and psychogenic seizures in veterans. *J Head Trauma Rehabil.* 2015;30(1):E65–E70.
33. Salinsky M, Parko K, Rutecki P, Boudreau E, Storzbach D. Attributing seizures to TBI: validation of a brief patient questionnaire. *Epilepsy Behav.* 2016;57(Pt A):141–144.
34. Defense and veterans Brain Injury Center. *DoD Numbers for Traumatic Brain Injury Worldwide 2000-2015.* http://dvbic.dcoe.mil/dod-worldwide-numbers-tbi.
35. Hudak AM, Trivedi K, Harper CR, et al. Evaluation of seizure-like episodes in survivors of moderate and severe traumatic brain injury. *J Head Trauma Rehabil.* 19(4):290–295.
36. Dworetzky B, Strahonja-Packard A, Shanahan C, Paz J, Schauble B, Bromfield E. Characteristics of male veterans with psychogenic nonepileptic seizures. *Epilepsia.* 2005;46:1418–1422.
37. Zatzick DF, Rivara FP, Jurkovich GJ, et al. Multisite investigation of traumatic brain injuries, posttraumatic stress disorder, and self-reported health and cognitive impairments. *Arch Gen Psychiatry.* 2010;67(12):1291–1300.
38. Carlson K, Kehle S, Meis L, et al. *The Assessment and Treatment of Individuals with History of Traumatic Brain Injury and Posttraumatic Stress Disorder: A Systematic Review of the Evidence.* Washngton, DC: Department of veterans Affairs (US); 2009. http://www.ncbi.nlm.nih.gov/books/NBK49144/.
39. Hoge CW, McGurk D, Thomas JL, Cox AL, Engel CC, Castro CA. Mild traumatic brain injury in U.S. soldiers returning from Iraq. *N Engl J Med.* 2008;358(5):453–463.

40. Polusny MA, Kehle SM, Nelson NW, Erbes CR, Arbisi PA, Thuras P. Longitudinal effects of mild traumatic brain injury and posttraumatic stress disorder comorbidity on post-deployment outcomes in National Guard soldiers deployed to Iraq. *Arch Gen Psychiatry.* 68(1):79–89.
41. Storzbach D, O'Neil ME, Roost S-M, et al. Comparing the neuropsychological test performance of Operation Enduring Freedom/Operation Iraqi Freedom (OEF/OIF) veterans with and without blast exposure, mild traumatic brain injury, and posttraumatic stress symptoms. *J Int Neuropsychol Soc.* 2015;21(5):353–363.
42. Institute of Education Sciences National Center for Education Statistics. *Students with disabilities.* https://nces.ed.gov/fastfacts/display.asp?id=64. Accessed December 1, 2016.
43. Duncan R, Oto M. Psychogenic nonepileptic seizures in patients with learning disability: comparison with patients with no learning disability. *Epilepsy Behav.* 2008;12(1):183–186.
44. Vedi K, Bernard S. The mental health needs of children and adolescents with learning disabilities. *Curr Opin Psychiatry.* 2012;25(5):353–358.
45. Lhatoo SD, Sander JW. The epidemiology of epilepsy and learning disability. *Epilepsia.* 2001;42:6–9.
46. Maulik PK, Mascarenhas MN, Mathers CD, Dua T, Saxena S. Prevalence of intellectual disability: a meta-analysis of population-based studies. *Res Dev Disabil.* 2011;32(2):419–436.
47. Murphy CC, Yeargin-Allsopp M, Decouflé P, Drews CD. The administrative prevalence of mental retardation in 10-year-old children in metropolitan Atlanta, 1985 through 1987. *Am J Public Health.* 1995;85(3):319–323.
48. Reuber M, Qurishi A, Bauer J, et al. Are there physical risk factors for psychogenic non-epileptic seizures in patients with epilepsy? *Seizure.* 2003;12(8):561–567.
49. Reuber M, Kral T, Kurthen M, Elger CE. New-onset psychogenic seizures after intracranial neurosurgery. *Acta Neurochir (Wien).* 2002;144(9):901–907; discussion 907.
50. Markoula S, de Tisi J, Foong J, Duncan JS. De novo psychogenic nonepileptic attacks after adult epilepsy surgery: an underestimated entity. *Epilepsia.* 2013;54(12):e159–e162.
51. Bazil CW, Legros B, Kenny E. Sleep structure in patients with psychogenic nonepileptic seizures. *Epilepsy Behav.* 2003;4(4):395–398.
52. Pavlova MK, Allen RM, Dworetzky BA. Sleep in psychogenic nonepileptic seizures and related disorders. *Clin EEG Neurosci.* 2015;46(1):34–41.
53. Bazil CW, Walczak TS. Effects of sleep and sleep stage on epileptic and nonepileptic seizures. *Epilepsia.* 1997;38(1):56–62.
54. Orbach D, Ritaccio A, Devinsky O. Psychogenic, nonepileptic seizures associated with video-EEG-verified sleep. *Epilepsia.* 2003;44(1):64–68.
55. Benbadis SR, Lancman ME, King LM, Swanson SJ. Preictal pseudosleep: a new finding in psychogenic seizures. *Neurology.* 1996;47:63–67.
56. Olafsson E, Benedikz J, Hauser WA. Risk of epilepsy in patients with multiple sclerosis: a population-based study in Iceland. *Epilepsia.* 1999;40(6):745–747.
57. Wong VS, Motika PV. Medications implicated in psychogenic seizures: insights from the open FDA initiative [abstract]. In: *American Epilepsy Society Annual Meeting.* 2014;Abst. 1.277.
58. Health care utilization following diagnosis of psychogenic nonepileptic seizures. Salinsky M, Storzbach D, Goy E, Kellogg M, Boudreau E. *Epilepsy Behav.* 2016;60:107–11.
59. Duncan R, Oto M, Martin E, Pelosi A. Late onset psychogenic nonepileptic attacks. *Neurology.* 2006;66(11):1644–1647.

60. American Psychiatric Association. *Diagnostic and Statistical Manual of Mental Disorders*, 5th edition *(DSM-5)*. Arlington, VA: American Psychiatric Association; 2013.
61. Turner MR, Kiernan MC. *Landmark Papers in Neurology*. Oxford: Oxford University Press; 2015.
62. Carson AJ. Do medically unexplained symptoms matter? A prospective cohort study of 300 new referrals to neurology outpatient clinics. *J Neurol Neurosurg Psychiatry*. 2000;68(2):207–210.
63. Hamilton J, Campos R, Creed F. Anxiety, depression and management of medically unexplained symptoms in medical clinics. *J R Coll Physicians Lond*. 1996;30(1):18–20.
64. Reuber M, Howlett S, Khan A, Grünewald RA. Non-epileptic seizures and other functional neurological symptoms: predisposing, precipitating, and perpetuating factors. *Psychosomatics*. 2007;48(3):230–238.
65. Bowman ES, Markand ON. Psychodynamics and psychiatric diagnoses of pseudoseizure subjects. *Am J Psychiatry*. 1996;153:57–63.
66. Mace CJ, Trimble MR. Ten-year prognosis of conversion disorder. *Br J Psychiatry*. 1996;169:282–288.
67. McKenzie P, Oto M, Russell A, Pelosi A, Duncan R. Early outcomes and predictors in 260 patients with psychogenic nonepileptic attacks. *Neurology*. 2010;74(1):64–69.
68. Ettinger AB, Devinsky O, Weisbrot DM, Ramakrishna RK, Goyal A. A comprehensive profile of clinical, psychiatric, and psychosocial characteristics of patients with psychogenic nonepileptic seizures. *Epilepsia*. 1999;40(9):1292–1298.
69. Pakalnis A, Paolicchi J. Frequency of secondary conversion symptoms in children with psychogenic nonepileptic seizures. *Epilepsy Behav*. 2003;4(6):753–756.
70. Gazzola DM, Carlson C, Rugino A, Hirsch S, Starner K, Devinsky O. Psychogenic nonepileptic seizures and chronic pain: a retrospective case-controlled study. *Epilepsy Behav*. 2012;25(4):662–665.
71. Ettinger AB, Devinsky O, Weisbrot DM, Goyal A, Shashikumar S. Headaches and other pain symptoms among patients with psychogenic non-epileptic seizures. *Seizure*. 1999;8(7):424–426.
72. Benbadis SR. A spell in the epilepsy clinic and a history of "chronic pain" or "fibromyalgia" independently predict a diagnosis of psychogenic seizures. *Epilepsy Behav*. 2005;6(2):264–265.
73. Shepard MA, Silva A, Starling AJ, et al. Patients with psychogenic non-epileptic seizures have a more severe form of migraine than patients with epilepsy. *Seizure*. 2016;34:78–82.
74. Kröner-Herwig B, Ruhmland M, Zintel W, Siniatchkin M. Are migraineurs hypersensitive? A test of the stimulus processing disorder hypothesis. *Eur J Pain*. 2005;9(6):661–671.
75. Baslet G. Psychogenic non-epileptic seizures: a model of their pathogenic mechanism. *Seizure*. 2011;20(1):1–13.
76. Binder LM, Kindermann SS, Heaton RK, Salinsky MC. Neuropsychologic impairment in patients with nonepileptic seizures. *Arch Clin Neuropsychol*. 1998;13(6):513–522.
77. Reuber M, Fernández G, Helmstaedter C, Qurishi A, Elger C. Evidence of brain abnormality in patients with psychogenic nonepileptic seizures. *Epilepsy Behav*. 2002;3(3):249–254.
78. Willment K, Hill M, Baslet G, Loring DW. Cognitive impairment and evaluation in psychogenic nonepileptic seizures: an integrated cognitive-emotional approach. *Clin EEG Neurosci*. 2015;46(1):42–53.
79. Gilbertson MW, Shenton ME, Ciszewski A, et al. Smaller hippocampal volume predicts pathologic vulnerability to psychological trauma. *Nat Neurosci*. 2002;5(11):1242–1247.

80. Werner NS, Meindl T, Engel RR, et al. Hippocampal function during associative learning in patients with posttraumatic stress disorder. *J Psychiatr Res.* 2009;43(3):309–318.
81. Bakvis P, Spinhoven P, Putman P, Zitman FG, Roelofs K. The effect of stress induction on working memory in patients with psychogenic nonepileptic seizures. *Epilepsy Behav.* 2010;19(3):448–454.
82. Gul A, Ahmad H. Cognitive deficits and emotion regulation strategies in patients with psychogenic nonepileptic seizures: a task-switching study. *Epilepsy Behav.* 2014;32:108–113.
83. Benbadis SR. How many patients with pseudoseizures receive antiepileptic drugs prior to diagnosis? *Eur Neurol.* 1999;41(2):114–115.
84. Meador KJ, Loring DW, Abney OL, et al. Effects of carbamazepine and phenytoin on EEG and memory in healthy adults. *Epilepsia.* 1993;34(1):153–157.
85. Salinsky MC, Storzbach D, Spencer DC, Oken BS, Landry T, Dodrill CB. Effects of topiramate and gabapentin on cognitive abilities in healthy volunteers. *Neurology.* 2005;64(5):792–798.
86. Breier JI, Fuchs KL, Brookshire BL, et al. Quality of life perception in patients with intractable epilepsy or pseudoseizures. *Arch Neurol.* 1998;55(5):660–665.
87. Elixhauser A, Leidy NK, Meador K, Means E, Willian MK. The relationship between memory performance, perceived cognitive function, and mood in patients with epilepsy. *Epilepsy Res.* 1999;37(1):13–24.
88. Boone KB, Lu PH. Impact of somatoform symptomatology on credibility of cognitive performance. *Clin Neuropsychol.* 1999;13(4):414–419.
89. Drane DL, Williamson DJ, Stroup ES, et al. Cognitive impairment is not equal in patients with epileptic and psychogenic nonepileptic seizures. *Epilepsia.* 2006;47(11):1879–1886.
90. Dodrill CB. Do patients with psychogenic nonepileptic seizures produce trustworthy findings on neuropsychological tests? *Epilepsia.* 2008;49(4):691–695.
91. Nimnuan C, Hotopf M, Wessely S. Medically unexplained symptoms. *J Psychosom Res.* 2001;51(1):361–367.
92. Dixit R, Popescu A, Bagić A, Ghearing G, Hendrickson R. Medical comorbidities in patients with psychogenic nonepileptic spells (PNES) referred for video-EEG monitoring. *Epilepsy Behav.* 2013;28(2):137–140.
93. McKenzie PS, Oto M, Graham CD, Duncan R. Do patients whose psychogenic non-epileptic seizures resolve, "replace" them with other medically unexplained symptoms? Medically unexplained symptoms arising after a diagnosis of psychogenic non-epileptic seizures. *J Neurol Neurosurg Psychiatry.* 2011;82(9):967–969.
94. Yunus MB. Central sensitivity syndromes: a new paradigm and group nosology for fibromyalgia and overlapping conditions, and the related issue of disease versus illness. *Semin Arthritis Rheum.* 2008;37(6):339–352.
95. Meeus M, Nijs J. Central sensitization: a biopsychosocial explanation for chronic widespread pain in patients with fibromyalgia and chronic fatigue syndrome. *Clin Rheumatol.* 2007;26(4):465–473.
96. So EL. Interictal epileptiform discharges in persons without a history of seizures: what do they mean? *J Clin Neurophysiol.* 2010;27(4):229–238.
97. Shelley B, Trimble M, Boutros N. Electroencephalographic cerebral dysrhythmic abnormalities in the trinity of nonepileptic general population, neuropsychiatric, and neurobehavioral disorders. *J Neuropsychiatry Clin Neurosci.* 2008;20(1):7–22.
98. Reuber M, Fernández G, Bauer J, Singh DD, Elger CE. Interictal EEG abnormalities in patients with psychogenic nonepileptic seizures. *Epilepsia.* 2002;43(9):1013–1020.

99. Knyazeva MG, Jalili M, Frackowiak RS, Rossetti AO. Psychogenic seizures and frontal disconnection: EEG synchronisation study. *J Neurol Neurosurg Psychiatry.* 2011;82(5):505–511.
100. Barzegaran E, Joudaki A, Jalili M, Rossetti AO, Frackowiak RS, Knyazeva MG. Properties of functional brain networks correlate with frequency of psychogenic non-epileptic seizures. *Front Hum Neurosci.* 2012;6:335.
101. Xue Q, Wang Z, Xiong X, Tian C, Wang Y, Xu P. Altered brain connectivity in patients with psychogenic non-epileptic seizures: a scalp electroencephalography study. *J Int Med Res.* 2013;41(5):1682–1690.
102. Devinsky O, Mesad S, Alper K. Nondominant hemisphere lesions and conversion non-epileptic seizures. *J Neuropsychiatry Clin Neurosci.* 2001;13(3):367–373.
103. Ley RG. An archival examination of an asymmetry of hysterical conversion symptoms. *J Clin Exp Neuropsychol.* 1980;2(1):61–69.
104. Neiman ES, Noe KH, Drazkowski JF, Sirven JI, Roarke MC. Utility of subtraction ictal SPECT when video-EEG fails to distinguish atypical psychogenic and epileptic seizures. *Epilepsy Behav.* 2009;15(2):208–212.
105. Spanaki MV, Spencer SS, Corsi M, MacMullan J, Seibyl J, Zubal IG. The role of quantitative ictal SPECT analysis in the evaluation of nonepileptic seizures. *J Neuroimaging.* 1999;9(4):210–216.
106. Arthuis M, Micoulaud-Franchi JA, Bartolomei F, McGonigal A, Guedj E. Resting cortical PET metabolic changes in psychogenic non-epileptic seizures (PNES). *J Neurol Neurosurg Psychiatry.* 2015;86(10):1106–1112.
107. Li R, Li Y, An D, Gong Q, Zhou D, Chen H. Altered regional activity and inter-regional functional connectivity in psychogenic non-epileptic seizures. *Sci Rep.* 2015;5:11635.
108. Ding J, An D, Liao W, et al. Altered functional and structural connectivity networks in psychogenic non-epileptic seizures. *PLoS One.* 2013;8(5):e63850.
109. van der Kruijs SJ, Jagannathan SR, Bodde NM, et al. Resting-state networks and dissociation in psychogenic non-epileptic seizures. *J Psychiatr Res.* 2014;54:126–133.
110. van der Kruijs SJ, Bodde NM, Vaessen MJ, et al. Functional connectivity of dissociation in patients with psychogenic non-epileptic seizures. *J Neurol Neurosurg Psychiatry.* 2012;83(3):239–247.
111. Allendorfer JB, Szaflarski JP. Contributions of fMRI towards our understanding of the response to psychosocial stress in epilepsy and psychogenic nonepileptic seizures. *Epilepsy Behav.* 2014;35:19–25.

5

Mechanisms of Possible Neurocognitive Dysfunction

Daniel L. Drane, PhD and Dona E. C. Locke, PhD

1. INTRODUCTION

Psychogenic nonepileptic seizures (PNES) have a long history in the annals of medicine.[1,2] The primary focus on this condition, however, has traditionally been placed on diagnostic methods for determining their occurrence and distinguishing them from epileptic seizures (ES). While associated cognitive dysfunction has been reported for many years, the investigation of such possible deficits has received limited attention.[3-5] Early research efforts suggested a strong likelihood of cognitive dysfunction, which was presumed to be rooted in structural brain impairments, perhaps resulting from associated traumas (e.g., head injury).[3] More recent PNES research following the advent of performance validity tests has suggested that such broad dysfunction may be of a transient nature, which may result from associated psychological and psychiatric factors, personality styles, medication effects, and an interaction of these previously latent variables.[6-8] Of note, however, is that while we can speculate about the possible etiological causes of such transient dysfunction, research is needed to definitively establish such mechanisms. Nevertheless, the good news of such findings is that cognitive dysfunction in PNES may be reversible in nature, rather than a chronic, unremitting consequence of a brain disease. The downside is that even a transient cognitive inefficiency can compromise daily function if the underlying causes are not recognized and remediated. Finally, much as physicians have long grappled with understanding functional neurological disorders in general (i.e., the psychological and possible neuropathological mechanisms that give rise to them), we still find ourselves uncertain as to whether or not there may be any cognitive deficits that reflect a diseased brain system. These two questions remain tightly interwoven.

We present the case that further research combining neuropsychological testing, psychological theory, neuroimaging analysis, and a thorough understanding of brain–behavior relationships will be required to unravel both questions. We believe the current weight of evidence suggests that transient dysfunction is the bigger problem for most individuals with PNES, yet such integrated research is required to establish or perhaps rule out a more focal neuropathological syndrome.

2. INITIAL ERA OF ASSESSING COGNITIVE FUNCTION IN PNES–COGNITIVE DEFICITS APPEARED EQUIVALENT TO THOSE OF EPILEPSY PATIENTS

Early neuropsychological research examining cognitive function in patients with PNES, completed during the 1970s through mid-1990s, suggested equivalent or greater dysfunction in patients with PNES as compared to those with epilepsy.[3,5,9–13] These studies tended to show general dysfunction that cut across multiple cognitive domains, with no indication of any consistent pattern of focal impairment. The alleged cause for cognitive impairment was typically presumed neurological injury, such as elevated rates of self-reported head trauma.[12]

Perhaps the most representative research of this era is the comprehensive studies conducted by Dodrill and colleagues.[3,9,11] These researchers demonstrated that cognitive deficits were highly similar across patients with PNES and those diagnosed with complex partial seizures on the basis of video-EEG evaluation. For example, Dodrill and colleagues demonstrated that both epilepsy and PNES patients were outside of normal limits on just over 50% of the tests from his Neuropsychological Battery for Epilepsy.[14] Deficits were general and covered widespread domains of cognition. Some investigators suggested that the presence of such dysfunction made patients with PNES poor candidates for psychotherapeutic interventions.

3. CURRENT ASSESSMENT OF COGNITION IN PNES: PERFORMANCE VALIDITY TESTING SUGGESTS COGNITIVE DYSFUNCTION RESULTS FROM NON-DISEASE VARIABLES

The introduction of performance validity tests (PVTs) has highlighted that task engagement is often poor in the PNES population.[6,8] PVTs are tasks designed to determine whether or not individuals are making adequate effort to comply with test parameters. More specifically, while they are usually designed to look difficult to perform, they include subcomponents that are quite easy even for patients with substantial cognitive disability to carry out. When minimum criteria are not met by the patient (i.e., they perform poorly on very easy tasks), one typically assumes that they are not putting forth adequate effort to meet minimum standards of task completion and may even be intentionally distorting their performance to make it look worse than they are capable of (i.e., faking bad).[15] While these measures were introduced in the legal arena with the primary goal of identifying malingering in forensic evaluations, their use with various neurological and psychiatric populations has suggested that there may be multiple reasons for their failure. Indeed, malingering is considered a rare reason for PVT failure in the PNES population.[6,8] Instead, PVT use has helped to identify many previously unrecognized variables that may have the potential to invalidate neuropsychological testing. These include the effects of interictal epileptiform discharges[16–18] and polypharmacy/medications.[19] A number of psychological variables (e.g., dissociative states, hyper- or hypoarousal associated with anxiety or post-traumatic stress disorder [PTSD]) have been proposed to potentially affect cognitive performance as well, and there is some evidence that they may do so.[20] Psychological variables have also been associated with poor PVT performance,[21] although this finding is usually interpreted to suggest that these data are simply invalid and that the psychological condition does not affect cognition when invalid data are removed. This argument is compelling in some patient groups, particularly when the subset of patients failing PVTs is restricted to those in litigation. Such patterns have rarely been explored in patients with functional neurological disorders. Some researchers have also suggested that cognitive dysfunction can at times represent a psychogenic state for some individuals (i.e., cogniform disorder).[22] Research on these potentially confounding latent variables remains in its infancy, and, particularly with regard to the psychological constructs, data are still lacking to establish if mental state can lead to suboptimal performance.

It should be noted that PVTs vary in their level of sensitivity and specificity. Some of these measures are low in sensitivity and will rarely pick up on potentially invalid cognitive data.[15] Others may be more prone to false-positive error due to low specificity (i.e., identifying data as invalid when they are not), which can be problematic, particularly if the PVT failure leads the examiner to infer poor motivation on the part of the patient. The use of different PVT measures will obviously lead to different conclusions about the proportion of invalid data in the research literature.

The work of Binder and colleagues assessing psychological and cognitive functions in PNES patients during the late 1990s introduced the idea that patients with PNES perform worse on PVT measures than do patients with epilepsy.[8] While the two groups performed very similarly on standard cognitive measures, the group with PNES performed much worse on a PVT measure. There was also a strong relationship between performance on PVT measures and cognitive tests in the PNES sample that was not observed in the epilepsy sample. Of note, however, is that the PNES patients failed the PVT measure at a rate of only 10%. This led the investigators to conclude that frank malingering was likely rare in this group. They felt that apparent neurocognitive impairment in the PNES group was more likely associated with emotional and psychological factors than with neuropathological (sic "structural") brain impairment. They also suggested that PNES patients lack the emotional resources to persist through a challenging test battery.

Drane and colleagues[6] replicated the work of Dodrill et al.[3,11] while extending the scope of this research by including PVT measures. They confirmed earlier findings that patients with PNES exhibited equivalent or greater cognitive dysfunction as compared to patients with epilepsy on a standard neuropsychological test battery. However, they also found that a much higher proportion of the PNES population failed PVT measures than did the epilepsy sample (i.e., 49% vs. 8%). As with the study by Binder et al.,[8] while there was little relationship between PVT failure and cognitive performance in the epilepsy sample, there was a strong relationship between these constructs in the PNES sample. The performance of patients with PNES passing PVT measures was most similar to that of healthy control subjects, while those failing PVT measures performed worse on cognitive tests than the majority of epilepsy patients (Figures 5.1 and 5.2). Many of these patients with PNES, a number of whom remained gainfully employed or at least lived independently, performed more poorly than patients with epilepsy who had severe cognitive disability (e.g., mild to moderate intellectual disability).

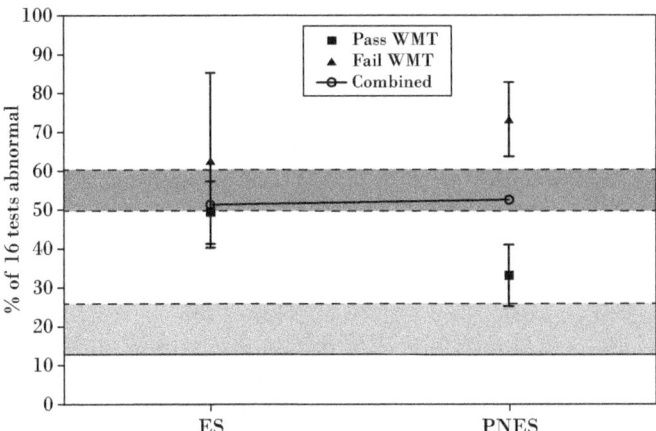

Figure 5.1 Mean Dodrill Discrimination Index (DDI) and 95% confidence intervals for patients with epileptic seizures (ES) and psychogenic nonepileptic seizures (PNES), stratified by performance on the effort-sensitive measures of the Word Memory Test (WMT). A higher DDI value indicates more impairment. Dotted line, mean level of performance for each group before stratifying for WMT performance. The uppermost (dark) shaded area is the 95% confidence interval of the DDI performance of 100 epilepsy patients,[9] whereas the lower (light) shaded area is the 95% confidence interval around the DDI performance of 50 normal control subjects.[14]

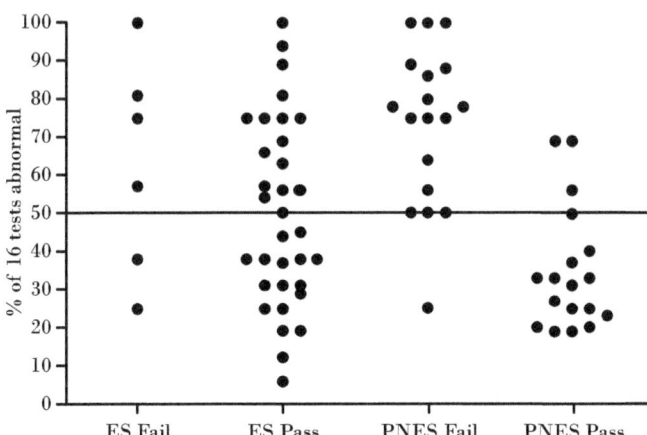

Figure 5.2 Scatterplot of Dodrill Discrimination Index (DDI) performance according to diagnostic group and Word Memory Test (WMT) performance. ES, epileptic seizure; PNES, psychogenic nonepileptic seizure. DDI: percentage of performances on 16 tests in the abnormal range; Pass, scored in the valid range on WMT effort-sensitive tests; Fail, scored in the invalid range on WMT effort-sensitive tests. The horizontal reference line at 50% denotes the typical mean level of overall impairment seen in both the current ES and PNES samples.

Dodrill later reported higher rates of PVT failure among epilepsy patients than other studies have found and attributed this to other studies excluding too many patients.[23] He felt that medications, recent seizures, and interictal discharges do not affect cognitive or PVT performance (see further discussion later in the chapter). Drane and colleagues have countered that leaving certain types of patients in studies (e.g., including those who have experienced a seizure in the last 24 hours) is potentially confounding,[1,24] as the cognitive function of such individuals may be transiently compromised.[16–18,25]

The use of PVT measures has become more commonplace in recent investigations of cognition in patients with PNES (Table 5.1). While the rates of PVT failure have been variable, a subset of patients with PNES routinely exhibit poor task engagement, which ranges from approximately 10% to 50% of the sample.[7,20,23,26] Variability in PVT failure range has been attributed to differences in PVT selection (sensitivity issues) and patient sampling.[24]

Table 5.1. Studies on PNES and Cognition

Study	Cognitive Findings	PVT Inclusion
Wilkus, Dodrill, & Thompson (1984)[3]	PNES patients had general deficits across all cognitive domains. No difference between the PNES and ES samples	No
Drake et al. (1993)[5]	PNES patients had higher IQ scores than ES patients and greater psychopathology.	No
Bortz et al. (1997)[75]	PNES patients failed to recognized target words (negative response bias) more often than epilepsy patients on a verbal list learning task, a pattern which was attributed to psychological factors.	No
Binder et al. (1998)[8]	PNES and ES samples showed general deficits compared to healthy controls. However, deficits in PNES were thought to be related to emotional factors, based on patterns observed on a PVT measure and a mood/personality inventory.	Yes Portland Digits Recognition Test[76]
Kalogjera-Sackellares & Sackellares (1999)[12]	Broad general deficits were observed in PNES patients that appeared equivalent to those observed in epilepsy patients.	No

Table 5.1. Continued

Study	Cognitive Findings	PVT Inclusion
Drane et al. (2006)[6]	Replicated Wilkus and Dodrill findings.[3,11] However, these findings were explained by poor task engagement, with PNES patients performing more like healthy controls after controlling for this factor.	Yes Word Memory Test (oral version)[77]
McNally et al. (2009)[80]	PNES patients exhibited deficits on a list-learning task equivalent to those of patients with temporal lobe epilepsy. However, signal detection theory suggested that PNES patients performed poorly owing to faulty decision-making strategies rather than genuine memory dysfunction.	No
Bakvis et al. (2010)[78]	Patients with PNES exhibited worse working memory functioning than controls when exposed to social or pain-induced stress.	No
Strutt et al. (2011)[79]	Women with PNES performed better on a wide range of tasks than did women with left temporal lobe epilepsy, with the exception of relative deficits in working memory and attention.	No
Williamson et al. (2012)[7]	Explored possible differences in PNES patients based on their performance on PVT measures. Failure on PVT measures was more likely to occur in patients with a self-reported history of abuse but was not related to disability status, financial decisions, or mood and personality assessment.	Yes Word Memory Test (oral version)[77]
Schonenberg et al. (2015)[74]	PNES patients exhibited greater alexithymia and theory-of-mind deficits as compared to healthy controls but were not impaired at recognizing facial expression.	No

The above studies represent a selection of studies of cognition in PNES patients but are not intended to be exhaustive. ES, epilepsy; PNES, psychogenic nonepileptic seizures; PVT, performance validity test.

4. POTENTIAL REASONS FOR PVT FAILURE IN PNES: GENERAL COGNITIVE TRANSIENT DYSFUNCTION

4.1. Medication Effects

Patients with PNES are often treated with a wide range of medications in an effort to manage their spells as well as their associated comorbidities. Many of these patients have comorbid psychiatric diagnoses, including mood disturbance, anxiety disorders, and trauma-related diagnoses (e.g., PTSD).[1,27] There are also elevated rates of chronic pain and fatigue issues,[28] which likely reflect the general somatic malaise from which they suffer. Therefore, it is not uncommon to find a given patient being treated with antiepileptic drugs (AEDs), analgesic medications, and a variety of psychotropic drugs (e.g., anxiolytics, antidepressants/mood stabilizers, antipsychotics, hypnotics).

Fortunately, once diagnosed, patients with PNES usually have their antiepileptic drugs discontinued, unless there is a secondary issue for which treatment is warranted (e.g., using an AED as a mood stabilizer).[29] Nevertheless, when cognitive status is assessed during a patient's initial workup, it is quite common for AEDs to still be a part of their medication regimen. Likewise, it is not uncommon for less informed clinicians in the broader community to restart AEDs when they are uncertain about the nature of a given patient's spells should they continue unabated. While the effects of AEDs are typically subtle and tolerable, it is well established that cognitive dysfunction does occur on these medications, particularly when polypharmacy is employed or when exceeding recommended drug dosages or standard therapeutic blood levels.[30,31] Likewise, some AEDs have greater effects on a subset of presumably vulnerable individuals (e.g., known effects of the decarboxylase inhibitors, such as topiramate and zonisamide, on verbal fluency).[32,33]

One recent study using a randomized, double-blind, crossover design with healthy controls demonstrated that a subset of drug-naïve individuals failed a commonly used PVT measure when given an acute dose of lorazepam.[19] Although the dose used in this study was fairly large (1 mg) in a drug-naïve group, this type of study raises the possibility that medications may at times cause transient cognitive dysfunction that can impact PVT results. Such impairment is explained by an identifiable neurobiological factor, but is also of a transient nature, and secondary to treatment rather than a feature of the diagnosed condition. While much more research is needed in this area, such findings suggest caution is warranted when trying to attribute a cause for invalid test data; such data are clearly invalid. However, unlike the forensic arena, studies such as those conducted by Drane and colleagues[17,18] suggest that PVT failure is not caused by malingering. Regardless of the reason for PVT failure, the only conclusions that can be drawn regarding performance on the remainder of the cognitive exam in such cases is that it represents a minimal standard of performance ability that likely underestimates optimal function.

Many psychotropic medications have proven negative effects on cognitive function.[34,35] For example, studies in the setting of depression have compared cognitive function in patients in remission but receiving ongoing treatment with an antidepressant versus those in remission with no pharmacological treatment and found impaired cognitive function in those receiving an antidepressant.[36] The effects of antidepressants can also vary by drug class, with differing profiles for different types of drugs (e.g., tricyclic antidepressants vs. SSRIs). Benzodiazepines, sometimes used for their anxiolytic and sedative properties, are known to cause disruption of memory processing and other select cognitive functions.[35,37-39] Sleep aids, such as trazodone and zolpidem, have been associated with cognitive and motor impairments.[40,41]

In summary, patients with PNES are highly likely to be treated with a large number of medications that act primarily on the central nervous system. A single study has been completed that demonstrated that patients with PNES were being treated with more medications than patients with epilepsy,[42] and PNES patients are more likely to be treated with benzodiazepines and narcotics. Although virtually no research has been conducted in a PNES sample to explore potential effects of medications as a cause of PVT failure and transient cognitive dysfunction, this possibility appears quite plausible.

4.2. Comorbid Psychiatric Conditions and Medically Unexplained Symptoms

As noted earlier, patients with PNES often present with multiple comorbid disorders.[1] These include mood disturbance,[43] anxiety disorders,[44] trauma-related disorders (e.g., PTSD),[20,45] chronic pain and chronic fatigue issues, fibromyalgia,[28] sleep disturbance,[46] and obesity.[47] Each of these conditions may contribute independently to the cognitive dysfunction reported by many with PNES. Chronic depression and its treatment, for example, have been associated with volumetric brain changes on neuroimaging and various neurocognitive limitations.[48] While not the focus of this chapter, one must remain mindful of comorbid conditions when attempting to sort out the etiology of cognitive dysfunction in PNES. It is also possible that PNES patients will experience comorbid neurological disease or injury related to cognitive dysfunction that is independent of their PNES condition, although this tends to affect a minority of such individuals (e.g., traumatic brain injury, multiple sclerosis, brain tumor).

4.3. Effect of General Psychological Variables

A variety of dysfunctional psychological profiles have been associated with PNES, and some researchers have speculated about the relationship between these psychological variables and reported cognitive dysfunction.[49] Once again, very little research has been completed exploring such traits and cognitive performance, but the plausibility of such a relationship is strong enough to engage in speculation in this area, if for no other reason than to spur on further research.

4.3.1. Somatoform/Conversion Personality Style

The one personality style that has been evaluated in terms of its contribution to PNES events and cognitive dysfunction is the presence of a somatoform or conversion personality style.[11] Many studies with formal personality measures have related this style to the development of PNES events and have even offered rules for classifying patients on these measures.[50-52] Of note, however, is that initial studies exploring a possible relationship between these PNES (conversion) profiles and cognitive dysfunction have been

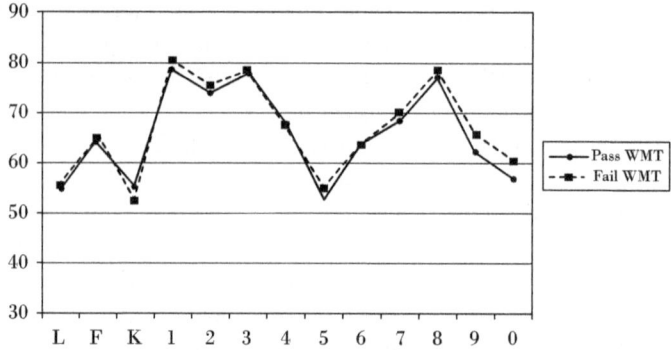

Figure 5.3 Minnesota Multiphasic Personality Inventory (2nd ed.) (MMPI-2) profiles of participants according to performance on the Word Memory Test (WMT) (oral version). Reprinted from Williamson et al.[7]

unfruitful.[7] Some have speculated that patients with somatoform tendencies might be more likely to present with cognitive dysfunction, perhaps due to a tendency to suppress internal emotional states at the expense of cognitive resources. However, this has not been borne out by objective analysis. Patients with PNES who failed PVT measures, for example, showed no personality style differences from patients with PNES who passed such measures.[7] This lack of difference between groups can be seen in Figure 5.3.

4.3.2. Alexithymia

Alexithymia is typically defined as an inability to recognize one's internal emotional state, difficulty labeling and articulating such internal emotions, and an external focus in terms of thinking that has been associated with some neurological (e.g., epilepsy, traumatic brain injury), psychiatric, and developmental conditions (e.g., schizophrenia, autism).[53,54] This condition can cause difficulty in social functioning and has been associated with difficulty empathizing with others. Some evidence exists that patients with alexithymia have limitations in verbal and sequencing abilities,[55] and that they often have difficulty recalling emotional material and recognizing emotional tone from faces. Therefore, some researchers have speculated that alexithymia may reflect, and contribute to, cognitive dysfunction in patients with PNES.[1]

Patients with PNES have a higher rate of alexithymia than healthy control subjects. Some studies have found greater rates of alexithymia in patients with PNES as compared to those with epilepsy,[56] although this difference has not always held up.[57,58] If both PNES and epilepsy patients experience alexithymia, this factor alone may not explain the difference in PVT performance typically found between these groups. However, more research is needed to explore potential differences in the mechanism underlying alexithymia in these two groups. For example, it is possible that epilepsy patients with temporal lobe seizure onset experience symptoms of alexithymia due to disturbance of the limbic system secondary to the effects of epileptiform discharges in this region. However, alexithymia in a PNES sample may be related to a stylistic approach to avoiding emotional content that was learned as a coping method for dealing with life trauma (although some would argue that the latter may lead to structural/functional brain changes in the limbic system as well). It could be that maintaining a subconscious, internal blocking of emotion compromises cognitive resources in a PNES patient, while alexithymia in a patient who experienced damage to the limbic system is simply a state of being. Currently, there are few data to support or refute these hypotheses.

4.3.3. Dissociation

Dissociative disorders have been reported to frequently occur in patients with PNES and are more common in patients with psychiatric backgrounds and precipitating experiences of trauma.[59,60] Dissociation occurs along a continuum, ranging from mild separation from one's immediate environment to severe detachment from physical and emotional experience. The patient does not lose the sense of reality completely, which would reflect a psychotic state. Both patients with PNES and those experiencing epilepsy experience elevated dissociative tendencies compared to healthy controls, with PNES patients tending to exhibit greater problems in this regard.[61] It has been suggested that patients who dissociate from their surroundings may be more likely to perform poorly on cognitive tasks, including PVT measures, as they are not fully engaged in their present situation.[1,7] Therefore, they may simply not be paying adequate attention to environmental information, which gives them the appearance of experiencing memory dysfunction. Some evidence of a relationship between dissociation and decreased cognitive performance has been reported in patients with PTSD and dissociative traits.[62] Patients experiencing dissociation have been shown to experience problems with speed of information processing, attention deficits, and verbal memory limitations.[62,63] Our group has also found that a self-report of abuse or trauma, one factor independently related to dissociation,[63] is related to poor PVT performance.[7,64]

4.3.4. Hypo-/Hypervigilant States Secondary to Anxiety and Trauma

In some individuals, PNES events appear to develop out of symptomatology related to anxiety and trauma. Baslet has suggested that such patients experience both intrusive and dissociative symptoms, which can result in recurrent somatic or cognitive experiences related to a specific event or a failure to adequately integrate some of these past experiences.[59] In such cases, it might be hypothesized that recurrent states of hypo- and hyperarousal may again contribute to a poor focus and disrupted cognitive processing. While research is lacking that examines PVT performance in relation to hypo- and hyperarousal states, some evidence exists that trauma and abuse may be related to PVT failure in general.[7]

4.3.5. Motivation/Malingering

Some physicians become skeptical when patients fail PVT measures and assume they are all performing suboptimally due to poor motivation or malingering. However, the

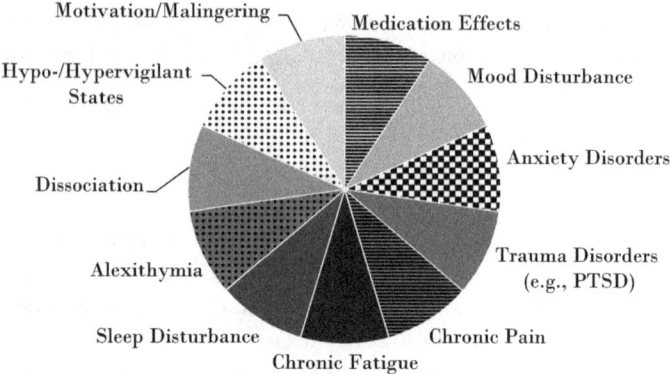

Figure 5.4 Potential factors affecting cognition in PNES. These are factors that have been proposed to affect cognition in PNES. However, such relationships have not been established in many cases. Some of these conditions have been related to cognitive functioning independent of PNES.

majority of practitioners working with patients with PNES believe that motivational issues tend to be observed in only a small subset of this group.[6,8] While we acknowledge that determining one's intent with certainty is beyond the current reach of psychometric methods, we are in agreement with this consensus.

In other patient populations with elevated rates of PVT failure (e.g., mild head trauma), financial incentive has been found to predict performance.[65,66] Therefore, we explored financial incentive in our PNES sample, attempting to determine if the presence of such incentive would predict a greater rate of PVT failure.[7] Our results did not find any relationship between financial incentive and PVT performance in patients with PNES. Instead, the only predictive factor appeared to be self-report of trauma. Figure 5.4 contains a list of proposed reasons for transient cognitive dysfunction occurring in PNES.

5. FUTURE RESEARCH

There are several clear objectives that need to be pursued by future research on PNES. One primary goal involves further attempts to determine if PNES involves a dysfunctional stylistic approach to dealing with life problems that avoids direct engagement with emotional content or whether this pattern is related to underlying brain neuropathology, perhaps resulting from trauma exposure. It is also possible that the etiology of PNES requires a diathesis stress model that incorporates both possibilities. Knowing more about the possible mechanisms of this condition will help us to focus our inquiry regarding cognitive performance in these individuals. Another means of honing our hypotheses about cognition in patients with PNES is to explore the findings from neuroimaging analysis of these patients. If consistent neuroimaging abnormalities emerge, this could help us focus our analyses on functions associated with the implicated brain regions.

Finally, an overarching concern in all cognitive function in PNES research is the need to adequately consider and control for the many confounding variables in this population (e.g., contribution of comorbid conditions, poor task engagement on formal testing).

5.1. Controlling for Confounding Variables in PNES Research on Cognition

As noted throughout this chapter, there are multiple confounding variables that can mislead our efforts to determine the nature and cause of cognitive dysfunction in PNES. These include an elevated rate of invalid test performances in this population,[6] a large number of common comorbidities (each with their own potential contribution to cognitive dysfunction or task engagement secondary to motivation issues),[27] and the possible effects of medications used in their care.[19]

We recommend that future studies make regular use of PVTs to recognize invalid test data when it occurs. Moreover, this occurrence may provide useful information to our understanding of cognition in this population, as failed performance validity testing may have meaningful underlying correlates in this subgroup of patients. For example, this group may turn out to have the most difficulty identifying internal emotional state and integrating it with cognitive processes.

Some groups have attempted to control for comorbidities by excluding various conditions from studies of cognitive performance in patients with PNES. However, as comorbidities are so common, this likely leads to a research sample that is not very representative of the vast majority of individuals with PNES. Instead, an alternative approach would be to include common comorbidities and then complete subgroup analyses to better determine the relative contribution of the additional disorders. Such an approach will require larger sample sizes to carry out meaningful statistical analysis, yet this may be more fruitful in the end. If done, the inclusion of psychiatric diagnostic interviews would also be useful. Finally, medications need to be carefully monitored in terms of type and dosage in order to control for this variable in the evaluation of cognition in PNES as well.

5.1.1. Examination of PNES Subgroups in Relation to Cognition

As PNES is believed to be a heterogeneous condition, it will be important to better determine subgroups of patients when conducting future research in this area. In general, patients with differing etiologies for their events may differ with regard to their cognitive status. Similarly, it may be possible to predict deficit types in subgroups. For example, it may prove to be the case that patients with PNES who exhibit dissociative tendencies may experience problems with primary attention, directed focus, and memory and learning ability. In contrast, patients with PNES who exhibit somatization tendencies may lack insight into their internal emotional state, may not be able to perceive emotional tone from facial expression alone, and may struggle to unite emotional and cognitive concepts of self. Dysfunction in the latter areas could represent areas of intervention to target in the development of treatment programs for working with functional neurological disorders.

Following up on the section on controlling for confounding variables, it may be possible that some potential confounds represent a subtype of PNES event (e.g., PTSD may be a central driver of one PNES subtype). Other confounds, such as depression, may have a major role in whether or not cognitive dysfunction is present, yet represent a result of PNES events rather than a cause. Such variables need to be controlled for, yet may need to be managed differently depending on whether they are true confounds or potential subtypes of populations. Myers and colleagues,[20] for example, recently demonstrated that patients with PNES who experienced PTSD exhibited problems with verbal memory (narrative recall) while those without PTSD did not. They argued that the comorbid PTSD group may represent a different subtype. As noted earlier, states of hypo- and hyperarousal have been associated with memory dysfunction, and this could reflect the underlying mechanism in the Myers sample. If so, this might yet reflect a remediable deficit that could recover with appropriate management of PTSD symptomatology. Once again, current data do not establish whether complaints of memory dysfunction in PTSD and similar conditions represent a primary neurological deficit or a transient epiphenomenon resulting from a pathological psychological state.

5.1.2. Neuroimaging and Lesion Analysis Studies in PNES Research on Cognition

Understanding whether the substrate for the development of PNES events is primarily neurological, psychological, or some interaction of the two could benefit from a greater focus on neuroimaging results and their relationship to cognitive performance. One potential problem in this area involves the difficulty involved in untangling the "cause and effect" of results. That is, are brain changes due to differences in psychological processes or do they lead to such differences?

A few studies have indicated that PNES events can develop after patients have undergone epilepsy surgery.[67,68] Some of these studies have reported that PNES events were more likely to develop after surgery involving the right temporal lobe than that in the left temporal lobe,[67] although this finding has not been consistently observed. These studies tend to be small and underpowered. The onset of postsurgical PNES events appears to occur in roughly 1.5% to 8.8% of epilepsy surgery patients, with the majority of these events representing de novo findings. These studies are also limited by being retrospective in nature and not designed to capture base rates. Overall, findings in these studies are representative of what is likely only a small subset of patients with PNES. They have also been confounded by not simultaneously exploring other explanatory variables (e.g., psychiatric variables). If "surgical lesions" or naturally occurring lesions could be linked to PNES, we might be able to learn something about the underlying disease mechanism. The relevance for cognitive function in PNES studies of such neurobiological findings would be to inform cognitive outcome research regarding possible substrates for dysfunction in these patients. Having targeted substrates would allow us to prospectively study the most relevant cognitive constructs rather than continuing to broadly sample all general domains of function. For example, if a subset of epilepsy surgery patients developed PNES after surgery involving the right anterior temporal lobe region, it might be useful to explore tasks assessing the ability of the patient to determine the positive or negative valence of emotional stimuli, to recognize emotional tone from faces, or to encode novel face and/or spatial information. The more refined our neurobiological theories of PNES, the more focused our cognitive and affective/emotional test batteries can become.

One study comparing patients with PNES ($n = 20$) and healthy controls ($n = 40$) using voxel-based morphometry (VBM) and cortical thickness analysis reported substantial differences between groups on these measures.[69] Using a region-of-interest approach and a whole-brain correlation approach, they found that patients with PNES exhibited abnormal cortical atrophy of the motor and premotor regions of the right hemisphere and the bilateral cerebellum. They also reported focal cortical thinning in the right precentral gyrus, right superior frontal gyrus, right precuneus, and right paracentral gyrus. However, they also reported an association between increasing depression scores and atrophy of premotor regions. Heightened depression was also related to cortical thinning of the right superior frontal gyrus and paracentral gyrus. Overall, the presence of depression in these patients somewhat confounds any interpretation of the data. In contrast, this study excluded patients with any current use of antipsychotic drugs, active psychiatric or neurological illness, or any history of substance abuse. These exclusions actually make this study more clear, but less applicable to real-world PNES samples. They also did not report on the length of time these patients had been treated with AEDs, which could be important, given the effects of such medications on cerebellar volume over time. While not directly studying cognition, such neuroimaging studies have relevance to this area of research, as they again potentially hone us in on brain regions and networks that may be abnormal, which, in turn, may drive our selection of cognitive and affective/emotional measures. Such research also provides insight into possible comorbid issues that may explain or even confound neurocognitive evaluation (e.g., the presence of depression).

A handful of research studies have reported abnormal functional connectivity using resting-state functional magnetic resonance imaging (fMRI) in patients with PNES and healthy controls.[70-72] Typically, areas reported to show differential connectivity (increased or decreased) include a number of regions important for emotional processing, executive control, attention, and sensorimotor areas. However, these studies remain few in number, often make numerous comparisons without adequate statistical correction, and sometimes fail to control for comorbidities that have the potential to contribute to functional connectivity problems independent of PNES status. While such functional imaging studies do not establish direct structure–function relationships,[73] they do highlight regions and networks that may be important to study in future work. As there are large numbers of cognitive constructs that can be assessed, and given that possible cognitive dysfunction in PNES may be limited to specific circumscribed brain networks, martialing all relevant neurobiological information to identify target areas of studies may be of great benefit.

A nice review of these early neuroimaging studies is provided by Perez and colleagues,[49] as well as a broader review of available data involving functional movement disorder, a condition that quite possibly reflects the same etiological substrate as PNES with a different behavioral expression. These investigators attempted to derive structure and function relationships from these neuroimaging studies. While such attempts are very much preliminary, the spirit of their efforts is exactly what future research requires. They suggested the following brain regions and related functions as hypothetically implicated in the pathophysiology of this disorder:

1) Regions mediating emotional processing, regulation and awareness—perigenual anterior cingulate cortex, ventromedal prefrontal cortex, insula, and amygdala
2) Regions supporting cognitive control—dorsolateral prefrontal cortex, dorsal anterior cingulate cortex, and inferior frontal gyrus
3) Regions involved in self-referential processing—temporoparietal junction, posterior cingulate cortex, and precuneus
4) Regions involved in motor planning—supplementary motor area

Overall, however, these suggested structure–function relationships remain tentative in functional neurological disorders, and substantial focused research is required to establish such patterns. They are derived from general ideas about these structures from broader research and the mixed results of a handful of neuroimaging studies from functional neurological disorders.[69–72] Recently, however, there have been a limited number of studies suggesting that patients with PNES exhibit some circumscribed deficits involving theory of mind and processing emotional valence from facial expression.[74] Pulling together the cognitive research and various neurobiological studies may yield better models of cognitive function in PNES and facilitate more useful prospective paradigms for studies in this area.

6. SUMMARY

- Initial research involving cognition in patients with PNES suggested that they have equivalent or greater deficits than those in people with epilepsy.[3] However, the use of PVT measures revealed that patients with PNES often show poor task engagement, which may result from a variety of factors, including treatment with medications, comorbid psychiatric and psychological variables, and motivational issues.[6–8]
- Future research should include the use of PVT measures to insure adequate task engagement, and an attempt should be made to control for the numerous secondary nuisance variables that can distort underlying relationships (e.g., comorbid psychiatric issues, medication effects). Many of these possible mechanisms for transient cognitive dysfunction in PNES remain theoretical, with only preliminary empirical support.[19,20]
- Patients with PNES showing poor task engagement appear to be experiencing general cognitive dysfunction of a pervasive but typically transient nature, which may be reversible if the cause of the dysfunction is identified and addressed. Management of PNES may result in improved cognitive performance in many cases, as it is possible that cognitive issues result from the poor integration of emotion and cognition that has been identified in this condition.[59]
- Whether or not PNES has a biological substrate (even in a subset of patients), and whether there are cognitive issues that may be related to this yet-to-be-identified substrate, remains an open question.
- PNES research should be informed by neuroimaging and lesion analysis studies directed toward identifying possible structure–function relationships and closely aligned with

cognitive testing and psychological theory. While neuroimaging of PNES remains in its infancy,[70,71] there are hints that there might be issues involving connectivity of regions important for emotion and affect processing (e.g., insula, amygdala, broader limbic system), attention, executive control, and sensorimotor regions.[49]
- Such research should guide our investigations of possible cognitive dysfunction in PNES, helping to guide test selection and underlying research hypotheses. If there are structural connectivity issues in these patients, then there may be focal limitations in aspects of emotional and affect processing, attention, and related cognitive constructs. Resolution of these questions will also shape our view of what we are calling functional (psychogenic) disorders and is a necessary step toward offering the most effective treatment.

REFERENCES

1. Drane DL, Coady E, Williamson DJ, Miller JW, Benbadis SR. Neuropsychological assessment of patients with psychogenic nonepileptic seizures. In: Schoenberg MR, Scott J, eds. *Black Book of Neuropsychology* (pp. 521–550). New York: Springer; 2011.
2. Reuber M, Elger CE. Psychogenic nonepileptic seizures: review and update. *Epilepsy Behav.* 2003;4(3):205–216.
3. Wilkus RJ, Dodrill CB, Thompson PM. Intensive EEG monitoring and psychological studies of patients with pseudoepileptic seizures. *Epilepsia.* 1984;25(1):100–107.
4. Devinsky O, Sanchez-Villaseñor F, Vasquez B, Kotahri M, Alper K, Luciano D. Clinical profile of patients with epileptic and nonepileptic seizures. *Neurology.* 1996;46:1530–1533.
5. Drake ME, Huber SJ, Pakalnis A, Phillips BB. Neuropsychological and event-related potential correlates of nonepileptic seizures. *J Neuropsychiatry Clin Neurosci.* 1993;5(1):102.
6. Drane DL, Williamson DJ, Stroup ES, et al. Cognitive impairment is not equal in patients with epileptic and psychogenic nonepileptic seizures. *Epilepsia.* 2006;47(11):1879–1886.
7. Williamson DJ, Holsman MN, Chaytor N, Miller JW, Drane DL. Abuse, not financial incentive, predicts non-credible cognitive performance in patients with psychogenic nonepileptic seizures. *Clin Neuropsychol.* 2012;26(4):588–598.
8. Binder LM, Kindermann SS, Heaton RK, Salinsky MC. Neuropsychologic impairment in patients with nonepileptic seizures. *Arch Clin Neuropsychol.* 1998;13(6):513–522.
9. Dodrill CB, Holmes MD. Psychological and neuropsychological evaluation of the patient with non-epileptic seizures. In: Gates JR, Rowan AJ, eds. *Non-epileptic Seizures*, 2nd ed. Boston: Butterworth-Heinemann; 2000 (pp. 169–181).
10. Hermann BP. Neuropsychological assessment in the diagnosis of non-epileptic seizures. In: Gates JR, Rowan AJ, eds. *Non-epileptic Seizures*. Boston: Butterworth-Heinemann; 2000 (pp. 221–232).
11. Wilkus RJ, Dodrill CB. Factor affecting the outcome of MMPI and neuropsychological assessments of psychogenic and epileptic seizure patients. *Epilepsia.* 1989;30(339–347).
12. Kalogjera-Sackellares D, Sackellares JC. Intellectual and neuropsychological features of patients with psychogenic pseudoseizures. *Psychiatry Res.* 1999;86:73–84.
13. Sackellares J, Giordani B, Berent S, et al. Patients with pseudoseizures: intellectual and cognitive performance. *Neurology.* 1985;35:116–119.
14. Dodrill C. A neuropsychological battery for epilepsy. *Epilepsia.* 1978;19(611–623).

15. Bashem JR, Rapport LJ, Miller JB, Hanks RA, Axelrod BN, Millis SR. Comparisons of five performance validity indices in bona fide and simulated traumatic brain injury. *Clin Neuropsychol.* 2014;28(5):851–875.
16. Drane DL. Can subclinical epileptiform activity impact symptom validity testing? Paper presented at the National Academy of Neuropsychology, November, 2012, Nashville, Tennessee.
17. Williamson DJ, Drane DL, Stroup ES, Wilensky AJ, Holmes MD, Miller JW. Recent seizures may distort the validity of neurocognitive test scores in patients with epilepsy. *Epilepsia.* 2005;46(8):74.
18. Drane DL, Ojemann JG, Kim M, et al. Interictal epileptiform discharge effects on neuropsychological assessment and epilepsy surgical planning. *Epilepsy Behav.* 2016;56:131–138.
19. Loring DL, Marino S, Drane DL, Parfitt D, Finney GR, Meador KJ. Lorazepam effects on Word Memory Test performance: a randomized, double-blind, placebo contolled, crossover trial. *Clin Neuropsychol.* 2011;25(5):799–811.
20. Myers L, Zeng R, Perrine K, Lancman M, Lancman M. Cognitive differences between patients who have psychogenic nonepileptic seizures (PNESs) and posttraumatic stress disorder (PTSD) and patients who have PNESs without PTSD. *Epilepsy Behav.* 2014;37:82–86.
21. Demakis GJ, Gervais RO, Rohling ML. The effect of failure on cognitive and psychological symptom validity tests in litigants with symptoms of post-traumatic stress disorder. *Clin Neuropsychol.* 2008;22(5):879–895.
22. Delis DC, Wetter SR. Cogniform disorder and cogniform condition: proposed diagnoses for excessive cognitive symptoms. *Arch Clin Neuropsychol.* 2007;22:589–604.
23. Dodrill CB. Do patients with psychogenic nonepileptic seizures produce trustworthy findings on neuropsychological tests? *Epilepsia.* 2008;49(4):691–695.
24. Williamson DJ, Drane DL, Stroup ES. Symptom validity tests in the epilepsy clinic. In: Boone K, ed. *Assessment of Feigned Cognitive Impairment.* New York: Guilford Publications; 2007.
25. Kleen JK, Scott RC, Holmes GL, et al. Hippocampal interictal epileptiform activity disrupts cognition in humans. *Neurology.* 2013;81(1):18–24.
26. Cragar DE, Berry DT, Fakhoury TA, Cibula JE, Schmitt FA. Performance of patients with epilepsy or psychogenic non-epileptic seizures on four measures of effort. *Clin Neuropsychol.* 2006;20(3):552–566.
27. Mokleby K, Biomhoff S, Malt UF, Dahlstrom A, Tauboll E, Gjerstad L. Psychiatric comorbidity and hostility in patients with psychogenic nonepileptic seizures compared with somatoform disorders and healthy controls. *Epilepsia.* 2002;43(2):193–198.
28. Benbadis SR. Association between chronic pain or fibromyalgia and psychogenic seizures. *Am J Pain Manage.* 2005;15(4):117–119.
29. Vasquez GH, Holtzman JN, Tondo L, Baldessarini RJ. Efficacy and tolerability of treatments for bipolar depression. *J Affect Disord.* 2015;183:258–262.
30. Drane DL, Meador KJ, ed. *Cognitive Toxicity of Antiepileptic Drugs.* Boston: Butterworth-Heinemann; 2002.
31. Aldenkamp AP, De Krom M, Reijs R. Newer antiepileptic drugs and cognitive issues. *Epilepsia.* 2003;44(Suppl 4):21–29.
32. Ojemann LM, Ojemann GA, Dodrill CB, Crawford CA, Holmes MD, Dudley DL. Language disturbances as side effects of topiramate and zonisamide therapy. *Epilepsy Behav.* 2001;2:579–584.

33. Mula M, Trimble MR, Thompson P, Sander JWAS. Topiramate and word-finding difficulties in patients with epilepsy *Neurology.* 2003;60(7):1104–1107.
34. Amado-Boccara I, Gougoulis N, Poirier Littre MF, Galinowski A, Loo H. Effects of antidepressants on cognitive functions: a review. *Neurosci Biobehav Rev.* 1995;19(3):479–493.
35. Stewart SA. The effects of benzodiazepines on cognition. *J Clin Psychiatry.* 2005;66(Suppl. 2):9–13.
36. Nagane A, Baba H, Nakano Y, et al. Comparative study of cognitive impairment between medicated and medication-free patients with remitted major depression: class-specific influence by tricyclic antidepressants and newer antidepressants. *Psychiatry Res.* 2014;218(1-2):101–105.
37. Duka T, Curran HV, Rusted JM, Weingartner HJ. Perspectives on cognitive psychopharmacology research. *Behav Pharmacol.* 1996;7:401–410.
38. Ghoneim MM, Mewaldt SP. Effects of diazepam and scopolamine on storage, retrieval and organizational processes in memory. *Psychopharmacologia.* 1975;44:257–262.
39. Loring DW, Marino SE, Parfitt D, Finney GR, Meador KJ. Acute lorazepam effects on neurocognitive performance. *Epilepsy Behav.* 2012;25(3):329–333.
40. Roth AJ, McCall WV, Liguori A. Cognitive, psychomotor, and polysomnographic effects of trazodone in primary insomniacs. *J Sleep Res.* 2011;20(4):552–558.
41. Verster JC, Vokerts ER, Schreuder AH, et al. Residual effects of middle-of-the-night administration of zaleplon and zolpidem on driving ability, memory functions, and psychomotor performance. *J Clin Psychopharmacol.* 2002;22(6):576–583.
42. Hantke NC, Doherty MJ, Haltiner AM. Medication use profiles in patients with psychogenic nonepileptic seizures. *Epilepsy Behav.* 2007;10(2):333–335.
43. Bowman ES. Etiology and clinical course of pseudoseizures. Relationship to trauma, depression, and dissociation. *Psychosomatics.* 1993;34:333–342.
44. Witgert ME, Wheless JW, Breier JI. Frequency of panic symptoms in psychogenic nonepileptic seizures. *Epilepsy Behav.* 2005;6:174–178.
45. Dworetzky BA, Strahonja-Packard A, Shanahan CW, Paz J, Schauble B, Bromfield EB. Characteristics of male veterans with psychogenic nonepileptic seizures. *Epilepsia.* 2005;46:1418–1422.
46. Pavlova MK, Allen RM, Dworetzky BA. Sleep in psychogenic nonepileptic seizures and related disorders. *Clin EEG Neurosci.* 2015;46(1):34–41.
47. Marquez AV, Farias ST, Apperson M, et al. Psychogenic nonepileptic seizures are associated with an increased risk of obesity. *Epilepsy Behav.* 2004;5(1):88–93.
48. Malykhin NV, Carter R, Seres P, Coupland NJ. Structural changes in the hippocampus in major depressive disorder: contributions of disease and treatment. *J Psychiatry Neurosci.* 2010;35(5):337–343.
49. Perez DL, Dworetzky BA, Dickerson BC, Leung L, Cohn R, Baslet G, Silberzweig DA. An integrative neurocircuit perspective on psychoenic nonepileptic seizures and functional movement disorders: Neural functional unawareness. *Clin EEG Neurosci.* 2015;46(1):4–15.
50. Cragar DE, Schmitt FA, Berry DTR, Cibula JE, Dearth CMS, Fakhoury TA. A comparison of MMPI-2 decision rules in the diagnosis of nonepileptic seizures. *J Clin Exp Neuropsychol.* 2003;25(6):793–804.
51. Cragar DE, Berry DTR, Fakhoury TA, Cibula JE, Schmitt FA. A review of diagnostic techniques in the differential diagnosis of epileptic and nonepileptic seizures. *Neuropsychol Rev.* 2002;12(1):31–64.
52. Derry PA, Mclachlan RS. The MMPI-2 as an adjunct to the diagnosis of pseudoseizures. *Seizure.* 1996;5:35–40.

53. Samur D, Tops M, Schlinkert C, Quirin M, Cuijpers P, Koole SL. Four decades of research on alexithymia: moving toward clinical applications. *Front Psychol.* 2013;4:1–4.
54. Sifneos PE. The prevalence of 'alexithymic' characteristics in psychosomatic patients. *Psychother Psychosom.* 1973;22:255–262.
55. Wood RL, Williams C. Neuropsychological correlates of organic alexithymia. *J Int Neuropsychol Soc.* 2007;13(3):471–478.
56. Kaplan MJ, Dwivdei AK, Privitera MD, Isaacs K, Hughes C, Bowman M. Comparisons of childhood trauma, alexithymia, and defensive styles in patients iwth psychogenic non-epileptic seizures vs. epilepsy: implications for the etiology of conversion disorder. *J Psychosom Res.* 2013;75(2):142–146.
57. Myers L, Matzner B, Lancman M, Perrine K, Lancman M. Prevalence of alexithymia in patients with psychogenic non-epileptic seizures and epileptic seizures and predictors in psychogenic non-epileptic seizures *Epilepsy Behav.* 2013;26:153–157.
58. Wolf LD, Hentz JG, Ziemba KS, et al. Quality of life in psychogenic nonepileptic seizures and epilepsy: the role of somatization and alexithymia. *Epilepsy Behav.* 2015;43:81–88.
59. Baslet G. Psychogenic non-epileptic seizures: a model of their pathogenic mechanism. *Seizure.* 2011;20(1):1–13.
60. Harden CL. Pseudoseizures and dissociatve disorders: a common mechanism involving traumatic experiences. *Seizure.* 1997;6:151–155.
61. Wagner EB, Drane DL. Evaluation of dissociation, self-efficacy, and rates of trauma in patients with psychogenic nonepileptic seizure (PNES) events or epilepsy. Paper presented at the American Epilepsy Society, 2015, Philadelphia, Pennsylvania.
62. Roca V, Hart J, Kimbrell T, Freeman T. Cognitive function and dissociative disorder status among verteran subjects with chronic posttraumatic stress disorder: a preliminary study. *J Neuropsychiatry Clin Neurosci.* 2006;18:226–230.
63. Guralnik O, Giesbrecht T, Knutelska M, Sirroff B, Simeon D. Cognitive functioning in depersonalization disorder. *J Nerv Ment Dis.* 2007;195:983–988.
64. Hebert M, Langevin R, Daigneault I. The association between peer victimization, PTSD, and dissocation in child victims of sexual abuse. *J Affect Disord.* 2016;193:227–232.
65. Grote CL, Kooker EK, Garron DC, Nyenhuis DL, Smith CA, Mattingly ML. Performance of compensation seeking and non-compensation seeking samples on the Victoria Symptom Validity Test: cross-validation and extension of a standardization study. *J Clin Exp Neuropsychol.* 2000;22(6):709–719.
66. Cottingham ME, Victor TL, Boone KB, Ziegler EA, Zeller M. Apparent effect of type of compensation seeking (disablity versus litigation) on performance validity test scores may be due to other factors. *Clin Neuropsychol.* 2014;28(6):1030–1047.
67. Devinsky O, Mesad S, Alper K. Nondominant hemisphere lesions and conversion nonepileptic seizures. *J Neuropsychiatry Clin Neurosci.* 2001;13:367–373.
68. Reuber M, Kral T, Kurthen M, Elger CE. New onset psychogenic seizures after intracranial neurosurgery. *Acta Neurochir (Wien).* 2002;144:901–907.
69. Labate A, Cerasa A, Mula M, et al. Neuroanatomic correlates of psychogenic nonepileptic seizures: a cortical thickness and VBM study. *Epilepsia.* 2012;53(2):377–385.
70. van der Kruijs SJ, Bodde NM, Vaessen MJ, et al. Functional connectivity of dissociation in patients with psychogenic non-epileptic seizures. *J Neurol Neurosurg Psychiatry.* 2012;83(3):239–247.
71. Ding J, An D, Lisao W, et al. Abnormal functional connectivity density in psychogenic non-epileptic seizures. *Epilepsy Res.* 2014;108:1184–1194.

72. Lee SH, Allendorfer JB, Gaston TE, et al. White matter diffusion abnormalities in patients with psychogenic non-epileptic seizures. *Brain Res.* 2015;1620:169–176.
73. Cole DM, Smith SM, Beckmann CF. Advances and pitfalls in the analysis and interpretation of resting-state fMRI data. *Front Syst Neurosci.* 2010;4(8):1–18.
74. Schonenberg M, Jusyte A, Hohnie N, et al. Theory of mind abilities in patients with psychogenic nonepileptic seizures. *Epilepsy Behav.* 2015;53:20–24.
75. Bortz JJ, Wong JL, Blum D, Prigatano GP, Fisher RS. Differential response bias patterns in patients with frontal lobe epilepsy vs. frontal lobe lesions. *Arch Clin Neuropsychol.* 1997;12(4):290.
76. Binder LM. Assessment of malingering afer mild head trauma with the Portland Digit Recogniton Test. *J Clin Exp Neuropsychol.* 1993;15:170–182.
77. Green P, Astner K. *Manual for the Oral Word Memory Test.* Durham, NC: CogniSyst; 1995.
78. Bakvis P, Spinhoven P, Putman P, Zitman FG, Roelofs K. The effect of stress induction on working memory in patients with psychogenic nonepileptic seizures. *Epilepsy Behav.* 2010;19(3):448–454.
79. Strutt AM, Hill SW, Scott BM, Uber-Zak L, Fogel TG. A comprehensive neuropsychological profile of women with psychogenic nonepileptic seizures. *Epilepsy Behav.* 2011;20(1):24–28.
80. McNally (2009). McNally, K. A., Schefft, B. K., Szaflarski, J. P., Howe, S. R., Yeh, H., Privitera, M. D. Application of signal detection theory to verbal memory testing to distinguish patients with psychogenic nonepileptic seizures from patients with epileptic seizures. *Epilepsy and Behav.* 2009;14(4):597–603.

6

The Neurobiology of PNES and Other Functional Neurological Symptoms

David L. Perez, MD and Valerie Voon, MD, PhD

1. INTRODUCTION

Patients with psychogenic nonepileptic seizures (PNES) and related functional neurological symptoms (FNS) are highly prevalent yet poorly understood on a neurobiological level. Patients with FNS were first described in ancient Greece using explanatory models of the "wandering womb"[1] and subsequent early formulations related to themes of demonic possession. The concept of FNS entered the medical literature as "hysteria," and leading neurologists in the 19th century, including Jean-Martin Charcot, viewed hysteria as an established neurological condition. Jean-Martin Charcot stated that "the neurological tree has its branches; neuroasthenia, hysteria, epilepsy, all the types of mental conditions, progressive paralysis, gait ataxia."[2] A paradigm shift occurred with Sigmund Freud, Austrian neurologist and developer of psychoanalysis, who transitioned the field toward conceptualizing FNS as a manifestation of psychological conflict. Freud wrote in *Studies on Hysteria* that the "etiology was to be sought in sexual factors" and used the term "conversion hysteria" to theorize that intolerable psychological conflicts were converted to physical symptoms.[3] Historically, clinical and research efforts aimed at understanding and treating PNES and other FNS have significantly lagged behind clinical neuroscience advancements in other neuropsychiatric conditions, including epilepsy, major depression[4] and post-traumatic stress disorder (PTSD).[5] Recent studies, however, have reported the high frequency with which clinicians encounter PNES and other FNS,[6] emphasizing a sizeable unmet medical need in this population. Furthermore, FNS are now identified by inspecting for "positive" signs and are no longer a diagnosis of exclusion. Advancing our neurobiological understanding of PNES is a critical step toward enabling neurologists, psychiatrists, psychologists, scientists, and allied professionals to develop an integrated biopsychosocial framework through which to conceptualize this population. Advancing our understanding of neurobiological mechanisms of disease for patients with PNES and other FNS will help destigmatize this enigmatic neuropsychiatric disorder and will catalyze research efforts to identify diagnostic, prognostic, and treatment response biomarkers.

In this chapter, systems-level neurobiological studies in PNES are reviewed.[7,8] Specific emphasis is given to structural and functional neuroimaging, electrophysiological, autonomic, and neuroendocrine investigations. Given a clinical overlap between PNES, other FNS populations,[7] PTSD, and dissociation, select findings from the clinical neuroscience literature on these populations will also be briefly discussed.[9-11] The importance of alterations in distributed neural networks mediating emotional processing, regulation and awareness, sense of agency, and bodily awareness will be examined as it pertains to the biology of PNES and related disorders.

2. NEUROIMAGING AND ELECTROPHYSIOLOGY STUDIES IN PNES

Observational and quantitative structural neuroimaging studies have been performed in patients with PNES. In a study of 206 patients with PNES alone and 123 patients with PNES and epileptic seizures, approximately 10% of individuals with isolated PNES displayed nonspecific brain magnetic resonance imaging (MRI) abnormalities.[12] Not surprisingly, this study showed that rates of such abnormalities were significantly higher among individuals with comorbid PNES and epileptic seizures (60%). The finding of nonspecific brain MRI abnormalities in PNES has also been independently replicated,[13] and one report suggested a possible association between right hemisphere lateralized brain lesions and PNES.[14] While more frequently associated with epileptic seizures, mesial temporal sclerosis has also been described in PNES,[15] highlighting the need to incorporate several aspects of the history and diagnostic evaluation when considering a diagnosis of PNES versus epileptic seizures. One possible interpretation of these non-specific structural MRI abnormalities in PNES is that their presence may result in a central nervous system vulnerability for the development of PNES, although more clinical research efforts are needed to clarify this further.

Specific structural brain abnormalities have been studied in PNES using quantitative MRI research techniques. Voxel-based morphometry (VBM), cortical thickness analyses, and diffusion tensor imaging (DTI) enable the investigation of regional and network-related brain abnormalities. VBM is a technique based in statistical parametric mapping (SPM) software and the general linear statistical model, which allows for the study of gray (and white) matter volumes.[16] Other automated MRI techniques provide in vivo cortical thickness measurements through the creation of inflated surface brain representations;[17] this approach has been validated in postmortem pathological[18] and MRI tracing studies.[19] A small study of 20 patients with PNES compared to 40 matched healthy controls, using VBM and cortical thickness analyses, showed that PNES was associated with reductions in gray matter volume in the right anterior cingulate cortex (ACC), supplementary motor area (SMA), middle frontal gyrus, precentral gyrus, and bilateral cerebellum.[20] Cortical thickness analyses similarly showed atrophy in the dorsomedial prefrontal cortex, right precentral gyrus, and precuneus in PNES. Additional within-group PNES analyses in this study probing brain–symptom relationships showed associations between increased depression scores and reductions in gray matter volume in the right dorsal premotor cortex. A study of adequate sample size in 37 subjects with PNES compared to 37 control subjects replicated the observation of bilateral precentral gyrus cortical thickness reductions in PNES and identified additional disease-associated increases in insular and orbitofrontal cortex cortical thickness.[21] Two recently published studies investigated white matter abnormalities in PNES using DTI. In a small cohort study (8 PNES patients vs. 8 matched healthy controls), a rightward asymmetry of the uncinate fasciculus (a fiber tract connecting the medial prefrontal and temporal cortices) was identified in patients with PNES compared to healthy subjects[22]. A separate study reported increases in fractional anisotropy in the left corona radiata, internal and external capsules, superior temporal gyrus, and uncinate fasciculus[23] in 16 patients with PNES compared to 16 matched healthy controls. Fractional anisotropy is a DTI-based quantitative measure of white matter microstructure integrity that is obtained by recording water diffusivity along white matter tracts. Taken together, these initial structural neuroimaging studies in PNES patients suggest possible gray matter abnormalities in the precentral gyrus (motor execution) and brain areas involved in motor planning (SMA), cognitive control, and the behavioral expression of mood states (ACC).[24] Structural neuroimaging studies, particularly DTI investigations, require larger sample-size investigations and replication. Furthermore, the variability in structural (and functional) neuroimaging findings may reflect that PNES is a heterogeneous disorder, potentially comprised of several incompletely overlapping disease subtypes. See Figure 6.1A for a plot of peak coordinates in the quantitative MRI studies just discussed (excluding DTI).

As a complement to structural MRI, resting-state functional connectivity neuroimaging techniques have also been used to investigate neural circuit alterations in PNES. As a brief introduction to this methodology, resting-state functional MRI (rs-fMRI) uses the intrinsic low-frequency oscillations in blood oxygen level–dependent (BOLD) signal to study brain connectivity. It has been previously well established that discrete neural networks at rest exhibit coherence in their BOLD oscillations, enabling the parcellation of frequency patterns into discrete brain networks[25]. Broadly speaking, rs-fMRI can be applied using region-of-interest "seed"-based techniques that evaluate whole-brain connectivity in relation to a given target region, or it can be implemented using data-driven computational approaches such as independent component analyses or graph-theory-based metrics. In the first of these studies in 11 patients with PNES compared to 12 healthy subjects, increased functional connectivity was observed between brain areas involved in movement (precentral sulcus), emotion processing (ACC, insula), and executive/attentional functions (inferior frontal gyrus, parietal cortex)[26] in PNES. Among several findings, increased coupling was observed between the left precentral sulcus, right perigenual ACC, and the insula. Functional connectivity strength between the precentral sulcus and posterior insula was associated with increased dissociation (measured using the Dissociative Experience Scale) in PNES. Several studies using data-driven approaches have shown widespread functional connectivity alterations in sensory-motor, emotion-processing, executive/attentional, and default-mode networks in PNES.[27-29] In addition to the dorsal ACC/middle cingulate cortex,[30] viscerosomatic, affective, and cognitive neural systems converge within the insula.[11,31] In a study that evaluated insular subregion connectivity, compared to healthy controls ($N = 20$), patients with PNES ($N = 18$) showed increased coupling among the left ventral anterior insula,

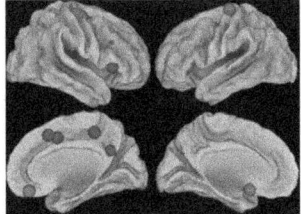

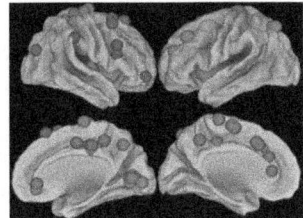

Figure 6.1 Display of volumetric and resting-state functional connectivity (FC) findings in psychogenic nonepileptic seizures (PNES) neuroimaging studies. Panel A displays peak coordinates of cortical thickness and voxel-based morphometry findings in PNES patients compared with healthy controls.[20,21] Panel B shows peak coordinates of abnormal resting-state FC in individuals with PNES compared with healthy controls.[26,27,32,33] Blue circles indicate decrease and red circles indicate increase. Evidence from neuroimaging studies, while requiring replication and further investigations, suggests that PNES may potentially develop in the context of alterations within and across brain networks implicated in sensory-motor (e.g., pre- and postcentral gyrus, premotor regions), emotion processing/regulation (e.g., anterior cingulate cortex [ACC], middle cingulate cortex [MCC], orbitofrontal cortex, insula), cognitive control (e.g., lateral prefrontal cortex, dorsal ACC, MCC), and multimodal integration functions (e.g., cingulate gyrus, posterior parietal cortex, precuneus). Only main findings are displayed using Caret 5. Cerebellar and basal ganglia foci and seed region coordinates are not shown. Modified from Perez and LaFrance (2016).[78]

left post-central gyrus, and bilateral SMA.[32] Additionally, the strength of resting-state connectivity between the left ventral anterior insula and the bilateral SMA positively correlated with PNES frequency. A similar positive association was observed between functional connectivity strength across the ACC-SMA and PNES event frequency in 18 patients.[33] A resting-state positron emission tomography (PET) study in 16 patients with PNES compared to 16 healthy subjects also showed hypometabolism in the bilateral ACC and the right inferior parietal lobule.[34] Hypometabolism of the right inferior parietal lobule is a notable finding given related literature on functional movement disorder (discussed later in the chapter) suggesting an association between hypoactivation of the right temporoparietal junction and deficits in awareness of self-agency.[35] The dorsal ACC and the temporoparietal junction are also higher-order multimodal integration regions,[36,37] which may help explain the complex and diverse nature of the viscerosomatic symptoms experienced by patients. See Figure 6.1B for a plot of peak coordinates for the resting-state fMRI studies discussed here.

In summary, resting-state neuroimaging studies in PNES, while requiring increased sample size, replication, and more adequate control of confounds (i.e., gender effects, psychiatric comorbidities, PNES subtype considerations, etc.), suggest disease-associated alternations in brain networks mediating sensory-motor, emotional processing/regulation, executive/cognitive, and multimodal integration functions. Specific associations have been observed regarding a relationship between PNES event frequency and heightened coupling between motor planning and paralimbic regions. The ACC and insula are paralimbic regions that form critically important parts of the salience network[38] (an intrinsic distributed brain network implicated in integrating highly processed viscerosomatic and affectively valenced information to detect the most homeostatically relevant inputs) and are particularly important regions for the convergence of negative emotion, viscerosomatic processing, interoception, and cognitive control.[30,39,40] These cortical regions, in conjunction with multimodal association areas, also play important roles in the internal representation of bodily states and prediction error.[41] Overall, the literature to date provides early evidence suggesting that abnormal interactions between emotion-processing and motor-control networks are implicated in the pathophysiology of PNES.

Quantitative electroencephalography (EEG) research techniques with better temporal resolution than that of neuroimaging modalities have also been used to study the pathophysiology of PNES. Similar to the nonspecific MRI abnormalities described previously, some patients with PNES also display interictal EEG abnormalities.[42] To increase regional specificity, one study applied multivariate phase synchronization mapping to high-density interictal EEG recordings in 13 PNES subjects compared to matched controls, showing that PNES event frequency was inversely associated with prefrontal and parietal cortical synchronization.[43] In a related study in the same cohort, graph-theory metrics applied to EEG data identified an association between decreased local network connectedness in the alpha band and PNES frequency.[44] In a study of 18 patients with PNES compared to 18 matched controls, quantitative EEG analyses demonstrated relative decoupling of corticosubcortical networks in PNES; additionally, reductions in paralimbic interhemispheric connectivity were also observed[45]. Other investigations using EEG and graph-theory metrics have also observed decreased connectedness between frontal and posterior regions.[46] In a unique case of PNES captured on intracranial recording, decreased power in the theta band was observed over the posterior parietal cortex.[47] These complementary electrophysiology findings add to the systems-level literature implicating the prefrontal cortex and posterior parietal cortex in the pathophysiology of PNES.

3. ABNORMALITIES OF AUTONOMIC FUNCTION AND THE HPA AXIS IN PNES

Consistent with neuroimaging and electrophysiology findings implicating neural circuit alterations in emotion processing and regulation circuits, there is early evidence for alterations in autonomic functions in PNES.[48] In a study of 67 epileptic seizures and 39 PNES events, epileptic seizures in comparison to PNES showed increased ictal and postictal heart rates.[49] Another study, however, reported that convulsive epileptic seizures and major motor PNES events were similarly associated with ictal heart rate increases; in this study only epileptic seizures were associated with postictal heart rate increases.[50] The latter study suggests that ictal heart rate increases in PNES may relate to the degree of PNES motor manifestations. Consistent with the lack of a differentiating ictal heart rate pattern, only preictal increases and postictal decreases in heart rate were observed in 42 patients with PNES compared to 46 individuals with complex partial seizures.[51] A separate study replicated preictal heart rate increases in PNES.[52] The finding of increases in heart rate preceding PNES events provides evidence implicating autonomic abnormalities in the pathophysiology of PNES and potentially provides a link between emotional stressors and PNES event frequency. This would also be consistent with the growing literature identifying an association between PNES and panic attacks (paroxysmal crescendo events of anxiety with somatic symptoms that may be untriggered).[7,53]

Heart rate variability, a measure of parasympathetic function, has also been used to study the biology of PNES.[54] One study observed that interictal heart rate variability was reduced in PNES patients compared to healthy subjects, but was not significantly different from variability in patients with refractory epilepsy.[55] During performance of an affectively valenced face-viewing task, heart rate variability did not differ between PNES, healthy subjects, and individuals with PTSD symptoms.[56] Consistent with findings of preictal heart rate increases in PNES, reductions in preictal heart rate variability (a marker of decreased parasympathetic tone) in the 5-minute interval before PNES (compared to the preceding 5 minutes) have also been reported in PNES.[52] By contrast, heart rate variability in the interictal and postictal period may be similar to that of healthy subjects.[57]

A few studies have characterized links between hypothalamic–pituitary–adrenal (HPA) axis function, specifically cortisol secretion, and PNES. A positive association was observed between attentional bias for threatening stimuli and baseline salivary cortisol levels in 19 unmedicated patients with PNES.[58] In a related study, 18 patients with PNES showed increased basal diurnal cortisol levels compared to levels in 19 matched healthy subjects; secondary analyses showed that this effect was driven particularly by those individuals who reported past sexual trauma. Positive associations have also been observed between deficits in stress-associated working memory performance and elevated cortisol levels in PNES.[59] Taken together, these results provide early evidence of heightened cortisol levels in PNES, with potential associations between increases in cortisol, history of sexual trauma, biased attention processing, and cognitive deficits.

4. PSYCHOLOGICAL TRAUMA, DISSOCIATION, AND OTHER FUNCTIONAL NEUROLOGICAL SYMPTOMS

Estimates suggest that up to three out of four adults with PNES report past traumatic experiences, with many specifically reporting sexual and/or physical abuse.[60,61] These associations between PNES and traumatic experiences provide important additional clues to the pathophysiology of PNES. In a large cohort of 148 healthy subjects, positive associations were identified between heightened amygdalar responses to threat-related facial expressions and the magnitude of previously experienced childhood trauma.[62] This finding of heightened amygdalar responses to threat, an indicator of biased attentional processing, fits well with the previously discussed observations of biased threat processing and increased cortisol secretion in PNES. In this same cohort, VBM analyses showed gray matter volume reductions in the ACC, insula, orbitofrontal cortex, caudate, and hippocampus that were associated with the severity of previously experienced childhood trauma. These findings denote important associations between past traumatic experiences and aberrant neuroplastic alterations in critical nodes of brain networks implicated in the pathophysiology of PNES. Convergent basic science studies in animal models used to study brain changes in response to chronic stress also suggest that the medial prefrontal cortex (including the ACC) and hippocampus exhibit dendritic spine density reductions following repeated stress.[63]

Non-military and military PNES populations show elevated rates of PTSD.[64] Patients with PTSD experience not only unwanted intrusive traumatic recollections, hyperarousal, and avoidance but also dissociative symptoms and emotional numbing.[65] *Dissociation* can be defined as fragmented processing of information related to the external world (derealization) and one's bodily experiences (depersonalization). As opposed to heighted traumatic recollection and other traditionally conceptualized PTSD symptoms, which are linked to increased amygdalar activity and decreased top-down engagement of regulatory prefrontal regions,[66] dissociative symptoms in PTSD may result from overmodulation of emotions, driven by abnormally increased top-down activation of regulatory circuits.[65] From a structural perspective, gray matter reductions in PTSD have been identified in the dorsal and perigenual ACC.[67] Structural and functional ACC alterations should be further investigated to clarify neurobiological associations between PNES subtypes with and without a history of PTSD. Furthermore, clarifying the neurobiological convergence with borderline personality disorder, which frequently also manifests with dissociative symptoms,[68] and other idiopathic dissociative disorders with the emerging biology of PNES will add important insights regarding the intersection of PNES and dissociation.

Approximately 50% of patients with PNES report other medically unexplained symptoms,[69] and trauma has been linked to the development of other medically unexplained symptoms in this population.[61] These observations suggest that there is likely a neurobiological overlap between PNES, other FNS, and somatic symptom disorders. While a comprehensive review of neuroimaging studies across functional neurological disorders (FND) is beyond the scope of this chapter and has been performed elsewhere,[7,8,10] select neuroimaging studies in functional movement disorders (FMD) will be highlighted, given increased recognition of a possible clinical overlap between these two functional neurological subtypes.[70] The influence of positive and negative arousal in 16 subjects with FMD was studied by Voon and colleagues using an emotionally valenced face-viewing paradigm.[71] Patients with FMD, compared to healthy controls, showed increased amygdalar activation to arousing stimuli and increased functional connectivity between the amygdala and the SMA (Figure 6.2). Findings of increased amygdala activations to emotionally valenced stimuli[72] and greater functional connectivity between the amygdala and SMA[73] have been replicated in other motor FND studies. Furthermore, task-based findings of heightened limbic–SMA connectivity are synergistic with the rsfMRI findings in PNES demonstrating increased paralimbic–motor/premotor connectivity, as shown previously among the anterior insula, anterior cingulate, and motor regions.[26,32,33] Further

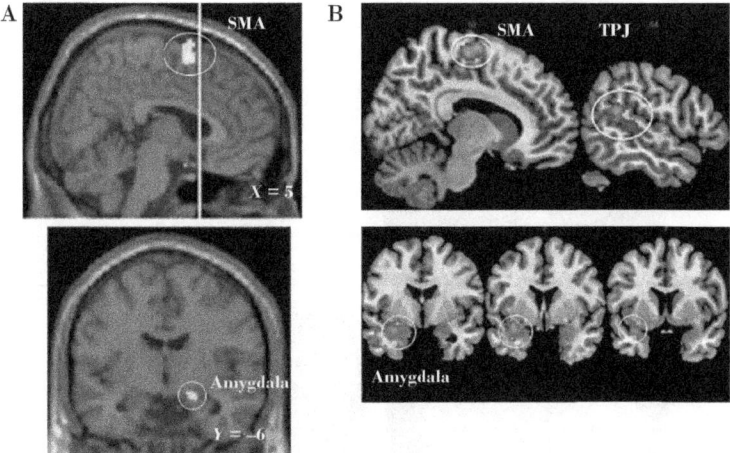

Figure 6.2 Limbic-motor functional connectivity in patients with motor functional neurological symptoms. A. Subjects with positive functional motor symptoms exposed to an affectively valenced face-viewing task show greater amygdala activity and task-based connectivity to the supplementary motor area (SMA) during both fearful and happy face processing, suggesting an effect of arousal.[71] B. Subjects with mixed motor symptoms exposed to recall of personalized traumatic episodes show enhanced supplementary motor complex activity to escape relative to non-escape traumatic memories with greater functional connectivity with the left amygdala to all traumatic memories.[73] TPJ, temporoparietal junction.

studies using similar resting-state and task fMRI designs in larger sample sizes would be useful to assess whether different networks may be implicated more specifically with particular motor FNS subtypes.

Patients with PNES have demonstrated hypometabolism of the right inferior parietal lobule, which may be contextualized, in part, through an fMRI study in patients with a positional functional tremor.[35] Using a within-subject design, hypoactivation of the right temporoparietal junction was identified in functional tremor movements, compared to voluntarily mimicked shaking (Figure 6.3). This pattern of right temporoparietal hypoactivation was also associated with reduced connectivity to sensory-motor and emotion-processing (ACC, ventral striatum) regions. Findings from the clinical neuroscience literature suggest important roles for the right inferior parietal lobule (and temporoparietal junction) in motor intention awareness and self-agency. Patients with right inferior parietal lobule lesions exhibit deficits in motor intention awareness.[74] The concepts of forward modeling or corollary discharge, developed on the basis of predictive coding concepts, suggest that sensory-motor regions provide the posterior parietal cortex with a "copy" of the expected sensory consequence of a given moment.[75,76] These corticocortical frontoparietal interactions are suggested to play important roles in one's sense of agency and action authorship of movement. A critical role for the inferior parietal lobule (including the temporoparietal junction) in awareness of motor intention and action authorship was further supported by an intraoperative

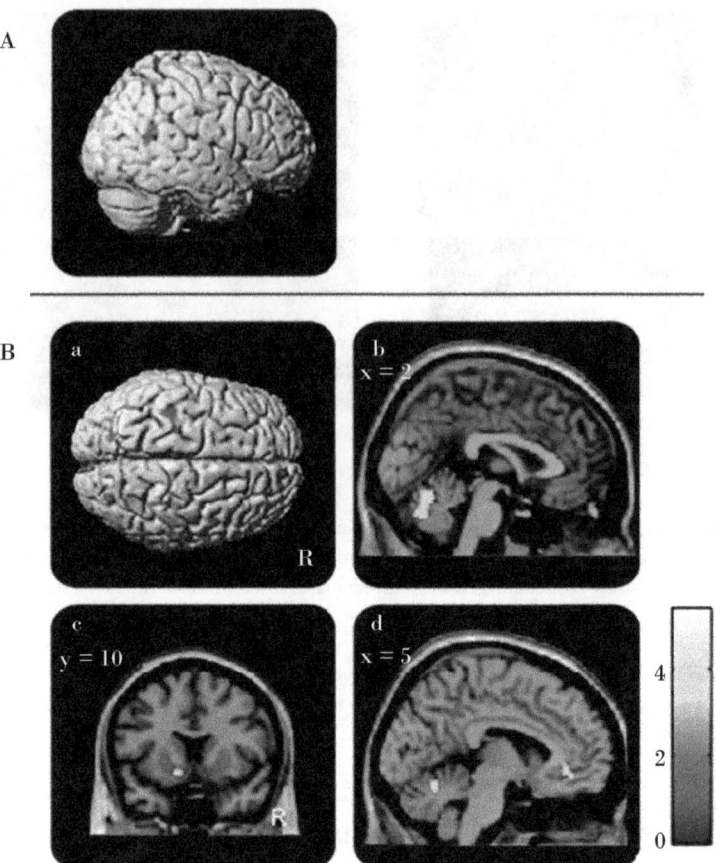

Figure 6.3 Involuntary functional movements are associated with aberrant activation and functional connectivity of the right temporoparietal junction. Display of select findings from Voon et al. (2010) investigating fMRI findings during functional (conversion) tremor versus voluntary mimicked tremor in eight patients with a positional functional tremor.[35] A. Right temporoparietal junction hypoactivation in the contrast of conversion tremor-rest compared with voluntary movement-rest (paired t test). The statistical parametric map image is shown at $p < 0.001$ uncorrected threshold >5 voxels. B. Temporoparietal junction connectivity map for the contrast of conversion versus voluntary tremor. The statistical parametric map shows decreased functional connectivity between the right temporoparietal junction (seed) and (a) left and right sensorimotor cortices, (b) bilateral cerebellar vermis, (c) left ventral striatum, and (d) bilateral ventral cingulate/medial prefrontal cortex during functional (conversion) tremor versus voluntary tremor.

cortical stimulation study in which patients endorsed the urge to move following low-intensity inferior parietal lobule stimulation and the experience of having moved (despite not moving) following high-intensity stimulation in this same region.[77] Given these findings, it may be theorized that deficits in right-lateralized inferior parietal lobule/temporoparietal junction function in PNES may contribute to the experience of patients having convulsive events "involuntarily" and outside of their control.

5. SUMMARY

PNES is a commonly encountered subtype of functional neurological disorder. Early systems-level neurobiology research suggests that PNES may develop in the context of alterations within and across brain networks mediating emotion processing, regulation and expression, cognitive control, multimodal integration, and sensory-motor functions (Figure 6.4). As the demarcations between neurology and psychiatry become increasingly blurred, continued clinical and research efforts are needed to incorporate biological models of PNES with psychosocial, developmental, and other predisposing, precipitating, and perpetuating factors (including neuroendocrine, autonomic, genetic, and epigenetic influences). An improved biological understanding of PNES may reduce the stigma commonly associated with this neuropsychiatric disorder and aid the development of biologically informed treatments and biomarkers of treatment response in this population.

- Functional MRI studies in PNES show that seizure frequency is positively associated with increased coupling of paralimbic regions to motor control networks.
- Studies in PNES suggest potential autonomic nervous system abnormalities and heightened cortisol levels.
- Chronic stress, one of several risk factors for PNES, has been shown in human and basic science studies to mediate neuroplastic brain changes in several brain areas implicated in the biology of PNES, including the anterior cingulate cortex and insula.
- Early systems-level neurobiology research suggests that PNES may develop in the context of alterations within and across brain networks mediating emotion processing, regulation and expression, cognitive control, multimodal integration. and sensory-motor functions.

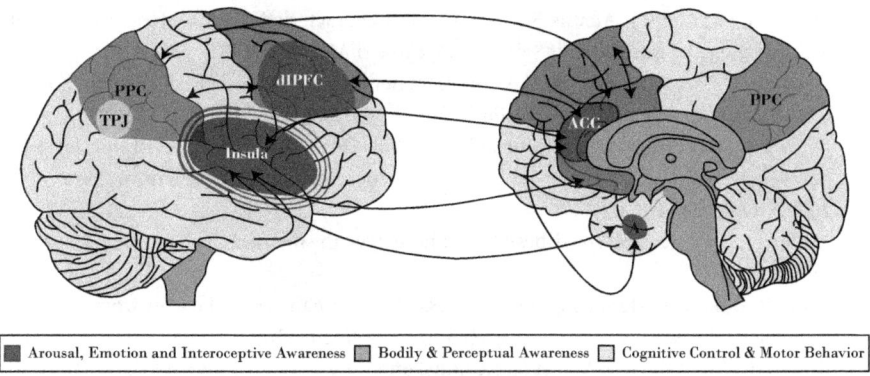

Figure 6.4 Model of an emerging neurobiology for PNES and related motor functional neurological symptoms (FNS). Evidence from neuroimaging studies suggest that PNES and related FNS may potentially develop in the context of alterations within and across brain networks implicated in 1) arousal, emotion, and interoceptive awareness; 2) bodily and perceptual awareness; and 3) cognitive control and motor behavior. A, amygdala; ACC, anterior cingulate cortex; dlPFC, dorsolateral prefrontal cortex; PPC, posterior parietal cortex; TPJ, temporoparietal junction. Updated model is based on original model put forth by Perez and colleagues (2012).[10] Subcortical components of cortico-subcortical connections are not displayed.

REFERENCES

1. Hurst LC. Freud and the great neurosis: discussion paper. *J R Soc Med.* 1983;76(1):57-61.
2. Charcot JM. Leðcons du mardi á la Salpãetriáere: policliniques, 1887-1888. Paris: Bureaux du Prográes Mâedical; 1887.
3. Breuer J, Freud S. *Studies on hysteria.* London: Hogarth Press; 1956.
4. Hamani C, Mayberg H, Stone S, Laxton A, Haber S, Lozano AM. The subcallosal cingulate gyrus in the context of major depression. *Biol Psychiatry.* 2011;69(4):301-308.
5. Pitman RK, Rasmusson AM, Koenen KC, et al. Biological studies of post-traumatic stress disorder. *Nat Rev Neurosci.* 2012;13(11):769-787.
6. Stone J, Carson A, Duncan R, et al. Who is referred to neurology clinics?—The diagnoses made in 3781 new patients. *Clin Neurol Neurosurg.* 2010;112(9):747-751.
7. Perez DL, Dworetzky BA, Dickerson BC, et al. An integrative neurocircuit perspective on psychogenic nonepileptic seizures and functional movement disorders: neural functional unawareness. *Clin EEG Neurosci.* 2015;46(1):4-15.
8. Voon V. Functional neurological disorders: imaging. *Neurophysiol Clin.* 2014;44(4):339-342.
9. Biswas J, Chu JA, Perez DL, Gutheil TG. From the neuropsychiatric to the analytic: three perspectives on dissociative identity disorder. *Harv Rev Psychiatry.* 2013;21(1):41-51.
10. Perez DL, Barsky AJ, Daffner K, Silbersweig DA. Motor and somatosensory conversion disorder: a functional unawareness syndrome? *J Neuropsychiatry Clin Neurosci.* 2012;24(2):141-151.
11. Perez DL, Barsky AJ, Vago DR, Baslet G, Silbersweig DA. A neural circuit framework for somatosensory amplification in somatoform disorders. *J Neuropsychiatry Clin Neurosci.* 2015;27(1):e40-e50.
12. Reuber M, Fernandez G, Helmstaedter C, Qurishi A, Elger CE. Evidence of brain abnormality in patients with psychogenic nonepileptic seizures. *Epilepsy Behav.* 2002;3(3):249-254.
13. Jones SG, O'Brien TJ, Adams SJ, et al. Clinical characteristics and outcome in patients with psychogenic nonepileptic seizures. *Psychosom Med.* 2010;72(5):487-497.
14. Devinsky O, Mesad S, Alper K. Nondominant hemisphere lesions and conversion nonepileptic seizures. *J Neuropsychiatry Clin Neurosci.* 2001;13(3):367-373.
15. Benbadis SR, Tatum WOt, Murtagh FR, Vale FL. MRI evidence of mesial temporal sclerosis in patients with psychogenic nonepileptic seizures. *Neurology.* 2000;55(7):1061-1062.
16. Ashburner J, Friston KJ. Voxel-based morphometry--the methods. *Neuroimage.* 2000;11(6 Pt 1):805-821.
17. Fischl B, Dale AM. Measuring the thickness of the human cerebral cortex from magnetic resonance images. *Proc Natl Acad Sci U S A.* 2000;97(20):11050-11055.
18. Rosas HD, Liu AK, Hersch S, et al. Regional and progressive thinning of the cortical ribbon in Huntington's disease. *Neurology.* 2002;58(5):695-701.
19. Salat DH, Buckner RL, Snyder AZ, et al. Thinning of the cerebral cortex in aging. *Cereb Cortex.* 2004;14(7):721-730.
20. Labate A, Cerasa A, Mula M, et al. Neuroanatomic correlates of psychogenic nonepileptic seizures: a cortical thickness and VBM study. *Epilepsia.* 2011;53(2):377-385.
21. Ristic AJ, Dakovic M, Kerr M, Kovacevic M, Parojcic A, Sokic D. Cortical thickness, surface area and folding in patients with psychogenic nonepileptic seizures. *Epilepsy Res.* 2015;11284-11291.

22. Hernando KA, Szaflarski JP, Ver Hoef LW, Lee S, Allendorfer JB. Uncinate fasciculus connectivity in patients with psychogenic nonepileptic seizures: a preliminary diffusion tensor tractography study. *Epilepsy Behav.* 2015;45:68–73.
23. Lee S, Allendorfer JB, Gaston TE, et al. White matter diffusion abnormalities in patients with psychogenic non-epileptic seizures. *Brain Res.* 2015;1620:169–176.
24. Etkin A, Egner T, Kalisch R. Emotional processing in anterior cingulate and medial prefrontal cortex. *Trends Cogn Sci.* 2011;15(2):85–93.
25. Raichle ME. Two views of brain function. *Trends Cogn Sci.* 2010;14(4):180–190.
26. van der Kruijs SJ, Bodde NM, Vaessen MJ, et al. Functional connectivity of dissociation in patients with psychogenic non-epileptic seizures. *J Neurol Neurosurg Psychiatry.* 2012;83(3):239–247.
27. Ding J, An D, Liao W, et al. Abnormal functional connectivity density in psychogenic non-epileptic seizures. *Epilepsy Res.* 2014;108(7):1184–1194.
28. Ding JR, An D, Liao W, et al. Altered functional and structural connectivity networks in psychogenic non-epileptic seizures. *PLoS One.* 2013;8(5):e63850.
29. van der Kruijs SJ, Jagannathan SR, Bodde NM, et al. Resting-state networks and dissociation in psychogenic non-epileptic seizures. *J Psychiatr Res.* 2014;54:126–133.
30. Shackman AJ, Salomons TV, Slagter HA, Fox AS, Winter JJ, Davidson RJ. The integration of negative affect, pain and cognitive control in the cingulate cortex. *Nat Rev Neurosci.* 2011;12(3):154–167.
31. Craig AD. How do you feel—now? The anterior insula and human awareness. *Nat Rev Neurosci.* 2009;10(1):59–70.
32. Li R, Liu K, Ma X, et al. Altered functional connectivity patterns of the insular subregions in psychogenic nonepileptic seizures. *Brain Topogr.* 2015;28(4):636–645.
33. Li R, Li Y, An D, Gong Q, Zhou D, Chen H. Altered regional activity and inter-regional functional connectivity in psychogenic non-epileptic seizures. *Sci Rep.* 2015;5:11635.
34. Arthuis M, Micoulaud-Franchi JA, Bartolomei F, McGonigal A, Guedj E. Resting cortical PET metabolic changes in psychogenic non-epileptic seizures (PNES). *J Neurol Neurosurg Psychiatry.* 2015;86(10):1106–1112.
35. Voon V, Gallea C, Hattori N, Bruno M, Ekanayake V, Hallett M. The involuntary nature of conversion disorder. *Neurology.* 2010;74(3):223–228.
36. Sepulcre J, Liu H, Talukdar T, Martincorena I, Yeo BT, Buckner RL. The organization of local and distant functional connectivity in the human brain. *PLoS Comput Biol.* 6(6):e1000808.
37. Sepulcre J, Sabuncu MR, Yeo TB, Liu H, Johnson KA. Stepwise connectivity of the modal cortex reveals the multimodal organization of the human brain. *J Neurosci.* 2012;32(31):10649–10661.
38. Seeley WW, Menon V, Schatzberg AF, et al. Dissociable intrinsic connectivity networks for salience processing and executive control. *J Neurosci.* 2007;27(9):2349–2356.
39. Touroutoglou A, Hollenbeck M, Dickerson BC, Feldman Barrett L. Dissociable large-scale networks anchored in the right anterior insula subserve affective experience and attention. *Neuroimage.* 2012;60(4):1947–1958.
40. Craig AD. Interoception: the sense of the physiological condition of the body. *Curr Opin Neurobiol.* 2003; 13(4):500–505.
41. Chanes L, Barrett LF. Redefining the role of limbic areas in cortical processing. *Trends Cogn Sci.* 2016;20(2):96–106.
42. Reuber M, Fernandez G, Bauer J, Singh DD, Elger CE. Interictal EEG abnormalities in patients with psychogenic nonepileptic seizures. *Epilepsia.* 2002;43(9):1013–1020.

43. Knyazeva MG, Jalili M, Frackowiak RS, Rossetti AO. Psychogenic seizures and frontal disconnection: EEG synchronisation study. *J Neurol Neurosurg Psychiatry.* 2011;82(5):505–511.
44. Barzegaran E, Joudaki A, Jalili M, Rossetti AO, Frackowiak RS, Knyazeva MG. Properties of functional brain networks correlate with frequency of psychogenic non-epileptic seizures. *Front Hum Neurosci.* 2012;6:335.
45. Barzegaran E, Carmeli C, Rossetti AO, Frackowiak RS, Knyazeva MG. Weakened functional connectivity in patients with psychogenic non-epileptic seizures (PNES) converges on basal ganglia. *J Neurol Neurosurg Psychiatry.* 2016;87(3):332–337.
46. Xue Q, Wang ZY, Xiong XC, Tian CY, Wang YP, Xu P. Altered brain connectivity in patients with psychogenic non-epileptic seizures: a scalp electroencephalography study. *J Int Med Res.* 2013;41(5):1682–1690.
47. Arzy S, Halje P, Schechter DS, Spinelli L, Seeck M, Blanke O. Neural generators of psychogenic seizures: evidence from intracranial and extracranial brain recordings. *Epilepsy Behav.* 2014;31:381–385.
48. Reinsberger C, Sarkis R, Papadelis C, et al. Autonomic changes in psychogenic nonepileptic seizures: toward a potential diagnostic biomarker? *Clin EEG Neurosci.* 2015;46(1):16–25.
49. Opherk C, Hirsch LJ. Ictal heart rate differentiates epileptic from non-epileptic seizures. *Neurology.* 2002;58(4):636–638.
50. Oliveira GR, Gondim Fde A, Hogan ER, Rola FH. Movement-induced heart rate changes in epileptic and non-epileptic seizures. *Arq Neuropsiquiatr.* 2009;67(3B):789–791.
51. Reinsberger C, Perez DL, Murphy MM, Dworetzky BA. Pre- and postictal, not ictal, heart rate distinguishes complex partial and psychogenic nonepileptic seizures. *Epilepsy Behav.* 2012;23(1):68–70.
52. van der Kruijs SJ, Vonck KE, Langereis GR, et al. Autonomic nervous system functioning associated with psychogenic nonepileptic seizures: Analysis of heart rate variability. *Epilepsy Behav.* 2016;54:14–19.
53. Hendrickson R, Popescu A, Dixit R, Ghearing G, Bagic A. Panic attack symptoms differentiate patients with epilepsy from those with psychogenic nonepileptic spells (PNES). *Epilepsy Behav.* 2014;37:210–214.
54. Ponnusamy A, Marques JL, Reuber M. Comparison of heart rate variability parameters during complex partial seizures and psychogenic nonepileptic seizures. *Epilepsia.* 2012;53(8):1314–1321.
55. Ponnusamy A, Marques JL, Reuber M. Heart rate variability measures as biomarkers in patients with psychogenic nonepileptic seizures: potential and limitations. *Epilepsy Behav.* 2011;22(4):685–691.
56. Roberts NA, Burleson MH, Weber DJ, et al. Emotion in psychogenic nonepileptic seizures: responses to affective pictures. *Epilepsy Behav.* 2012;24(1):107–115.
57. Mungen B, Berilgen MS, Arikanoglu A. Autonomic nervous system functions in interictal and postictal periods of nonepileptic psychogenic seizures and its comparison with epileptic seizures. *Seizure.* 2010;19(5):269–273.
58. Bakvis P, Spinhoven P, Roelofs K. Basal cortisol is positively correlated to threat vigilance in patients with psychogenic nonepileptic seizures. *Epilepsy Behav.* 2009;16(3):558–560.
59. Bakvis P, Spinhoven P, Putman P, Zitman FG, Roelofs K. The effect of stress induction on working memory in patients with psychogenic nonepileptic seizures. *Epilepsy Behav.* 2010;19(3):448–454.

60. Myers L, Perrine K, Lancman M, Fleming M, Lancman M. Psychological trauma in patients with psychogenic nonepileptic seizures: trauma characteristics and those who develop PTSD. *Epilepsy Behav.* 2013;28(1):121–126.
61. Duncan R, Oto M. Predictors of antecedent factors in psychogenic nonepileptic attacks: multivariate analysis. *Neurology.* 2008;71(13):1000–1005.
62. Dannlowski U, Stuhrmann A, Beutelmann V, et al. Limbic scars: long-term consequences of childhood maltreatment revealed by functional and structural magnetic resonance imaging. *Biol Psychiatry.* 2011;71(4):286–293.
63. Leuner B, Shors TJ. Stress, anxiety, and dendritic spines: What are the connections? *Neuroscience.* 2013;251:108–219.
64. Chen DK, Izadyar S. Characteristics of psychogenic nonepileptic events among veterans with posttraumatic stress disorder: an association of semiology with the nature of trauma. *Epilepsy Behav.* 2010;17(2):188–192.
65. Lanius RA, Vermetten E, Loewenstein RJ, et al. Emotion modulation in PTSD: clinical and neurobiological evidence for a dissociative subtype. *Am J Psychiatry.* 2010;167(6):640–647.
66. Etkin A, Wager TD. Functional neuroimaging of anxiety: a meta-analysis of emotional processing in PTSD, social anxiety disorder, and specific phobia. *Am J Psychiatry.* 2007;164(10):1476–1488.
67. Kuhn S, Gallinat J. Gray matter correlates of posttraumatic stress disorder: a quantitative meta-analysis. *Biol Psychiatry.* 2013;73(1):70–74.
68. Vermetten E, Spiegel D. Trauma and dissociation: implications for borderline personality disorder. *Curr Psychiatry Rep.* 2014;16(2):434.
69. Duncan R, Razvi S, Mulhern S. Newly presenting psychogenic nonepileptic seizures: incidence, population characteristics, and early outcome from a prospective audit of a first seizure clinic. *Epilepsy Behav.* 2011;20(2):308–311.
70. Mula M. Are psychogenic non-epileptic seizures and psychogenic movement disorders two different entities? When even neurologists stop talking to each other. *Epilepsy Behav.* 2013;26(1):100–101.
71. Voon V, Brezing C, Gallea C, et al. Emotional stimuli and motor conversion disorder. *Brain.* 2010;133(Pt 5):1526–1536.
72. Aybek S, Nicholson TR, O'Daly O, Zelaya F, Kanaan RA, David AS. Emotion-motion interactions in conversion disorder: an FMRI study. *PLoS One.* 2015;10(4):e0123273.
73. Aybek S, Nicholson TR, Zelaya F, et al. Neural correlates of recall of life events in conversion disorder. *JAMA Psychiatry.* 2014;71(1):52–60.
74. Sirigu A, Daprati E, Ciancia S, et al. Altered awareness of voluntary action after damage to the parietal cortex. *Nat Neurosci.* 2004;7(1):80–84.
75. Blakemore SJ, Goodbody SJ, Wolpert DM. Predicting the consequences of our own actions: the role of sensorimotor context estimation. *J Neurosci.* 1998;18(18):7511–7518.
76. Wolpert DM, Ghahramani Z, Jordan MI. An internal model for sensorimotor integration. *Science.* 1995;269(5232):1880–1882.
77. Desmurget M, Reilly KT, Richard N, Szathmari A, Mottolese C, Sirigu A. Movement intention after parietal cortex stimulation in humans. *Science.* 2009;324(5928):811–813.
78. Perez DL, LaFrance WC, Jr. Nonepileptic seizures: an updated review. *CNS Spectr.* 2016;21(3):239–246.

Section III
Diagnostic Procedures

7

Diagnostic Challenges for the Neurologist

Jigar Rathod, MD and Selim R. Benbadis, MD

1. INTRODUCTION

Psychogenic nonepileptic seizures (PNES) resemble epileptic seizures and pose several diagnostic challenges for the neurologist.[1] A quarter to a third of patients evaluated at epilepsy monitoring units end up being diagnosed with PNES, making this condition a frequent diagnostic possibility in busy comprehensive epilepsy centers.[2] While epileptologists have specialized training focused on making this diagnosis carefully and correctly, there are nevertheless many challenges that regularly arise and must be skillfully navigated if we are to improve outcomes for these patients. Challenges occur when the neurologist failed to suspect the diagnosis because events were controlled or infrequent, there was no apparent psychopathology, or the EEG was "abnormal." Conversely, if the neurologist was biased by the presence of psychopathology, this could lead to a misdiagnosis of PNES. That is, there was premature closure. Challenges may also occur when there is a failure to establish the diagnosis because events evade capture. Additionally, it can be very challenging to effectively communicate a diagnosis of PNES. In this chapter, we divide the challenges facing neurologists into those occurring during the initial encounter, when it is key to suspect the diagnosis; those that occur when it is difficult to establish the diagnosis even when it is strongly suspected; and the significant challenge of skillfully communicating the diagnosis for the best possible treatment outcome.

2. SUSPECTING THE DIAGNOSIS

2.1. History

When presented with an uncertain diagnosis, it is always best to begin a careful assessment with a detailed history. This is of critical importance in the diagnosis of PNES. Historically, patients who present to the ambulatory clinic or emergency department with "refractory seizures" and who have tried multiple antiepileptic drugs (AEDs) with multiple negative evaluations for epilepsy, especially repeatedly normal electroencephalograms (EEGs), should raise suspicion for a PNES diagnosis. This is important, because an earlier recognition of PNES leads to less exposure to AEDs, fewer hospitalizations, and better outcomes.[3] When a patient presents with a history of at least two uncontrolled seizures per week and has tried at least two AEDs at therapeutic doses without improvement and has a history of two or more normal EEGs, then one must consider a diagnosis of PNES. This has been referred to as the "rule of two's" and can be a helpful phrase when suspecting the diagnosis.[4] A history of prior "abnormal EEGs" may delay the diagnosis.[5] Often the EEGs in question will not be available for review at the initial visit, and the neurologist will need to focus on the history and on collecting further data to make the correct diagnosis.

The appearance of certain medical comorbidities increases the suspicion for PNES. Chronic pain syndromes; including "fibromyalgia," tension headaches, and migraines along with chronic fatigue syndrome, irritable bowel syndrome, asthma, gastroesophageal reflux disease, and a history of multiple allergies have a high positive predictive value and specificity for a diagnosis of PNES.[6-8] A history of psychiatric comorbid disorders may further increase the likelihood of PNES; however, such a history can also be present with epileptic seizures (ES). Depressive and anxiety disorders occur more commonly in patients with PNES and ES than in the general population. However, a closer evaluation of personality disorders can provide valuable information when suspecting PNES. Cluster B personality disorders (antisocial, borderline, histrionic, and narcissistic) coexist more commonly with PNES than with ES. Cluster C personality disorders (avoidant, dependent, and obsessive-compulsive) coexist more commonly with ES than with PNES.[9] However, clinicians assessing patients with suspected PNES should not *assume* that the presence of psychiatric comorbidities automatically imply a diagnosis of PNES, since many patients with intractable ES have similar psychiatric disorders. Therefore, certain psychiatric comorbidities may raise the suspicion but do not establish the diagnosis of PNES.

In addition to the medical and psychiatric history, a detailed social history can also provide hints about the diagnosis. Patients with PNES report prior traumatic experiences, such as sexual or physical abuse, school or family-related difficulties, and medical trauma in greater numbers than patients with epilepsy.[10] As a consequence, high rates of post-traumatic stress disorder (PTSD) are seen in PNES.[11] Overall, women are affected more commonly than men in multiple studies.[12] The history provided by the patient and witnesses is of key importance in helping the clinician suspect the diagnosis of PNES.

2.2. Observations

After evaluating the history, the clinician must look for clues for the diagnosis of PNES during the initial visit. In the ambulatory setting, patients with PNES may have an event in the waiting room or in the clinical exam room, which can be observed by the clinician. Events occurring in the office setting increase the likelihood of a diagnosis of PNES.[6] The physical exam generally is normal, but subtle clues during the exam, such as give-way weakness, Hoover's sign, and tremor entrainment, may help the clinician confirm the presence of other functional neurological symptoms or signs, which therefore increases the likelihood of a diagnosis of PNES, as they frequently coexist.

Provoking an event in the ambulatory setting (clinic or while obtaining a routine EEG) can be helpful for clinicians without access to video-EEG (vEEG) monitoring.[13]

In one study, compression of the temple region effectively provoked a PNES event, with a sensitivity of around 65% and specificity of 100%. Other reported and controversial methods of induction included verbal suggestion, tuning fork application, placing a torch light 10 cm away from the line of sight, and injecting saline into the antecubital vein, which has largely been abandoned because of ethical concerns.[13] Some acceptable methods of provocation are hyperventilation (HV) or photic stimulation while patients are connected to EEG in order to show lack of epileptic correlate to the episodes. Since these methods provoke epileptic and nonepileptic seizures alike and are part of any routine EEG, they are not considered deceptive to the patient. If the "typical" or habitual episode occurs with an induction method in the ambulatory setting, then this strongly suggests a diagnosis of PNES, keeping in mind that typical absence seizures can be triggered by HV, and convulsive seizures can be triggered by photic stimulation.

With increasing use of technology and cell phone video recording, events that are rather frequent may be captured by the patient's significant other or family members, making it easier for the clinician to directly view the incident. Based on the recorded clinical features, a neurologist may be able to have a strong clinical suspicion for PNES. Even if the patient does not have a video of the habitual event, the information about the semiology of the events provided by the patient or witness often leads to suspecting the diagnosis of PNES.

3. ESTABLISHING THE DIAGNOSIS

Long-term vEEG monitoring that captures a typical episode without associated EEG changes and not fitting any other epileptic or physiological characteristics remains the gold standard for the diagnosis of PNES. Long-term vEEG monitoring traditionally takes place during an admission to the inpatient epilepsy monitoring unit (EMU), where simultaneous recording of the EEG and the video is done 24 hours a day.

Prior to referring the patient for long-term vEEG monitoring, it is good practice to discuss with the patient that PNES is one of several possible diagnoses in consideration so that delivery of the diagnosis in the EMU does not amount to a "surprise diagnosis" just prior to hospital discharge. While some neurologists may be concerned that a patient will not show for diagnostic testing, we believe that honest dialogue shared between doctor and patient will help prepare the patient for the diagnosis in a gentler manner. In other areas of medicine, it would be regarded as negligent to not ready the patient for an unexpected or unwelcome diagnosis. Regardless, any patient who continues to experience frequent seizures despite adequate AED treatment should undergo long-term vEEG monitoring with the goal of recording a typical event simultaneously on video and on EEG.[14]

3.1. Diagnostic Challenges

Several challenges exist in establishing the diagnosis of PNES. The most important of these is the inability to capture a typical event. There are several reasons for an event not being captured: a typical episode may not occur while the patient is hooked up to vEEG monitoring; monitoring may not be possible because it is not covered by insurance;

Table 7.1. Diagnostic Levels of Certainty for Psychogenic Nonepileptic Seizures

Diagnostic Level	History	Witnessed Event	EEG
Possible	+	By witness or self-report/description	No epileptiform activity in routine or sleep-deprived *interictal* EEG
Probable	+	By clinician who reviewed video recording or in person, showing semiology typical for PNES	No epileptiform activity in routine or sleep-deprived *interictal* EEG
Clinically established	+	By clinician experienced in diagnosis of seizure disorders (on video or in person) showing semiology typical for PNES, while not on EEG	No epileptiform activity in routine or ambulatory *ictal* EEG during a typical ictus/event in which the semiology would make ictal epileptiform EEG activity expectable during an equivalent epileptic seizure
Documented	+	By clinician experienced in diagnosis of seizure disorders, showing semiology typical of PNES, while on video EEG	No epileptiform activity immediately before, during, or after ictus captured on ictal video EEG with typical PNES semiology

Adapted from LaFrance WC, Baker GA, Duncan R, Goldstein LH, Reuber M. Minimum requirements for the diagnosis of psychogenic nonepileptic seizures: A staged approach. *Epilepsia.* 2013;54(11):2005–2018.

or this type of testing may not be available or accessible. LaFrance and colleagues have addressed this challenge in a recent publication where they establish levels of diagnostic certainty for PNES (Table 7.1).[15] Where this becomes challenging for the neurologist is in navigating the different reports for the typical event (self-report versus witness report versus video from recorded event or from vEEG). When the patient is referred to the EMU for vEEG, the clinician must be fully aware of the typical or habitual events that need to be captured in order to make the correct diagnosis. Patients with PNES may have multiple event semiologies (for instance, staring spells and shaking events). The clinician must make sure that each event type is characterized in the history and, preferably, captured on vEEG.

Other difficult challenges in making a PNES diagnosis include the existence of concurrent epilepsy and the need to reverse or overturn a prior incorrect diagnosis. Approximately 10% of patients diagnosed with PNES may have comorbid epilepsy.[16] The possibility of the episodes being other (non-psychogenic) seizure mimics, such as migraine, syncope, or sleep-related movements, should also be considered.[17] Finally, another particularly difficult challenge is overturning a prior diagnosis of "epilepsy" (whether due to an abnormal EEG in the past or from a prior treatment team). We address these challenge in subsequent sections of this chapter.

3.2. Semiology

3.2.1. Preictal Evaluation

Experienced neurologists pay attention to changes that occur before (preictal), during (ictal), and after (postictal) a seizure or seizure-like episode and will carefully interpret the EEG and the video in the context of each other during these different phases. A solid rule is that episodes that occur out of EEG-verified sleep are not psychogenic or, stated differently, PNES should not occur out of sleep. However, when patients *report* that episodes occur during sleep, such episodes often occur out of "pseudo-sleep." Preictal pseudo-sleep resembles sleep clinically; however, the EEG shows evidence of wakefulness with a normal posterior dominant rhythm. One study showed that pre-ictal pseudo-sleep was able to predict PNES at a sensitivity of 56% and a specificity of 100%.[18]

3.2.2. Ictal Evaluation

During the ictal phase patients may experience subjective sensations, such as a perception of "feeling funny," numbness, olfactory changes, micropsia, or dizziness, which are seen in about 22% of patients with PNES.[19] Overall, the helpfulness of these subjective complaints remains limited because of minimal or no change in the EEG even if they represent an epileptic phenomenon (i.e., these limited symptoms may occur due to discharges limited to a very small region in the brain and may represent a simple partial seizures, which may not show changes in the EEG). Evaluation of motor manifestations during the ictal phase is crucial. Eye closure during the ictal phase occurs in about 75% of patients with PNES, while eye opening during the ictal phase points more to an ES.[19,20] Both patients with PNES and those with ES *report* injuries during their habitual event; however, *significant* injuries such as burns or bone fractures are more typically found in patients with ES.[19] Evaluation of tongue biting shows anterior tip of the tongue involvement in PNES, while ES tend to involve the lateral aspect of the tongue, which occurs during the clonic phase in generalized tonic-clonic seizures.[19] Other common motor manifestations include out-of-phase limb movements and side-to-side head shaking, and PNES episodes are more likely to be prolonged in duration.[19] Pelvic thrusting during the ictal phase generally points toward a diagnosis of PNES in events described as "thrashing"; however, it also occurs in frontal lobe epilepsy in about 20 to 25% of the cases.[21] Apart from the classical "convulsive" movements and limp attacks, when a patient with PNES is unresponsive and motionless, the ictal event may include weeping, ictal vocalization with grunting, moaning, uttering words, and resistant behavior such as opposing forced eye opening.[19,20] In a study by Peguero and colleagues, urinary incontinence was reported in 44% of PNES patients and 57% of ES patients.[22] Therefore, urinary incontinence may not be an entirely useful measure to differentiate between the two. Table 7.2 summarizes the semiological differences between PNES and ES. These different semiological features can be strongly suggestive of one type of spell versus the other, but they do not confirm the diagnosis. Also, when comparing age groups, children and adolescents present with fewer motor manifestations than do adults with PNES.[23]

Table 7.2. Comparison of Findings in PNES and Epileptic Seizures (ES)

	PNES	ES
Occurs out of sleep	No (pseudo-sleep)	Can occur
Sensation of dizziness, olfactory sensation, or numbness	Can be seen	Can be seen
Eyes	More commonly closed	More commonly opened
Significant bodily injury (broken bones, burns, etc.)	Not common	Yes
Tongue biting	Anterior tip of the tongue	Lateral aspect of the tongue
Pelvic thrusting	Can be seen	Can be seen (frontal lobe seizures)
Duration	Can be prolonged	Short if frontal lobe
Ictal weeping	Yes	Unlikely
Urinary incontinence	Can be seen	Can be seen

3.2.3. Postictal Evaluation

The postictal clinical evaluation can also help differentiate PNES from ES. Patients with ES report a higher incidence of a postictal headache and postictal fatigue after a generalized tonic-clonic seizure compared to patients with PNES.[19] This poses a diagnostic challenge when these symptoms are reported by a patient for whom there is suspicion for PNES and who should undergo further diagnostic testing to confirm the diagnosis, that is, prolonged vEEG monitoring.[24] Further, the absence of postictal findings in patients with PNES presents a diagnostic challenge in distinguishing PNES from frontal lobe seizures, as they both can end abruptly with minimal to no postictal phase.[24] However, frontal lobe seizures tend to occur out of sleep, rather than pseudo-sleep as in PNES, with vocalization, tonic limb posturing, or hypermotor activity different from the flailing and thrashing movements seen with PNES.[25-27] If the question of epilepsy remains in doubt and the EEG is normal, the neurologist should remove AEDs during the inpatient monitoring in hopes of capturing a secondarily generalized tonic-clonic seizure to definitively diagnose epilepsy of frontal lobe origin (Table 7.3).

3.3. EEG

The EEG in PNES, by definition, should remain normal during the clinical event or at least show no epileptiform change. However, limitations do exist when interpreting the EEG, as the EEG may be obscured by muscle or movement artifact during the event. Therefore, paying attention to the video and the EEG are of utmost importance. In instances where patient awareness appears altered, maintenance of a normal posterior dominant rhythm, including at the end of the event, is quite informative and suggestive

Table 7.3. Comparison between PNES and Frontal Lobe Seizures

	PNES	*Frontal Lobe Seizures*
Seizure duration	Tend to be prolonged (>5 minutes)	Short (<30 seconds)
Events out of EEG-verified sleep	Never	Common
Flipping (supine to prone or prone to supine)	Can be seen	Almost never
Eyes	Closed	Open
Eye deviation	Geotropic*	Versive
Pelvic thrusting	Can be seen	Very rare
Opisthotonic posturing	Common	Never
Bicycling/kicking	Can be seen	Very rare
Side-to-side head shaking	Common	Almost never
Tonic posturing	Not seen	Common
Clonic movements	Not seen	Common
Ictal grasping	Rare	May be seen
Intact awareness with bilateral motor activity	Common	Rare

*Geotropic eye movements occur when eyes deviate downward toward the side that the head is turned.

of PNES (Figure 7.1). Further, certain types of seizures, as mentioned before, may not manifest on EEG, such as frontal lobe seizures, simple partial seizures, and some temporal lobe seizures with deep origins. Therefore, not all normal EEGs during an episode establish a definitive diagnosis of PNES.[27,28] For instance, a sensation of déjà vu, fear, or brief tonic posturing may represent an epileptic seizure and not PNES.[28] Therefore, it is critical to interpret the EEG and video in the context of each other. The episodes could also represent other nonepileptic paroxysmal symptoms, such as sleep disorders (parasomnias, restless legs syndrome, hypnic jerks, periodic limb movements of sleep), movement disorders, or syncope (including convulsive syncope).[27]

A very challenging situation for the neurologist is when a patient has both epilepsy and PNES; this occurs in about 10% of patients with PNES.[16] In these instances, there should be *at least two different* types of events described by the patient or witness. Of note, epileptiform abnormalities can occur in about 2% of asymptomatic adults, but with a history supportive of epileptic seizure, these suggest a diagnosis of epilepsy.[29,30] Therefore, when the interictal EEG has epileptiform abnormalities, the importance of analyzing the EEG during the event in question is particularly crucial. The neurologist should make every effort to capture each event type described by the patient during the initial clinic visit to confirm the diagnosis of PNES.

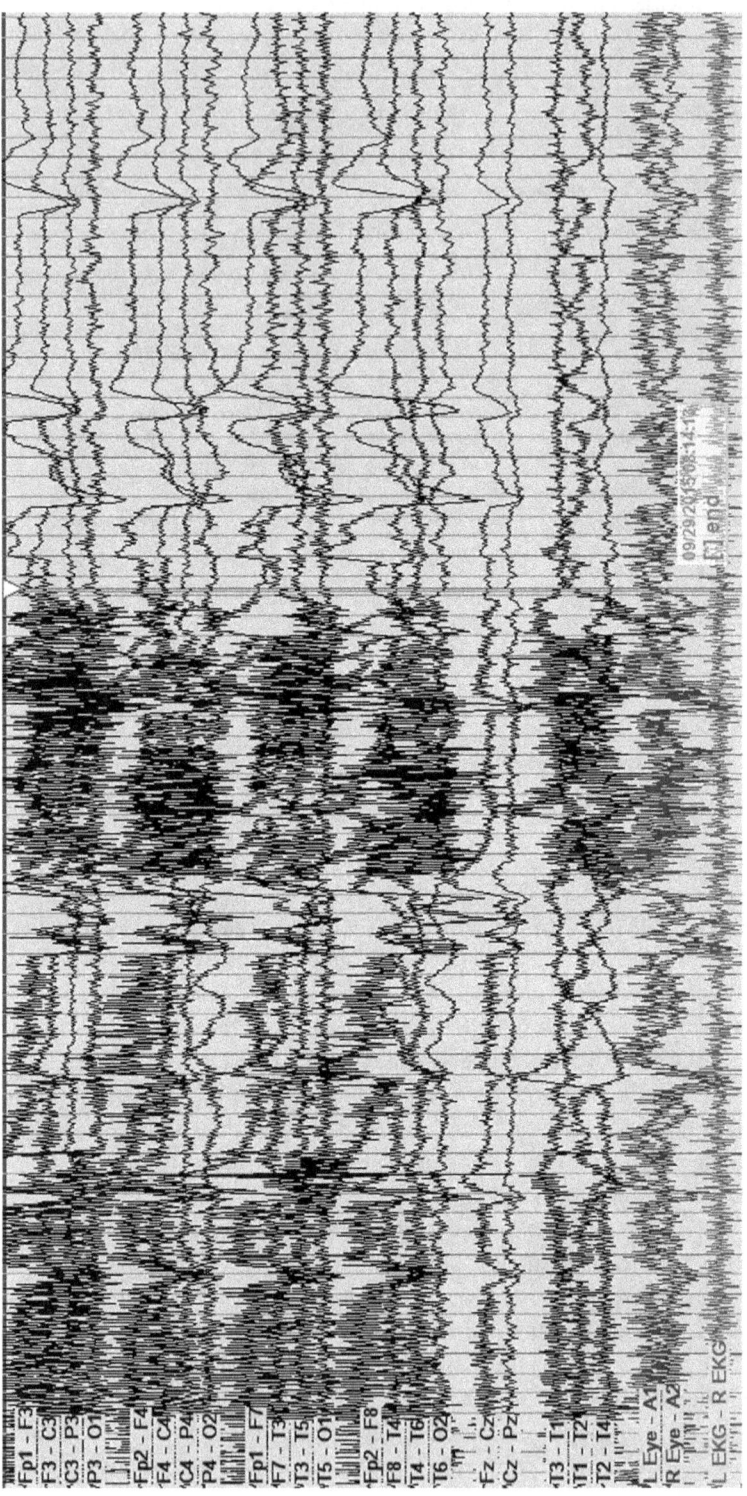

Figure 7.1 Depiction of how the EEG is obscured by artifact initially but later shows a normal posterior dominant rhythm at the end, in a patient with PNES.

3.4. What to Do If the Event Is Not Captured or Diagnosis Remains Unclear?

In many cases, it is not possible to capture all event types reported by a patient during a long-term monitoring admission. This can be quite challenging for the neurologist as well as for the patient. It can be very helpful to ask the patient to have a family member record the event type not captured during the admission so that the neurologist can review it at the follow-up appointment. This may require the patient to remain on an AED for a longer period, which is less than ideal if suspicion for PNES is high. In the vast majority of cases, in the hands of experienced epileptologists, the diagnosis of PNES with vEEG is not difficult, but a handful of difficult cases account for the only moderate inter-rater reliability.[31] Fortunately, experienced epileptologists are aware of the pitfalls of vEEG.

If an epilepsy center or epileptologist are not accessible, such as in a rural area, there may be a role for the neurohumoral marker prolactin to help distinguish convulsions or complex partial seizures from PNES. In 2005, the American Academy of Neurology evaluated the use of serum prolactin in the diagnosis of ES and found one class I and seven class II studies (level B evidence). They found that when prolactin levels were measured 10 to 20 minutes after a seizure, it could be a useful adjunct in differentiating generalized tonic-clonic or partial seizure with loss of awareness from PNES. Prolactin was not useful in differentiating a syncopal spell from PNES. Additionally, prolactin varies with the circadian cycle, and a baseline level unrelated to the seizure episode must be checked at the same time of day. A normal prolactin level assay by itself is insufficient to confirm a diagnosis of PNES or to exclude generalized tonic-clonic seizures or a complex partial seizure, due to its low sensitivity, low negative predictive value,[32,33] and high false-positive rate.[34] A recent study concluded that prolactin is not a useful test in the EMU.[34]

If the episodes do not occur spontaneously while the patient is in the EMU, or the diagnosis remains uncertain even after a captured clinical episode, then provocation or induction methods may help facilitate a typical episode. Hoepner et al. demonstrated increased success in capturing PNES during an EEG if the patient was informed about the potential reduction in seizure threshold when performing photic stimulation and hyperventilation.[35] In situations where the EEG is not useful (obscured or symptoms consistent with a type of seizures where EEG changes are not always present), the very presence of suggestibility (an event is triggered by a placebo maneuver) is the main argument supporting a psychogenic origin. Suggestibility is, in fact, used as a main criterion in psychogenic movement disorders.[36] However, such conclusion should be drawn with much caution and sound clinical judgment, as it could also be a coincidence that the episode in question occurred with activation procedures. As has been already emphasized, the diagnosis of PNES is not based solely on a normal EEG and the event being provoked by activation procedures, but in combination with the supportive history and physical examination.[27]

The use of provocation may raise ethical concerns if not done appropriately. It is best used in a patient who does not have an event in the allotted days of monitoring and not just in those who are suspected of having PNES. Clinicians must keep in mind the ethical concept of doing well toward the patient (beneficence) and doing no harm (malfeasance).

Overall, missing or delaying the diagnosis of PNES may be more harmful, as it causes socioeconomic, psychological, and medical consequences, including inappropriate treatment, low self-esteem, economic loss, and disability.[13] Therefore, induction methods used appropriately in the EMU can help the neurologist make a definitive diagnosis.

For captured events that were possibly considered physiological nonepileptic paroxysms (such as movement disorders, sleep disorders, syncope, etc.), triggering an event with provocation may also suggest a psychogenic origin.[28] When there is suspicion of a nonepileptic physiological paroxysm as the explanation of the event, we recommend referral to a specialist (for example, in the case of tremors, to a movement disorder specialist, or in the case of a sleep disorder, to a sleep specialist) with communication to that specialist regarding what was discovered on vEEG.

3.5. Navigating Other Diagnostic Options

Not infrequently, despite several days of vEEG monitoring, none of the patient's typical events have been captured, which poses a diagnostic dilemma with regard to the next step in diagnosis and management (Figure 7.2). One could consider repeating the long-term vEEG monitoring with the hope that a typical event would be captured, perhaps during a period with maximum event frequency. One study showed that repeating a vEEG yielded diagnosis in more than 80% of cases.[37] However, this may pose a challenge, as patients may not want or be able to return for vEEG monitoring, as it may mean missing more time from work or school. Furthermore, insurance companies may not cover another EMU admission.

If a repeat inpatient vEEG is not feasible, an ambulatory (take-home) recording of 24 hours or more is an option, as long as the episodes are very frequent. The diagnosis hinges on capturing the typical event on EEG and having the patient or family member signal the episode by pressing a button. These studies are most helpful if a definitive

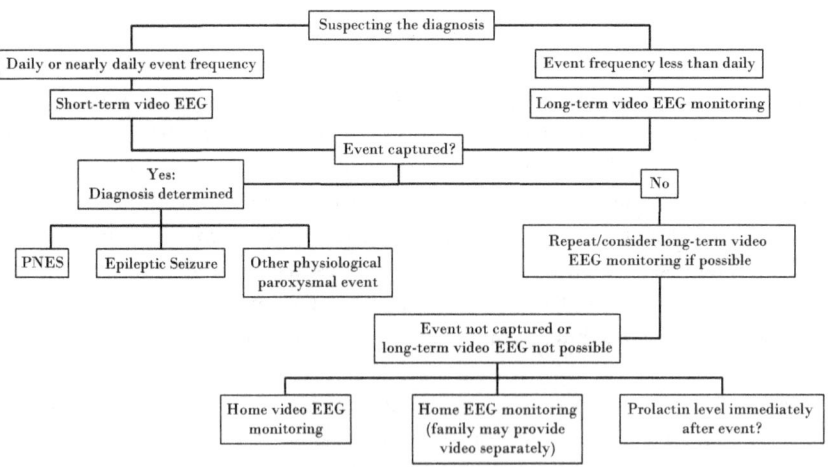

Figure 7.2 A possible algorithm for navigating of diagnostic testing in PNES.

epileptic seizure is captured. Encouraging patients and families to provoke an episode while the EEG is hooked up adds to the success of capturing an event. Even if ambulatory EEG is performed without video, family members may be able to capture unsynchronized but nevertheless helpful video of the episode during the EEG recording. There are also ambulatory EEGs performed with video; however, if the patient is not in front of the camera during the event or if the equipment malfunctions, the data is less useful. A study in which patients were given camcorders along with ambulatory EEG facilitated the interpretation of the ambulatory EEG in about one third of patients.[38]

The advantage of using ambulatory EEG (with or without video) is to have patients in their regular and, in some cases, more stressful environment, which may facilitate the events in question. It is also less expensive than vEEG. The disadvantages are mainly logistical as staff and equipment are required in the setup. Further, patients are unable to be evaluated by the multidisciplinary team, including a psychiatrist, who can be very helpful in transitioning the patient from formulating the diagnosis in psychological terms to getting them ready for treatment. Another disadvantage is the safety issue related to withdrawal of AEDs without nursing staff immediately available, as is the case in the inpatient setting. In a small study using ambulatory EEG, the recording quality of the video was comparable to inpatient vEEG monitoring and the rate of habitual seizures was fairly equal.[39]

However, even after using alternative methods for establishing the diagnosis, the habitual events may still not be captured. If vEEG attempts fail to record events, it is best to not draw a firm conclusion and to keep an open mind. It is probably safest to continue the prescribed AED and for the neurologist to continue to follow the patient so that a firm diagnosis can be made, with the ultimate goal being to refer the patient for mental health treatment. As mentioned earlier, La France et al. proposed classifying PNES diagnosis as probable, possible, clinically established, or documented PNES (Table 7.1), and it is helpful to share with the patient and family what the degree of confidence is when making the diagnosis.[15]

With several test options available in the neurologist's tool box for making the diagnosis of PNES, one challenge is to decide which particular monitoring test to use. Prolonged vEEG monitoring in the inpatient setting is the gold standard for patients on AEDs. However, when this is not feasible or the patient is on no medication to withdraw, an ambulatory vEEG may suffice. A short-term EEG can be performed in the EEG lab over an hour or more if events are extremely frequent.

4. DATA FROM OUTSIDE PROVIDERS

The vast majority of patients with PNES referred to epilepsy centers have been labeled with a diagnosis of epilepsy, mostly because of an abnormal EEG. Once the diagnosis of PNES is made, the question becomes whether there is a coexisting diagnosis of epilepsy. It then is extremely helpful to review the actual prior "abnormal" EEG(s) on disk or paper (not just the printed report), as they will usually turn out to be normal studies misinterpreted as abnormal, also known as "over-reads."[40,41] Most of the time the over-read patterns consist of benign normal variants such as "benign temporal sharp transients of sleep," "small sharp spikes," or even more commonly "wicket" rhythms and simple fluctuations of sharply contoured waveforms.[41] The reason for the high frequency of misinterpreted EEG is multifactorial, but largely it is the limited training and experience with EEG among neurologists.[41] Obtaining the prior EEG or EEGs that were read as "abnormal" can pose a significant challenge because they may not be available or the software between clinics is incompatible, but this is a critical step and well worth the effort.

If the "abnormal" EEG is reviewed and reread as normal, this needs to be discussed with the patient, which may prove to be difficult. This is especially true for patients treated for many years as if they had epilepsy or if the doctor who made the initial incorrect diagnosis is well liked and trusted by the patient. Letting the patient know that it is common to have irregularities on the EEG that are not necessarily indicative of epilepsy can be quite helpful. Communicating with the trusted doctor, if at all possible, can be even more helpful, as this integrates the team who will follow the patient after diagnosis and lets the patient know that you respect their doctor. Removing the diagnosis of epilepsy is often easier if done in the inpatient setting, as many patients are quite fearful of coming off their AEDs and are unwilling to try this on their own at home. The greatest challenge a neurologist can face is when the typical episodes are clearly PNES, but the prior "abnormal" EEG does indeed show suspicious or clearly abnormal epileptiform discharges. In these cases, the history plays an important role in determining whether a diagnosis of coexisting epilepsy can also be confirmed. Again, collaboration with the provider who has been treating the patient will be vital, as it will reinforce the patient's trust in the diagnostic process.

5. WHAT TO DO IF THE EPISODES CHANGE?

Once the patient is diagnosed with PNES and appropriately treated, different episodes with new semiology may occur or new neurological symptoms may develop. If the event is similar to the original semiology, then it is recommended to discuss the diagnosis again and reconnect with the treating mental health provider to reinforce the diagnosis. However, if the history provides information that the episodes have changed or new types of episodes are occurring, then it is up to the neurologist to make certain that these new episodes do not represent ES, which may require another evaluation with vEEG monitoring. The more the treating team is integrated (neurologist and mental health team in communication), the less confusing it will be for the patient to navigate these complex scenarios. More detailed discussion about the role of the neurologist after the diagnosis is established can be found in Chapter 15.

6. DELIVERING THE DIAGNOSIS

Once the diagnosis of PNES is established, the neurologist is responsible for communicating the diagnosis to the patient (see Chapter 10). The diagnosis needs to be given clearly and definitively, in language easy for the patient to understand. Protocols for this are discussed in Chapter 10. Effective communication of the diagnosis is important, as the patient and family may feel embarrassed or stigmatized by a diagnosis of PNES. Sensitivity on the part of the neurologist regarding the implications of this message to the patient is key. The patient's understanding of the psychological mechanism and its significance may be aided by having a mental health provider involved early in this process, as well as by establishing good rapport with the patient prior to the diagnosis being conclusively delivered.

A good patient–physician relationship is essential and can make a challenging conversation about the diagnosis proceed more smoothly, especially if the patient has carried the diagnosis of epilepsy for many years. In this scenario, the neurologist is removing a diagnosis that has led to turmoil and disability and replacing it with a psychological diagnosis, which for many patients is quite difficult to accept. Therefore, it can be helpful to coordinate this discussion with the mental health provider who has evaluated the patient, if that can be arranged. At the same time, the neurologist should try to coordinate the team and make sure everyone (including the mental health provider) is on the same page with the diagnosis. This can be challenging when the mental health worker or psychiatrist is from another healthcare setting and may disagree with the conclusions of the vEEG monitoring.[42]

Once the diagnosis is delivered, the neurologist needs to discuss follow-up with the patient—with whom and when. Getting the patient to follow up with a mental health provider for further management is critical, but this may take some time. Until then, the patient should continue to follow up with a neurologist to reinforce the diagnosis and engagement in treatment (see Chapter 15). If, during treatment, the patient develops new somatic symptoms, such as abdominal pain, weakness, or headache, continued follow-up with mental health providers is recommended. The primary care provider can firmly conclude that those symptoms do not represent a coexisting medical diagnosis. In the case of new neurological symptoms, such as weakness or gait abnormalities, the neurologist who is familiar with the patient should help re-establish the diagnosis of a functional disorder. Of course, if the presentation exceeds the expertise of the practitioner, collaboration with specialty providers should be pursued. Having one main provider as the go-to person can be quite helpful in avoiding a collection of doctors treating the patient as well as unnecessary medications or procedures.

7. CONCLUSION

The diagnosis of PNES should be considered at the initial visit with the patient. The history, physical exam, and the ability to induce an episode help facilitate the diagnosis; however, long-term video EEG capturing of all typical episodes allows for definitive diagnosis. The challenges discussed in this chapter are among the most common that are faced by the neurologist, but these are not the only ones. Open dialogue with the patient, family, and team of providers can ease some of these challenges and ready the neurologist for the work that lies ahead when episodes are not captured, when they recur, or when the patient fails to follow up with treatment.

8. SUMMARY

- The diagnosis of PNES begins with a careful detailed history of the patient's event or events, followed by long-term video EEG monitoring to capture those events on video and EEG concurrently.

- If the patient's events are not captured with long-term video EEG monitoring, then induction methods and suggestibility can be used to help facilitate an event in order to get a clear diagnosis.
- If the patient's events are not captured during long-term video EEG monitoring, the clinician can consider using outpatient short-term video EEG monitoring or ambulatory EEG with or without video (cell phone videos can be useful).
- If the patient has a diagnosis of epileptic seizures due to a prior "abnormal EEG," then it is important for the epileptologist to obtain the EEG on paper or CD for review, to clarify the diagnosis.
- The use of a multidisciplinary team and good rapport with the patient make the challenge of delivering a diagnosis easier and may help the patient adhere to treatment recommendations.

REFERENCES

1. Baslet G. Psychogenic non-epileptic seizures: a model of their pathogenic mechanism. *Seizure*. 2011;20:1–13.
2. Benbadis SR, Hauser WA. An estimate of the prevalence of psychogenic non-epileptic seizures. *Seizure*. 2000;9:280–281.
3. LaFrance WC, Benbadis SR. Avoiding the cost of unrecognized psychological nonepileptic seizures. *Neurology*. 2006;66:1620–1621.
4. Davis BJ. Predicting nonepileptic seizures utilizing seizure frequency, EEG, and response to medication. *Eur Neurol*. 2004;51:153–156
5. Benbadis SR, Tatum WO. Overinterpretation of EEGs and misdiagnosis of epilepsy. *J Clin Neurophysiol*. 2003;20(1):42–44.
6. Benbadis SR. A spell in epilepsy clinic and a history of "chronic pain" or "fibromyalgia" independently predict a diagnosis of psychogenic seizures. *Epilepsy Behav*. 2005;6:264–265.
7. Dixit R, Popescu A, Bagic A, Ghearing G, Hendrickson R. Medical comorbidities in patients with psychogenic nonepileptic spells referred for video-EEG monitoring. 2013;28:137–140.
8. Benbadis SR. Nonepileptic behavioral disorders: diagnosis and treatment. *Continuum*. 2013;19(3):715–729.
9. Direk N, Kulaksizoglu IB, Kadriye A, Gurses C. Using personality disorders to distinguish between patient's with psychogenic nonepileptic seizures and those with epileptic seizures. *Epilepsy Behav*. 2012;23:138–141.
10. Fleisher W, Staley D, Krawetz P, Pillay N, Arnett J, Maher J. Comparative study of trauma-related phenomena in subjects with pseudoseizures and subjects with epilepsy. *Am J Psychiatry*. 2002;159:660–663.
11. Auxemery Y, Hubsch C, Fidelle G. Psychogenic non epileptic seizures: a review. *Encephale*. 2011;37(2):153–158.
12. Thomas A, Preston J, Scott RC, Bujarski KA. Diagnosis of probable psychogenic nonepileptic seizures in the outpatient clinic: does gender matter? *Epilepsy Behav*. 2013;29:295–297.
13. Goyal G, Kalita J, Misra UK. Utility of different seizure induction protocols in psychogenic nonepileptic seizures. *Epilepsy Res*. 2014;108:1120–1127.

14. Benbadis SR, LaFrance WC. Clinical features and video EEG. In: Schachter SC, LaFrance WC, eds. *Gates and Rowan's Nonepileptic Seizures*, 3rd ed. New York: Cambridge University Press; 2010:38–50.
15. LaFrance WC, Baker GA, Duncan R, Goldstein LH, Reuber M. Minimum requirements for the diagnosis of psychogenic nonepileptic seizures: a staged approach, a report from the International League against Epilepsy Nonepileptic Seizures Task Force. *Epilepsia*. 2013;54(11):2005–2018.
16. Benbadis SR, Agrawal V, Tatum WO. How many patients with psychogenic nonepileptic seizures also have epilepsy? *Neurology*. 2001;57(5):915–917.
17. Smith D, Defalla BA, Chadwick DW. The misdiagnosis of epilepsy and the management of refractory epilepsy in a specialist clinic. *QJM*. 1999;92:15–23.
18. Benbadis SR, Lancman ME, King LM, Swanson SJ. Preictal pseudosleep: a new finding in psychogenic seizures. *Neurology*. 1996;47:63–67.
19. Mostacci B, Bisulli F, Alvisi L, Licchetta L, Baruzzi A, Tinuper P. Ictal characteristics of psychogenic non-epileptic seizures: what we have learned from video/EEG recordings—a literature review. *Epilepsy Behav*. 2011;22:144–153.
20. Patidar Y, Gupta M, Khwaja GA, Chowdhury D, Batra A, Dasgupta A. Clinical profile of psychogenic non-epileptic seizures in adults: a study of 63 cases. *Ann Indian Acad Neurol*. 2013;16(2):157–162.
21. Geyer JD, Payne TA, Drury Ivo. The value of pelvic thrusting in the diagnosis of seizures and pseudoseizures. *Neurology*. 2000;54:227.
22. Peguero E, Abou-Khalil B, Fakhoury T, Matthews G. Self-injury and incontinence in psychogenic seizures. *Epilepsia*. 1995;36:586–591.
23. Alessi R, Vincentiis S, Rzezak P, Valente KD. Semiology of psychogenic seizures: age-related differences. *Epilepsy Behav*. 2013;27:292–295.
24. Ettinger A, Weisbrot DM, Nolan E, Devinsky O. Postictal symptoms help distinguish patients with epileptic seizures from those with non-epileptic seizures. *Seizure*. 1999;8(3):149–151.
25. Kanner AM, Moris HH, Luders H, et al. Supplementary motor seizures mimicking pseudoseizures: some clinical differences. *Neurology*. 1990;40(9):140–147.
26. Jobst BC, Williamson PD. Frontal lobe seizures. *Psychiatr Clin North Am*. 2005;28(3):635–651.
27. LaFrance WC, Benbadis SR. Differentiating frontal lobe epilepsy from psychogenic non-epileptic seizures. *Neurol Clin*. 2011;29:149–162.
28. Benbadis, SR. The EEG in nonepileptic seizures. *J Clin Neurophysiol*. 2006;23(4):340–352.
29. Zivin L, Ajmone-Marsan C. Incidence and prognostic significance of epileptiform activity in the EEG of nonepileptic subjects. *Brain*. 1968;91:751–778.
30. Ajmone-Marsan C, Zivin L. Factors related to the occurrence of typical paroxysmal abnormalities in the EEG records of epileptic patients. *Epilepsia*. 1970;11:361–381.
31. Benbadis SR, LaFrance WC, Papandonatos GD, Korabathina K, Lin K, Kraemer HC. Interrater reliability of EEG-video monitoring. *Neurology*. 2009;73:843–846.
32. Chen DK, So YT, Fisher RS. Use of serum prolactin in diagnosing epileptic seizures: report of the Therapeutics and Technology Assessment Subcommittee of the American Academy of Neurology. *Neurology*. 2005;65(5):668–675.
33. Alving J. Serum prolactin levels are elevated also after pseudo-epileptic seizures. *Seizure*. 1998;7:85–89.
34. Abubakr A, Wambacq I. Diagnostic value of serum prolactin levels in PNES in the epilepsy monitoring unit. *Neurol Clin Pract*. 2016;6:116–119.

35. Hoepner R, Labudda K, Schoendienst M, May TW, Bien CG, Brandt C. Informing patients about the impact of provocation methods increases the rate of psychogenic nonepileptic seizures during EEG recording. *Epilepsy Behav*. 2013;28:457–459.
36. Hallett M, Weiner WJ, Kompoliti K. Psychogenic movement disorders. *Parkinsonism Relat Disord*. 2012;18S1:S155–S157.
37. Muniz JC, Benbadis SR. Repeating prolonged EEG-video monitoring: why and with what results? *Epilepsy Behav*. 2010;18:472–473.
38. Goodwin E, Kandler RH, Alix JJP. The value of home video with ambulatory EEG: a prospective service review. *Seizure*. 2014;23:480–482.
39. Brunnhuber F, Amin D, Nguyen Y, Goyal S, Richardson MP. Development, evaluation and implementation of video-EEG telemetry at home. *Seizure*. 2014;23:338–343.
40. Benbadis SR. "Just like EKGs!" Should EEGs undergo a confirmatory interpretation by a clinical neurophysiologist? *Neurology*. 2013;80(Suppl 1):S47–S51.
41. Benbadis SR. The tragedy of over-read EEGs and wrong diagnoses of epilepsy. *Expert Rev Neurother*. 2010;10(3):343–346.
42. Harden CL, Burgut FT, Kranner AM. The diagnostic significance of video EEG monitoring findings on pseudoseizures patients differs between neurologist and psychiatrist. *Epilepsia*. 2003;44(3):453–456.

8

Diagnostic Challenges for the Mental Health Team and Psychiatrist

Lorna Myers, PhD and John J. Barry, MD

1. INTRODUCTION

Working with patients suspected of having PNES during the diagnostic phase poses a number of interesting challenges and opportunities for the mental health team and psychiatrist to contribute to the diagnosis and outcome.

From the moment the psychiatrist or mental health professional greets the patient, a therapeutic alliance can begin developing, which facilitates the patient to be more receptive when the diagnosis of PNES is presented. Mental health professionals assess patients with suspected PNES in a multiplicity of settings, including inpatient epilepsy monitoring units, outpatient epilepsy clinics, and general mental health clinics. For a subset of patients with PNES, simply learning that their events are psychogenic may result in the elimination of seizures.[1] However, for the majority, psychological therapy, with or without psychopharmacology, is the indicated form of treatment. Maximizing patient receptivity to the diagnosis and to recommended treatments is essential.

Therapy refusal is defined as failure to follow up with the first therapy session after an initial psychiatric screening interview and is unfortunately a common problem in general psychiatry. Failure to attend the first psychotherapy session after completing an initial psychiatric or psychological assessment ranges anywhere from 32.6% to 49%.[2-4] Missed first psychiatry appointments are estimated to be twice as high as the rate for other medical specialties and represent a major challenge in the proper management of psychiatric conditions.[5] This problem is equally troubling in PNES.[6]

2. CLINICIAN CHARACTERISTICS

An array of clinician characteristics and interventions can potentially play a role during the first contact with the patient (Table 8.1). The circumstances of the first contact may also impact rapport, especially when a psychiatric inpatient consult is requested by the diagnostic team without clearly providing a rationale for this to the patient. In this type of situation, it can be useful to introduce oneself as part of the diagnostic team, explaining

Table 8.1. Clinician Factors That Can Affect Patient–Clinician Connection

Clinician Factors Associated with Therapeutic Alliance	Connection-Promoting Factors	Connection-Preventing Factors
Empathy	Warm, empathetic	Cold
Quality of listening	Actively listening	Not listening, firing questions
Quality of session content	Responses that combine cognitive-emotional content	Lack emotional content, general information and impersonal advice
Level of engagement	Engaged, asking follow-up questions	Disengaged
Choice of words	Use words similar to those the patient uses	Use words dissimilar to those the patient uses
Use of terminology	Using terms patient naturally understands	Overly technical and academic language
First half of session	Patient initially decides salient themes	Clinician dominates the interview
Second half of session	Clinician becomes active	Clinician remains passive
Clinician flexibility/rigidity	Flexibility	Dogmatism and dominance
Intervention types	Nurturing, collaborative, insight-oriented	Cold, dominating, impersonal, advice giving
Length of session	Longer is more impactful	Short, rushed
Clinician knowledge	Clinician is educated about PNES	Clinician lacks education on PNES
Illness perception	Internal locus of control, illness is involuntary, unconscious	External locus of control, illness can be voluntarily controlled

that psychological issues can be present in seizure disorders and that as part of a comprehensive evaluation emotional well-being is also being assessed.

Clinician characteristics typically fall along two dimensions: those that are externally observable (i.e., age, gender, ethnicity, professional background, and interventions) and inferred qualities (i.e., values, beliefs, attitudes, and philosophy about therapy).[7] Therapy outcome research consistently underscores that there is a strong relationship between therapeutic alliance and therapy outcome. The depth of patient–clinician connection is largely established in the first session, and patient–therapist connection and patient personality characteristics account for more than 50% of the variance in alliance ratings.[8] In early sessions, connections have been described as deeper with clinicians who are warm, actively listening, and responding with a combination of cognitive-emotional content.[9]

High alliance sessions tend to have fewer topic changes, more listening, and a greater degree of early patient therapeutic work, while clinicians who provide general information or advice rather than personally relevant information tend to have weaker connections. The effects of an alliance developed during the initial psychiatric assessment have been found to persist across the course of treatment.[10–12] Feeling liked and respected appears to play a major role in patients' decision to continue treatment after their initial interview.[13] Mental health clinicians might find it helpful to engage more with patients by viewing themselves in the very unique position of being able to assist those with PNES in bridging the mind–body gap by facilitating verbal expression of distress.

Relying on words that the client might naturally and effortlessly use to define experiences and ideas, rather than technical and scholarly terms, can also solidify the connection. Therefore, if the patient is describing the presenting problem as "seizures," the clinician might initially choose to use the patient's idiosyncratic terminology rather than introducing novel terms such as "events" or "episodes."

It is useful at the outset of the interview to "give the patients the floor" by asking open-ended questions and encouraging them to initiate salient themes regarding their distress and concerns. Patients should be invited to speak about what brought them to the interview (i.e., their seizures and their theories and speculations regarding the onset and maintenance of this condition). Features occurring before, during, or after the seizure and symptoms of anxiety, panic, or pain should be discussed. What does the seizure look like? Is awareness preserved? Is the onset abrupt? Are eyes open? What is the postictal period like? Typically, in the first half of the interview, the clinician will choose to give feedback that closely matches the patient's preconceptions, but by the second half of the interview, the patient is presented with information that is progressively more discrepant from initial concepts of self and pathology. For example, the interviewer may begin introducing "episodes" to replace "seizures" or can begin providing psychological explanations, if relevant, about the process of dissociation or stress response. As the interview progresses, the clinician can move on to other concrete difficulties associated with the presenting problem, such as changes in cognitive functioning and daily life activities. It has been reported that patients who drop out after their initial screening interview tend to view the clinician as more passive.[13] Therefore, as the interview progresses, the clinician must essentially become a more active and explorative participant, introducing associations and connections between the patients' histories and their present predicament. The clinician can then "expand time," clarifying the association between emotional triggers and the events themselves. In this way, the clinician can help challenge automatic cognitive schemas and provide greater awareness of the connection between psychosocial events and somatic language. The clinician will need to assess for psychiatric comorbidities (e.g., depression, anxiety, somatization, trauma and PTSD, dissociation, and suicidality) as well as defensive tendencies and significant family characteristics. The clinician may choose to introduce interpretations (i.e., adding motivation to action) and assess the level of introspective abilities of the patient. This information may provide a window into the patient's ability to use more psychodynamic principles in the treatment to follow. Clinician flexibility will be necessary in this stage, as dominant and dogmatic stances typically impact outcome in a negative fashion.[14]

Examples of how comorbidities can be reviewed include questions such as the following:

"What has been your reaction to having seizure activity?"
"What have you had to give up?"
"Do you ever get sad?"
"How bad does that sadness get?"
"Ever get to the point of not wanting to live anymore?"
"Do you have trouble concentrating?"
"Have you stopped enjoying activities?"
"Do you get anxious?"
"Have there been fluctuations in your mood?"

If there are symptoms of depression, a timeline should be obtained, and it would be important to note if there is an association between mood and somatic symptoms. The presence of other disease states frequently associated with somatization also provide useful information, such as fibromyalgia, chronic fatigue syndrome, Lyme disease, or chronic pain. As the alliance deepens, the interviewer can begin to ask about trauma, neglect and abuse, and episodes of dissociation, but details are unnecessary at this point. If the patient is distrustful or anxious and insecure, this investigation can take place during a second interview. However, if a sentinel traumatic episode has been described, the clinician might consider asking if any legal issues are pending. Clinicians who are perceived as empathetic, convey warmth, and appear to be actively listening are likely to connect better and have better outcomes.[7] Although taking notes or typing into a computer during the interview is not recommended, if it is necessary, pausing to make eye contact is a necessity. Patients who feel that the clinician is genuinely concerned about their welfare even if the clinician disapproves of the patient's activities or behaviors (e.g., use of substances or self-harm) tend to engage better. Nonverbal communication (e.g., facial expressions that are concordant with the patient's verbal content and nodding) and brief verbal utterances can help cement positive rapport. Other highly useful tools in fostering the therapeutic alliance include frequently summarizing what the patient appears to be saying with the adage, "Let me see if I have this clear. This is what I heard you say.... Is that correct?"

Clinicians who are involved in impactful and longer first sessions are more likely to engage the patient. When assessing a patient with confirmed or suspected PNES, it is recommended to schedule the interview allowing extra time if needed. This serves several purposes, including facilitation of comprehensive information gathering and communicating to patients that they are important and deserving of the professional's time. In the event of a delay in the session secondary to a psychogenic episode occurring during the interview, having more time allows for the intake to be completed. Of note: when the patient has a seizure during the interview, the clinician is provided with useful information regarding triggers (e.g., was the topic being discussed when the episode started potentially stressful?) and regarding modifications that may be needed in future sessions, depending on seizure characteristics (e.g., will safety measures be needed and will "grounding techniques" and "suggesting recovery" after a reasonable amount of time be feasible?).

Treatment refusal has been linked to perceived lack of expertise, trustworthiness, and understanding of the clinician. For example, using the outdated term "pseudoseizures" or obstinately digging for a trauma history (despite the facts that approximately 20% of adult patients diagnosed with PNES deny such a history and that trauma is not as common a risk factor for PNES in pediatric cases as it is in adult cases) can stifle positive rapport. Therefore, it is essential that clinicians are well informed about PNES, including the typical etiological and prognostic factors, psychiatric comorbidities, and treatment options. It is also helpful to let the patient's history evolve without preconceived notions of probable causality. Over time, the pieces of the puzzle will come together.

When the time comes to address the condition's etiology and treatment expectations, contradictory conceptualizations by the clinician and patient can present an important hurdle.[15] Most neurologists consider PNES a disorder related to psychological difficulties or "stress," for which psychotherapy is the most appropriate treatment.[16-18] In contrast, many patients with PNES tend to see their condition as physical in etiology and deny or diminish significant non-health stressors in their lives.[19] The clinician will need to work to help the patient understand that internal locus of control does not translate to "voluntary" or "feigned." More importantly, the clinician may choose to communicate that there is a wealth of new perspectives about PNES as a functional disease rather than as a "mental" illness. Discussing other conditions that fall along these dual lines (ulcers and stress, heart disease and depression) can further solidify these concepts.

One final and very important clinician-based challenge is that some clinicians still view PNES as a voluntary consciously produced disorder with secondary gain. This view significantly damages rapport and clinician effectiveness. Education of professionals is needed so that clinicians are aware that malingering represents a very small proportion of patients suspected of having PNES.[20] Moreover, clinicians are urged to examine the exact wording they use with these patients, since at times even the most well-meaning clinician unintentionally communicates the concept of faking (e.g., your events are not "real seizures").[21]

Clinicians' attitudes regarding PNES and related disorders are further explored in Chapter 11. A summary of clinician characteristics that can impact rapport is found in Table 8.1.

3. PATIENT CHARACTERISTICS

Patients' psychiatric and other health comorbidities, characteristics of PNES (semiology, duration, severity, etc.), and prior experiences with health professionals (e.g., emergency medical personnel, neurologists, mental health professionals) can impact the interview. A checklist for clinicians interviewing a patient with suspected PNES can be found in Table 8.2. An array of patient characteristics can potentially play a role during the first psychiatric contact (Table 8.3).

Table 8.2. Checklist of Elements Clinicians Should Assess When Screening a Patient with Suspected PNES

Element to be Assessed	Details of Assessment
Seizure characteristics	Semiology, duration, severity, frequency, identifiable triggers
Patients' prior experiences with health/mental health professionals	Positive, trusting vs. negative, distrusting; requires patience to build rapport
Presence of family during interview	Preferably family is not included; if family is present, the clinician observes quality of interactions
Principal psychiatric comorbidities to assess	Mood disorders, potential for suicide, anxiety disorders, trauma history and PTSD, dissociative and somatization tendencies
Other health comorbidities	Fibromyalgia, chronic fatigue, Lyme disease, pain syndromes, mild traumatic head injury
Intellectually disabled patients	Assess for environmental triggers, developmental issues, psychotic symptoms
Malingering	Assess carefully for secondary gain
Factitious disorders	Assess for "sick role" and reinforcing factors
Difficult patients	Clinicians should allow patient to vent and should genuinely "hear" complaints, but set reasonable limits to conduct a comprehensive evaluation
Patients with incapacitating seizures	Inpatient treatment should be sought, but if unavailable an outpatient multispecialty team can be assembled

It is often recommended to start the interview with the adult patient separated from the family unless there is significant resistance. If the latter occurs, the session can begin collectively and as the patient grows more comfortable, they can be separated. While they are together, watching any interactive pattern between family members is extremely useful. For example, how dependent is the patient? Do physical complaints dictate family response? Is the patient's independence invalidated by the family? Understanding the family system is crucial to discerning the secondary and primary unconscious reinforcement that the patient's symptoms may serve in the family unit. In addition, interviewing family members separately is useful because they are often reluctant to talk in front of their relatives. However, free from restrictions, an assessment of exacerbating and ameliorating factors can take place, and a clearer picture of the patient's response to their illness may become evident.

Cluster analysis of emotion regulation profiles in PNES subjects has identified two major subgroups. The undermodulating subgroup is characterized by heightened

Table 8.3. Patient and Family Characteristics to Evaluate in Those with Suspected PNES

Domain Assessed	Characteristics of PNES Patients/Families and Recommendations for Clinicians
Family's response to independence in patient	Encourages dependence
Family's regard for somatic complaints and explanations	Overvalues somatic complaints, invalidates cognitive-emotional explanations
Patient's emotional expression tendencies (undermodulating)	Clinician should aim to relieve patient's concern of being "just a psych case"
Patient's emotional expression tendencies (overmodulating)	Tendency toward emotional avoidance, controlled behavior, somatization, and less obvious psychiatric comorbidity
Patient's emotional awareness	Clinician should initially avoid emotionally laden content with alexithymics
Patient's cognitive flexibility/introspective capacity	Cognitively rigid/not introspective

emotional reactivity, poor tolerance to arousal, difficulty controlling affect, impaired quality of life, and numerous psychiatric comorbidities. However, because these patients often have had multiple encounters with mental health professionals, chances are high that some of these previous interactions have been negative experiences, which might affect this encounter. Patients may sense that their psychiatric history is "water under the bridge" and independent of the seizures. In the meantime, the interviewing clinician may feel flooded by the extensive psychiatric history being provided. These patients may use very primitive defenses, such as splitting, projection, idealization, and devaluation, and this practice may be associated with the clinician feeling overwhelmed, which may result in the induction of a significant countertransference in the examiner. It will also be necessary to pay attention to discrepancies in affect during the interview—for example, a display of *la belle indifference* associated with a description of significant trauma. These patients will need interventions that focus on modulation and control of affective lability.

An example of an interview with an undermodulating patient follows.

Psychiatric Interview with Undermodulating Patient during Admission to Epilepsy Monitoring Unit

Patient: Believe me, I know I had trauma and was diagnosed with depression, anxiety, post-traumatic stress disorder, and have an eating disorder. I have worked on it for years in therapy and I have come to grips with it. These seizures are different and I don't want to be discarded as a "psych case" just because I have a psych history.

Clinician: I agree, this is why we are doing all of these tests and why you are on this unit. We want to make sure we get to the right diagnosis. However, trauma can have some very serious consequences, one of which is called psychogenic nonepileptic seizures, and we need to assess for that as well. We are not closing our minds to any possibility; rather, we are keeping our minds open and reviewing the problem from several different but complimentary angles. In the future, we may change our perspective, but we will never give up on searching for all causes.

In this example, the clinician is not challenging the patient but rather presenting a collaborative and educational stance, which has the best chance of creating a lasting positive working alliance.

The second subgroup, characterized by emotion overregulation, typically presents with emotional avoidance, excessively controlled behavior, a tendency toward somatization, and less obvious psychiatric comorbidity. These individuals tend to be less aware of or reluctant to identify and/or accept emotional distress. When working with this patient type, it is especially important for the interviewer to use language that is similar to the one used by the patient and to avoid emotionally laden vocabulary while collecting evidence of psychosocial stressors and history that can later be constructed into a rational and hypothetical explanation once the diagnosis of PNES is confirmed. The beginning of the interview should include a complete evaluation of the patients' chief complaint, the seizures. This detailed investigation solidifies the therapeutic alliance.

In the following example, the patient is met where she can start naturally (e.g., seizure and somatic complaints). The investigation of psychological stressors continues with the patient's "somatic" vocabulary by asking about post-event *cognitive complaints*. This opens the door to discussing employment, for example, which appears to be a source of physical and emotional stress. Subsequently, the clinician can begin to introduce psychological components and draw connections between events and circumstances and stress and the effect of stress on health. The patient might argue that this stressful job has been part of her life for years and that the seizures just began. This provides the clinician with the opportunity to speak about the potential cumulative effect of stress over time.

Psychiatric Interview with Overmodulating Patient Resistant to Possible Psychological Precipitants to Seizures

After discussing seizure semiology and associated characteristics in detail, the clinician can introduce the following:

Clinician: You mentioned that you are having up to 10 seizures a day. Sometimes a high frequency of seizures is accompanied by other problems—for example, cognitive difficulties in your daily activities. Have you noticed any of this?

Patient: Absolutely, my memory is gone; it's like I'm demented. And I have trouble speaking. . . . I don't know how long my boss will keep me on if this keeps on like this.

> *Clinician:* What's your job?
>
> *Patient:* I am a store manager. I have 10 employees under my charge. I usually work 10 hours a day, but when the holidays roll around, we sometimes start at 2 AM.
>
> *Clinician:* That sounds exhausting and stressful. How long have you been at this position and how has your health been while there?

Sometimes, contrary to expectation, the psychogenic events do not happen during obvious stressful situations but only when the patient lets his or her guard down and relaxes. The clinician can underscore that often people are able to get through an emergency and then suffer the consequences when it is over (like after a final exam).

The presence of alexithymia has been noted in the literature as a frequent harbinger of PNES. It is important to note if the patient has difficulty describing emotions. From the patient's interactive style, does he or she form secure or ambivalent attachments? How does the patient describe people in his or her life? Are their descriptions colorful, inclusive of both positive and negative qualities or bland and monosyllabic? Even the patient's description of the seizure itself can be an important diagnostic indicator. Plug et al [22] noted that patients with PNES often describe their events with imprecision, and some patients may exhibit extreme "avoidance," simply stating when asked about their seizures, "I don't know what happens during my seizure, ask my spouse or parent."

4. SPECIAL PATIENT GROUPS

4.1. Intellectually Disabled Patients

Patients with intellectual disability (ID) can display both epilepsy and PNES and may have a higher frequency of seizures than their cognitively intact counterparts. In one review [23] of 746 video EEG–monitored children, of the 57 with developmental disability, 45% had PNES. These patients present different levels of difficulty for the evaluator. Patients with ID often display their distress by somatization, and the anxiety they experience and display is often a result of a "system" dysfunction. Thus a comprehensive evaluation requires a full investigation of the patient's environment. Are patients reacting to a conflict in their group home? Are their parents getting divorced? Do they have a friend that has moved away? Is one of the patient's siblings accomplishing something (e.g., graduating from college, getting married) that the patient is struggling with owing to his or her cognitive delay? These unmet developmental milestones may highlight the patient's limitations. In addition, it is important to ask about neurovegetative signs of depression or the internal preoccupation that can be seen with a psychotic event. It can be very challenging to help a patient with ID understand the association between psychological factors and psychogenic seizures. A focus on caregiver education and psychological support may be extremely helpful.

> **Interview with ID Patient that Shifts to Body-Based Focus When Emotional Content Not Understood**
>
> *Patient:* I feel fine, I just have seizures, that's it. I don't feel nervous.
> *Clinician:* You just said that your parents are getting divorced and that you don't know what this might mean for your future.
> *Patient:* Yeah, they are getting divorced, but I am ok. All I have are the seizures. I am not nervous at all.
> *Clinician:* Let's try something different. I am going to teach you a breathing exercise, is that ok?
> (Practice deep breathing for a couple of minutes.) Tell me how it felt to breathe deeply. How did it feel in your body?
> *Patient:* Yeah, when I breathe out, it's like good.
> *Clinician:* This is a relaxation exercise. A lot of people find that when they breathe like this, tension leaves their body and their muscles relax. Sometimes we think we aren't tense, but when you breathe like this, it helps show you that you may be a little tense. Does that make sense? And sometimes we think that nothing is bothering us, but we do actually have some worries.

In this example, the focus of the interview is shifted to a body-based exercise to illustrate to the patient that he may in fact be feeling tension. The clinician uses the patient's somatic vocabulary to connect. Clinician flexibility is necessary to help the patient recognize the connection between anxiety and the psychogenic events.

4.2. Factitious Disorder and Malingering

One of the first records of seizures and malingering came from *The Journal of Insanity*, in 1880.[24] Feigned symptoms can be seen in those who are malingering and in patients with factitious disorder. In the former, intentionally produced symptoms are consciously reproduced to obtain external rewards. In the latter, the motive is to attain the sick role, but again the symptoms are intentionally produced. Clear examples of these situations are rare in the setting of PNES evaluations, but the possibility must always be kept in mind. Typically, during the interview, the clinician is collecting information regarding potential secondary gain that might work against recovery. There are screening questionnaires, the Structured Interview of Reported Symptoms Test and the Miller Forensic Assessment of Symptom Test, that have demonstrated good efficacy at identifying these situations.[25] If a patient is thought to be malingering, honestly discussing reasons why this is suspected and how treatment would be an effortful and likely ineffective endeavor needs to be addressed. If the patient is diagnosed with factitious disorder, the clinician will need to employ a much more complex and lengthy approach to reduce the patient's identification with the sick role and the reinforcing factors while highlighting and strengthening the patient's healthy qualities.

4.3. The Difficult Patient

Projected anger may be apparent during the initial psychiatric interview with certain patients, and this can make it especially difficult for the clinician to engage. These patients may quickly become disliked by all on the unit or in the office and seem generally unlikable. A useful approach can be to allow the patient to vent about all the "injustices and indignities" that have occurred since arriving at the epilepsy center. This allows the patient to feel that he or she has been heard and to release his or her anger. Then the clinician can proceed or negotiate a subsequent interview. In a seminal article [26] on the topic, Groves broke this group into categories; the underlying theme of all of these groups being a fear of abandonment. Setting firm limits for the patient (e.g., making it clear to the patient that the diagnostic team will need to complete a comprehensive evaluation, including a psychiatric assessment) can also be helpful when it is coupled with the reassurance that the neurologist will continue to follow the patient's care in the future, regardless of whether a psychiatric condition is determined to be causative.

Interview with Resistant and Oppositional Patient Who Does Not Want to Engage with Clinician

Patient: Oh great, now they went and called psych in to see me, do they think I'm crazy!? I don't see why I need to speak to you. I am here for a medical condition and have no psychological problems!

Clinician: I'm not here to see you because people think you are crazy or in lieu of your medical issues, but rather because often seizure disorders are accompanied by problems with quality of life, stressors, and, yes, sometimes depression or anxiety. We are hoping to get the best use of your time spent in the hospital, and that includes providing a comprehensive assessment, which includes psychological issues as well. I want to assure you that we never stop the medical evaluation, but we do need to investigate your symptoms from all possible perspectives.

In this example, the clinician meets the patient on the common ground of seizures and explains that "psych" has been called in because psychological issues might exist in any form of seizure disorder. The clinician can now tentatively continue to explore symptoms and their triggers with the patient.

4.4. Patients with Incapacitating Events

Occasionally, patients with PNES present to an evaluation unit with events that are numerous and/or intense and result in severe disability. A transfer to an inpatient psychiatric unit can be considered at that time. Comprehensive inpatient treatment including hypnosis, occupational and physical therapy, and group and individual therapy may be very useful.[27,28] However, sometimes inpatient units do not wish to accept these patients because of liability concerns, lack of education about PNES, or the psychogenic diagnosis is questioned. In these cases, the referring center should be prepared to speak with the receiving clinicians to share information regarding PNES and brainstorm necessary adjustments to ensure safety. If an inpatient option is unavailable, an alternative is to organize an outpatient treatment team that would likely include psychiatry, psychology, other therapists, home health aides, and practical support from family and friends. Initially, this team may require coordination and consultation with the referring center. Safety precautions will be similar to those employed in treating a patient with epilepsy.

5. SETTING UP A TREATMENT TEAM AFTER DIAGNOSIS CONFIRMATION

Some final words are warranted regarding patients who are discharged after being given a diagnosis of PNES. Local patients should receive treatment whenever possible within the same epilepsy center where the evaluation and diagnosis was made, to avoid the risk of early dropout.[29] When it is not possible to provide all services at one institution, the referring clinician should be prepared to consult with outside clinicians. A follow-up appointment with the diagnosing neurologist is also recommended. A follow-up phone call might be a useful secondary approach for patients with severe logistical concerns (e.g., residing far from the hospital). An in-house support group is a valuable resource for local patients, and a phone-in support group could represent a good resource for patients who have limited transportation options. Teletherapy may be another useful alternative to consider.

6. SUMMARY

- A positive therapeutic alliance counts significantly toward psychological or psychiatric treatment retention and effectiveness.
- Clinician behaviors (e.g., empathy, choice of words, flexibility, knowledge of the condition, and illness perception) can improve or obstruct the therapeutic alliance in evaluations of patients with PNES.
- Searching for comorbidities during the interview, including mood disorders, anxiety disorders, dissociative and other trauma-related disorders, is recommended.
- Associated medical illnesses are also commonly seen with functional neurological disorders, such as Lyme disease, chronic fatigue syndrome, and pain syndromes.
- Patient characteristics need to be observed, especially the presence of under- and overmodulated emotional expression. Overmodulating patients, those with alexithymic and highly avoidant tendencies, require distinct and flexible approaches to the evaluation process. Undermodulated patients may require approaches to help regulate overwhelming affect and to limit primitive defenses.
- Special considerations are needed when encountering unique populations (e.g., developmentally disabled, those incapacitated by event frequency, hostile patients) with suspected PNES.

REFERENCES

1. Hall-Patch L, Brown R, House A, et al. Acceptability and effectiveness of a strategy for the communication of the diagnosis of psychogenic nonepileptic seizures. *Epilepsia.* 2010;51(1):70–78.
2. Sue S, McKinney HL, Allen DB. Predictors of the duration of therapy for clients in the community mental health system. *Community Ment Health J.* 1976;12(4):365–375.
3. Phillips EL, Fagan PJ. Attrition: focus on the intake and first therapy interviews. Paper presented at the 90th annual convention of the American Psychological Association, Washington, DC, 1982.
4. Akhigbe S, Morakinyo O, Lawani A, James B, Omoaregba J. Prevalence and correlates of missed first appointments among outpatients at a psychiatric hospital in Nigeria. *Ann Med Health Sci Res.* 2014;4:763–768.
5. Killaspy H, Banerjee S, King M, Lloyd M. Prospective controlled study of psychiatric outpatient non-attendance characteristics and outcome. *Br J Psychiatry.* 2000;176(2):160–165.
6. Baslet G, Prensky E. Initial treatment retention in psychogenic non-epileptic seizures. *J Neuropsychiatry Clin Neurosci.* 2013;25(1):63.
7. Beutler L, Machado P, Neufeldt A. Therapist variables. In: Bergin A, Garfield S, eds. *Handbook of Psychotherapy and Behavior Change.* New York: John Wiley & Sons; 1994:229–269.
8. Sexton H, Littauer H, Sexton A, Tømmerås E. Building an alliance: early therapy process and the client–therapist connection. *Psychother Res.* 2005;15(1-2):103–116.
9. Sexton H. Process, life events, and symptomatic change in brief eclectic psychotherapy. *J Consult Clin Psychol.* 1996;64(6):1358.
10. Bachelor A. Clients' perception of the therapeutic alliance: a qualitative analysis. *J Counsel Psychol.* 1995;42(3):323.
11. Hilsenroth MJ, Peters EJ, Ackerman SJ. The development of therapeutic alliance during psychological assessment: patient and therapist perspectives across treatment. *J Pers Assess.* 2004;83(3):332–344.
12. Huber D, Henrich G, Brandl T. Working relationship in a psychotherapeutic consultation. *Psychother Res.* 2005;15(1-2):129–139.
13. Mohl PC, Martinez D, Ticknor C, Huang M, Cordell L. Early dropouts from psychotherapy. *J Nerv Ment Dis.* 1991;179(8):478–481.
14. Myers L. *The Relation of Interviewer Ethnic, Cultural, and Interpersonal Characteristics to Patient Dropout.* New York: City University of New York; 1999.
15. Bohart AC, Graves WA. The client in psychotherapy. In: Lambert MJ, ed. *Bergin and Garfield's Handbook of Psychotherapy and Behavior Change*, 6th ed. New York: Wiley; 2011:219–257.
16. LaFrance WC, Rusch MD, Machan JT. What is "treatment as usual" for nonepileptic seizures? *Epilepsy Behav.* 2008;12(3):388–394.
17. Mayor R, Smith PE, Reuber M. Management of patients with nonepileptic attack disorder in the United Kingdom: a survey of health care professionals. *Epilepsy Behav.* 2011;21(4):402–406.
18. Whitehead K, Kandler R, Reuber M. Patients' and neurologists' perception of epilepsy and psychogenic nonepileptic seizures. *Epilepsia.* 2013;54(4):708–717.
19. Stone J, Binzer M, Sharpe M. Illness beliefs and locus of control: a comparison of patients with pseudoseizures and epilepsy. *J Psychosom Res.* 2004;57(6):541–547.

20. Dodrill C. Do patients with psychogenic nonepileptic seizures produce trustworthy findings on neuropsychological tests? *Epilepsia*. 2008;49(4):691.
21. Dworetzky BA. What are we communicating when we present the diagnosis of PNES? *Epilepsy Curre*. 2015;15(6):353–357.
22. Plug L, Sharrack B, Reuber M. Conversation analysis can help to distinguish between epilepsy and non-epileptic seizure disorders: a case comparison. *Seizure*. 2009;18:43–50.
23. Montenegro MA, Sproule D, Mandel A, et al. The frequency of non-epileptic spells in children: results of video–EEG monitoring in a tertiary care center. *Seizure*. 2008;17(7):583–587.
24. Mac Donald CF. Feigned epilepsy. *Am J Insanity*. 1880;37(1):1–22.
25. Zubera A, Raza M, Holaday E, Aggarwal R. Screening for malingering in the emergency department. *Acad Psychiatry*. 2015;39(2):233–234.
26. Groves J. Taking care of the hateful patient. *N Engl J Med*. 1978;298(16):883–887.
27. Moene FC, Spinhoven P, Hoogduin KA, van Dyck R. A randomised controlled clinical trial on the additional effect of hypnosis in a comprehensive treatment programme for in-patients with conversion disorder of the motor type. *Psychother Psychosom*. 2002;71(2):66–76.
28. Acton EK, Tatum WO. Inpatient psychiatric consultation for newly-diagnosed patients with psychogenic non-epileptic seizures. *Epilepsy Behav*. 2013;27(1):36–39.
29. Baslet G, Prensky E. Initial treatment retention in psychogenic non-epileptic seizures. *J Neuropsychiatry Clin Neurosci*. 2013;25(1):63.

9

Practical and Diagnostic Challenges for the Neuropsychologist

Kim Willment, PhD and David Loring, PhD

1. INTRODUCTION

This chapter presents an overview of the practical challenges facing clinicians during the neuropsychological assessment of patients with psychogenic nonepileptic seizures (PNES). The chapter serves as to guide decision-making in this process. The neuropsychology of PNES and potential mechanisms for neurocognitive impairment are reviewed in detail in Chapter 5. Clinical decision-making is predicated on the goal(s) of the neuropsychological evaluation, which varies based on a number of factors, including clinical setting, patient characteristics, and treatment/intervention resources. In addition, there is no standard approach that neuropsychologists take to address the concerns presented in this chapter. Our objective in presenting the following practical challenges and clinical decision points is to guide neuropsychologists in refining their approach to this patient population by developing a plan for a consistent response to these challenges. This chapter will focus on the challenges faced and neuropsychological objectives implemented in a hospital setting where the neuropsychologist functions as a member of an interdisciplinary team within an epilepsy program. As such, there may be some benefit to developing an integrated team-based plan for neuropsychological decision-making. The *neuropsychological evaluation*, as it is defined in this chapter, refers to a comprehensive assessment of cognition, psychological functioning, personality, and behavior through standardized objective tests and self-report inventories.

This chapter also outlines multiple diagnostic challenges related to the complexity of the neuropsychological evaluation in PNES. The heterogeneity of the PNES population has made characterization of neuropsychological profiles challenging, and this is reflected in the sometimes conflicting reports on cognitive findings in PNES samples. While it is generally accepted that many PNES patients have objective abnormalities or weaknesses on cognitive testing,[1-5] these findings are not specific to the PNES population. In addition, the PNES population is also characterized by psychopathological heterogeneity,[6] and PNES subtyping based on psychopathology or emotion regulation style still requires further research.

The final focus of this chapter relates to the therapeutic goals of the neuropsychological evaluation. Particular emphasis is placed on the integration of neuropsychological findings during delivery of the diagnosis and on promoting cognitive self-efficacy.

2. DEFINING OBJECTIVES OF NEUROPSYCHOLOGICAL EVALUATION IN PNES

In the hospital epilepsy team-based context, the objective of the neuropsychological evaluation in PNES is often less focused on diagnosis, since video-EEG monitoring is the diagnostic gold standard.[7] However, it may be that a typical event is not captured on video-EEG prior to a patient's discharge. Therefore, it is generally recommended that the neuropsychological evaluation address the factors in a patient's neuropsychological profile that increase or decrease the risk for PNES, which includes the patient's profile of cognitive strengths and weaknesses and psychological and personality functioning. This allows the team to rely on the neuropsychological evaluation to inform the direction of care or treatment after discharge, as well as to keep the patient engaged with the provisional PNES diagnosis in the absence of video-EEG confirmation.

Another objective of the neuropsychological evaluation in PNES is to support the patient's understanding of the diagnosis and associated symptoms. PNES patients often present with cognitive complaints that contribute significantly to functional impairment. Providing psychoeducation regarding the overlap of neural systems that mediate their cognitive, physical, and emotional symptoms provides a unified explanation for their presence. The therapeutic aspects of the neuropsychological evaluation are discussed in greater detail later in this chapter.

The neuropsychological evaluation is also a valuable tool to inform treatment planning in a number of different ways. For example, the patients' personality and behavioral profiles can be utilized to identify treatment targets for psychotherapy. With better understanding of the heterogeneity of the PNES population, it is hoped that subgroup definition will facilitate the development of empirically supported treatments and the ability of the neuropsychologist to direct patients to the most effective treatment based on their neuropsychological profile. Finally, for patients who are highly focused on their subjective cognitive concerns, providing psychoeducation about their cognitive profile and helping them implement compensatory strategies to improve everyday functioning may be useful. While there are no formal research studies on cognitive rehabilitation in PNES, this treatment modality has been shown to beneficially affect outcomes in a range of other psychiatric disorders.[8–13] The objectives described here for the neuropsychological evaluation in PNES are summarized in Table 9.1.

Table 9.1. Objectives of Neuropsychological Evaluation in PNES

---

1) Identify factors in the neuropsychological profile that increase or decrease the risk for PNES.
2) Provide evidence to support the patient's understanding of the diagnosis and associated symptoms.
3) Inform treatment planning and direct patients to effective treatments.

---

3. PRACTICAL CHALLENGES

Many factors may impact the ability to accurately characterize a PNES patient's neuropsychological profile, including inadequate effort or test engagement, performance validity test failures, testing environment, and the sequelae of medications, including antiepileptic drugs (AEDs). Many of the practical challenges outlined are not specific to PNES and relate more generally to issues that prompt clinical decision-making on the part of the neuropsychologist. As mentioned earlier, there is no standard protocol for how neuropsychologists are expected to respond to these challenges. In general, if the neuropsychologist is functioning as a member of an interdisciplinary epilepsy team, it is recommended that an integrated team-based plan or protocol is developed that balances the following threats to validity and the team's patient care mission.

3.1. Performance Validity Test Failures

Neuropsychological testing typically includes formal measures to determine whether examinees are sufficiently engaged so that results are credible and can be considered to reflect true ability levels.[14] Although these tests are often characterized as measures of effort or motivation, they are increasingly referred to as performance validity tests (PVTs), since the underlying reason for poor performance cannot always be correctly inferred.[14] In addition to volitional factors, PVTs may be influenced by true ability levels.[15] Furthermore, failure criteria, including performance thresholds to infer invalid responding, have been incompletely established (discussed more below).

PVT failure rates tend to be higher among PNES patients (at 28% or greater) than among patients with epilepsy (8%) and in the general medical population (8%).[16,17] Malingering, which reflects the volitional manipulation of performance for secondary gain, is not a significant factor in the etiology of PNES[18] or the main source of variability in PVT findings unless there are incentives for obtaining (or maintaining) disability benefits due to impaired cognition. When poor PVT scores are obtained, they are typically ascribed to internal factors not under a patient's direct volitional control (e.g., emotional conflict, psychiatric severity/complexity, distress).

While there is often a dichotomous pass/fail description based on suggested performance thresholds, there are more nuanced ways of interpreting PVT findings, particularly outside the context of medicolegal evaluations. "Failing" scores typically range from just below the failure cutoff to significantly lower performance levels. These two PVT "failure" categories are described next. We also present a model for clinical decision-making for PVT failures in PNES (Figure 9.1).

3.1.1. Below Failure Cutoff But Well Above Chance Performance—"Just Fail"

This category represents an intermediate group; while technically a PVT failure is characterized by a score less than a specified cutoff, performance is still well above chance.[19] It has been argued that certain neurological and neuropsychiatric conditions may impact PVT performance,[20] leading to scores that represent a "just fail." For example, part of illness or sickness behavior may be a feeling that anything that requires sustained attention is burdensome [21] and may play a major factor in cognitive test performance, including performance on PVTs. Consistent with these ideas, a conceptual model of cognition in PNES suggests that PVT failures result from dysregulation in attentional deployment.[6] That is, PNES patients may alternate between states of hyper- and hypoarousal,[6] as has been observed in individuals with emotional trauma histories.[22] This pattern of alternation between attentional states may lead to periods of fixation or compulsivity and periods of distractibility and disengagement. As such, variability in the cognitive profile, particularly on tests of sustained attention, would be expected. Thus, reduced PVT performance may not invalidate neuropsychological data collected in this population; instead, it may capture an important psychopathological phenomenon reflecting current, though potentially modifiable, cognitive difficulties.

3.1.2. Below Chance Performance

Significantly less than chance performance reflects active intent to avoid the correct answer, and with clearly identifiable external incentive, malingering can be comfortably inferred. When malingering is suspected, as reflected by performances below chance on forced-choice validity measures, and there is a clear external incentive, the patient's cognitive and personality profiles are largely uninterpretable and constructive treatment targets based on formal assessment cannot be established. Without clear external motivating factors, intentional manipulation of performance may represent "elaboration" or "exaggeration" of symptoms, to ensure that what the patient identifies as an interfering and distressing symptom is detected by the neuropsychologist.

3.1.3. Clinical Decision-Making around PVT Failures

There is no standard response that neuropsychologists employ when faced with a PVT failure.[23,24] It can be beneficial for the neuropsychologist to develop a clinical decision-making protocol to address PVT failures with input from the multidisciplinary epilepsy team. For example, if the team's approach is founded in the conceptual model that predicts PVT failures as a result of dysregulation in attentional deployment related to the psychopathological phenomena of PNES,[6] the decision-making plan in Figure 9.1 may represent the agreed-upon balance between ensuring performance validity and a patient care approach. The plan outlined in Figure 9.1 reflects a high threshold for discontinuing testing when individuals perform below a specific cutoff on a PVT but still perform well above chance—the "just fail" category. This leniency allows for variable performance that may result from attentional dysregulation in PNES.

Some neuropsychologists choose to confront patients regarding validity findings. There are advantages and drawbacks to confronting patients, as well as logistical impracticalities. In terms of advantages, addressing performance concerns may motivate or energize a patient to exert more effort to focus or engage, improving the overall validity of the patient's cognitive profile. In this way, confrontations can function as brief interventions and may even prompt the patient to change his or her approach to test-taking and symptom endorsement on self-report inventories. The drawbacks are that patients may respond negatively to even the most patient-sensitive approach to confrontation on PVT findings, potentially leading to a rupture in the alliance with

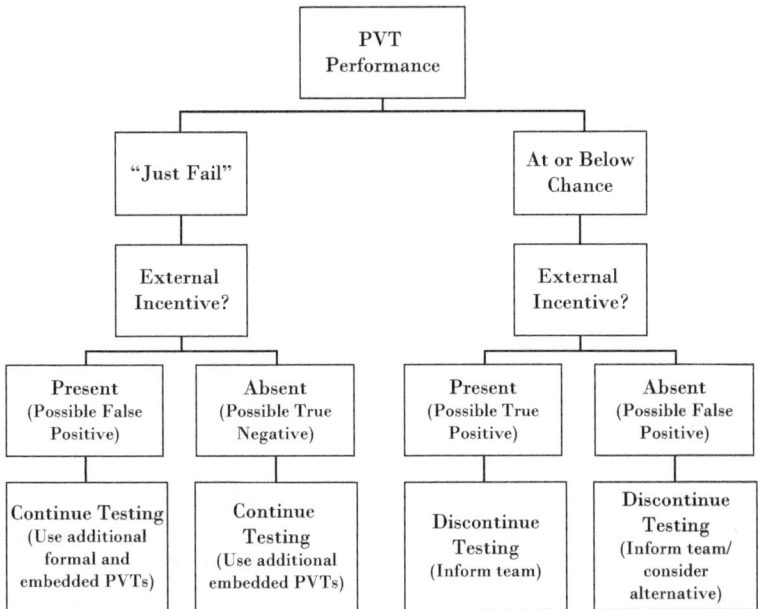

Figure 9.1 Performance validity test (PVT) clinical decision-making model (adapted from Marcopulos et al., 2014[24]).

the provider or the treatment team more broadly. In addition, discussing failed PVTs may compromise test security (i.e., if a discussion occurs immediately after a failed PVT, then the patient may learn to identify that measure as one reflecting validity or task engagement, decreasing its utility in possible future assessments). In terms of logistical challenges, when testing is done by a technician rather than the psychologist, results of PVTs are not always readily available in real time and testing may not be halted.

3.2. Clinical Environment

Neuropsychological tests are developed in settings that allow for the control of external factors that have the potential to impact the interpretation of findings. Matching the standardized testing environment ensures the validity of conclusions that can be drawn based on normative data samples. It is generally more feasible to replicate standardized testing environments in the outpatient setting. However, many PNES patients are tested as inpatients when they are admitted for video-EEG monitoring. The pros and cons of inpatient testing are outlined next.

3.2.1. Inpatient Testing–Pros

1) Patients are typically admitted for video-EEG monitoring for several days and often have ample time to complete a comprehensive neuropsychological evaluation.

2) Performing testing while an individual is an inpatient ensures that information regarding subjective cognitive concerns can be incorporated into the presentation of the PNES diagnosis.
3) In the event of a negative response to receiving the PNES diagnosis, patients may be lost to follow-up, missing an opportunity to provide them with valuable input to inform their care and engage them in treatment.

3.2.2. Inpatient Testing–Cons

1) Inpatient testing is generally not ideal from a standardized testing perspective given the risk of multiple environmental distractions.
2) Other factors that relate to an inpatient admission may also pose a challenge to accurately characterizing the patient's current cognitive abilities (particularly attention and executive functioning). These factors include measures undertaken to provoke events, such as sleep deprivation and medication withdrawal (see next section for more details). While we realize that there may be other hospital demands, the timing of the neuropsychological evaluation and the delivery of the diagnosis of PNES should be coordinated to limit the impact of the patient response on test performance. It is generally beneficial to delay the diagnosis until the neuropsychological evaluation is complete.
3) The hospital setting can also be quite emotionally and physically stressful and result in PVT failures. For example, patients with certain trauma histories may find being restricted and tethered to a bed emotionally triggering, resulting in a heightened emotional state that is not representative of their everyday functioning (see later discussion for more information regarding testing a patient in acute distress). If the neuropsychologist is serving as part of an interdisciplinary team, he or she may benefit from the input of team members (particularly psychiatry or social work) to better understand how the patient is responding to the inpatient environment and monitoring. If team input is not available, assessing the patient's response to the inpatient admission should be included as part of the clinical interview.

3.3. Medications with Known Cognitive Sequelae

As is the case with all neuropsychological evaluations, the patient's medication regimen may have cognitive sequelae. PNES patients often undergo unnecessary AED treatment, which has risks of cognitive side effects.[25] The neuropsychologist must make a clinical decision regarding whether the patient's medicated or nonmedicated state can provide clinically useful information to inform care. Several points for consideration in guiding decision-making are detailed next.

3.3.1. Does the Patient Attribute Cognitive Difficulties to AED Side Effects?

It can often be helpful to consider whether the patient attributes all or some of his or her cognitive difficulties to medication side effects. Understanding patient beliefs regarding the impact of AEDs on cognitive functioning is particularly relevant in the inpatient setting, where patients are typically tapered off their AEDs in order to provoke typical episodes. If the patient does not identify a correlation between medications and cognitive difficulties, then the neuropsychologist should feel comfortable moving forward with testing in the context of medication discontinuation. However, if it is important to demonstrate the influence of an AED that cannot be removed (perhaps for mood stabilization), then deferring testing to a point when the patient is stable on medications may be more clinically useful. This may be accomplished by performing testing later in an inpatient admission when AED medications are reintroduced or referring the patient for outpatient testing.

3.3.2. Is There a Change in Patient Status with Medication Discontinuation?

Discontinuing medication may result in a change in patient status—at times with cognitive improvement and at other times negatively impacting physical, cognitive, or emotional functioning. In cases of cognitive improvement, the neuropsychologist should feel comfortable proceeding with testing, unless it is important to demonstrate the impact of a medication that cannot be removed. In cases of medical, cognitive, or emotional worsening, neuropsychologists may choose to defer testing if they believe testing will cause undue stress and discomfort that will be detrimental to patient care. For example, this may occur when a patient is experiencing symptoms that are the direct result of a medication withdrawal, such as headache or other physical discomfort, fatigue, uncharacteristic mood lability, or severe psychiatric symptoms such as psychosis or suicidal ideation. Brief or abbreviated cognitive screens may be most helpful in these situations, with outpatient follow-up for more comprehensive testing.

3.4. Acute Psychological Distress

In both the inpatient and outpatient settings, individuals can present for neuropsychological evaluation in acute psychological distress. Initial assessment of the patient should attempt to identify factors contributing to the acute response, as well as the presence of any safety concerns. Active suicidal ideation with intent and plan would certainly preclude moving forward with a neuropsychological evaluation.

Prior to testing, a neuropsychologist may choose to initiate a discussion of the factors contributing to psychological distress and help the patient develop a therapeutic plan for managing the factors and/or their response to the factors. For example, the neuropsychologist may choose to contact the patient's outpatient mental health professional after the evaluation to schedule an earlier follow-up visit or help a patient not currently engaged in treatment find a mental health clinician.

The neuropsychologist may choose to move forward with the evaluation in the context of acute psychological distress if state-based measurement of cognitive function will inform clinical care. Such an evaluation may be helpful for patients who are chronically prone to labile fluctuations in mood and distress levels. If there is minimal concern about losing the patient to follow-up, a multisession testing plan can be developed to evaluate the patient at different time points, with the hope of characterizing cognitive and emotional function across various psychological states, including the resolution of acute distress.

Some neuropsychologists would argue that it is not clinically useful to conduct an evaluation on a patient in acute psychological distress in the context of an atypical emotional response or uncharacteristic provoking factor (e.g., death of a close relative). The ability of the neuropsychologist to make this determination may depend on the patient's level of insight (e.g., the patient reports not feeling like him- or herself), knowledge of the patient's history from medical records, and/or ability to communicate with the patient's clinicians (which is more feasible when working in a team setting).

Finally, acute psychological distress has been associated with reductions on performance validity measures in some clinical populations.[26] As mentioned earlier, some neuropsychologists may choose to discontinue testing in the context of PVT failures.

3.5. Comprehensive Evaluations versus Brief Screens

Some neuropsychologists may feel that the threats to accurately characterizing a patient's neuropsychological profile are too high when a PNES patient is admitted for inpatient monitoring and choose to conduct a brief neurocognitive screen.

3.5.1. Comprehensive Neuropsychological Evaluations

It is generally the goal of a comprehensive neuropsychological evaluation to capture a relatively stable picture of a patient's recent neuropsychological status. This is the optimal scenario that allows the neuropsychologist to address several questions posed by referring providers and the subjective concerns of patients, as well as more readily adapt testing in response to patient performance. An example comprehensive neuropsychological battery for use in patients with PNES is detailed in Table 9.2. The tests chosen for inclusion in this battery were selected on the basis of our current understanding of neurocognitive functioning in PNES (see Chapter 5 for more detail).

3.5.2. Brief Neuropsychological Screens

It is recommended that brief screens consist of an abbreviated neuropsychological battery that samples the range of cognitive domains (i.e., attention/executive functioning, memory, language, visuospatial skills, performance validity). There are a number of commercially available batteries that can be used for this purpose, including the Repeatable Battery for the Assessment of Neuropsychological Status (RBANS[48]), and while computerized cognitive batteries are still largely restricted to research, they may soon be available for clinical use. Some neuropsychologists choose to develop their own abbreviated battery in order to customize it to their preferences and clinical objectives. An example brief neuropsychological screen is presented in Table 9.3.

Implementing the brief neuropsychological screen approach allows for some cognitive information to be available to the team when delivering the PNES diagnosis and can also inform clinical decision-making upon discharge from a long-term video-EEG

Table 9.2. Comprehensive Neuropsychological Battery

Attention—refers to a number of processes that allow an individual to selectively direct or orient cognitive resources to a target while decreasing the allocation of cognitive resources to unwanted or irrelevant inputs.[27]

Basic attention span/ Registration	Wechsler Adult Intelligence Scale—Fourth Edition (WAIS-IV)[28] Digit Span Subtest
Sustained attention	Conners' Continuous Performance Test (CPT-II)[29]
Selective/Focused attention	Conners' Continuous Performance Test (CPT-II)[29]
	Brief Test of Attention[30]

Executive Functioning—These skills encompass a wide range of higher-level cognitive and behavioral capacities that allow an individual to pursue goal-directed behavior. Examples of executive functioning skills include working memory, response inhibition, problem-solving, and reasoning.

Working memory	Wechsler Adult Intelligence Scale—Fourth Edition (WAIS-IV) Working Memory Index (WMI; Digit Span, Arithmetic)[28]
Processing speed	WAIS-IV Processing Speed Index (PSI; Coding, Symbol Search)[28]
Flexibility—set-shifting	Trail-Making Test B[31]
Flexibility—response inhibition	Stroop Color-Word Interference Test[32]
Flexible problem solving	Wisconsin Card Sorting Test[33]
Abstract reasoning	WAIS-IV Subtests Similarities, Matrix Reasoning[28]

Memory—refers to the process of encoding, storing, and retrieving information.

Verbal memory	Rey Auditory Verbal Learning[34]
	Wechsler Memory Scale—Fourth Edition (WMS-IV)[35] Subtest—Logical Memory
Nonverbal memory	Brief Visuospatial Memory Test –Revised (BVMT-R)[36]

Language—Neuropsychological evaluation of language skills typically involves, at the very least, a screen of basic linguistic functioning (e.g., comprehension, repetition, reading, writing) and an account of higher-order language abilities (e.g., confrontation naming, verbal fluency).

Confrontation naming	Boston Naming Test[37]
Verbal fluency	Controlled Oral Word Association—Phonemic and Semantic Fluency[34]

(continued)

Table 9.2. Continued

Visuospatial Functioning—measurement of visual-perceptual skills, visuospatial processing (e.g., mental rotation, line judgment), and visual constructional skills.	
Construction skills	WAIS-IV Subtest Block Design[28]
	Rey Osterrieth Complex Figure Copy[31]
Motor Functioning—In PNES, reductions in motor speed may be related to a number of factors, including antiepileptic medications, psychomotor retardation, or factors specific to PNES that have not been fully characterized.	
Speed of fine-motor dexterity	Lafayette Grooved Pegboard[38]
Psychopathology (Self-Report)	
Psychiatric comorbidities	Beck Depression Inventory—Second Edition (BDI-II)[39]
	Beck Anxiety Inventory (BAI)[40]
	Generalized Anxiety Disorder (GAD-7)[41]
	Psychiatric Diagnostic Screening Questionnaire (PDSQ)[42]
Dissociation	Dissociative Experiences Scale (DES)[43]
Personality	Personality Assessment Inventory (PAI)[44]
Validity, Effort, Motivation—It is generally recommended that formal, stand-alone measures of performance validity and performance measures embedded in traditional tests be interwoven throughout neuropsychological assessments.[45]	
Formal measure	Test of Memory Malingering (TOMM)[46]
Embedded measures	Reliable Digit Span[47] using the WAIS-IV Digit Span subtest
	Personality Assessment Inventory (PAI) Negative Impression and Positive Impression Management subscales[44]

admission. A neurocognitive screen can serve as a triage to identify patients that would benefit from more extensive neuropsychological characterization as an outpatient. For example, a young adult who is functionally impaired and performs below expectation on a neuropsychological screen may benefit from a comprehensive neuropsychological evaluation in the outpatient setting to further characterize his or her cognitive profile and to determine what compensatory strategies may be most useful to improve functioning and ability to engage in treatment.

4. DIAGNOSTIC CHALLENGES

The heterogeneity of the PNES population has posed a significant challenge to characterizing the neuropsychological profiles in the research literature. This is reflected in the

Table 9.3. Brief Neuropsychological Screen

Attention	
Basic attention span/ Registration	Wechsler Adult Intelligence Scale—Fourth Edition (WAIS-IV)[28] Digit Span Forward Subtest
Executive Functioning	
Working memory	Wechsler Adult Intelligence Scale—Fourth Edition (WAIS-IV)[8] Digit Span Backward Subtest
Flexibility—set-shifting	Trail-Making Test B[31]
Memory	
Verbal memory	Rey Auditory Verbal Learning[34]
Language	
Verbal fluency	Controlled Oral Word Association—Phonemic and Semantic Fluency[34]
Visuospatial Functioning	
Construction skills	Rey Osterrieth Complex Figure Copy[31]
Psychopathology (Self-Report)	
Psychiatric comorbidities	Beck Depression Inventory—Second Edition (BDI-II)[39]
	Beck Anxiety Inventory (BAI)[40]
Validity, Effort, Motivation	
Embedded measures	Reliable Digit Span[47] using the WAIS-IV Digit Span subtest

sometimes conflicting reports on cognitive findings in PNES samples and the range of psychopathological mechanisms that have been linked to the disorder.

4.1. Nonspecific Cognitive Profiles

While it is true that PNES patients often perform outside of normal limits on formal neurocognitive measures,[1-5] focal and lateralized profiles have not been reported in the neuropsychology literature. Altered attention is perhaps the most consistent finding reported in individuals with PNES,[7,49] and it has been suggested that impaired attention plays the primary role in cognitive deficits in PNES.[50] *Altered attention*, as the term is used here, generally describes attention regulation difficulties that may impact a person's ability to initiate, divide, shift, or sustain focus. The PNES literature has found evidence for different forms of attention regulations difficulties, ranging from heightened vigilance (diminished ability to filter out irrelevant sensory stimuli),[51] to impaired response inhibition and divided attention (visuomotor set-shifting on Trailmaking Test B),[27,52] to weakness in working memory and cognitive flexibility.[27] Diminished executive function in PNES, most notably on a visuomotor sequencing and set-shifting task, has been associated with earlier age of symptom onset and greater PNES event frequency.[27] Attention and executive functioning difficulties have also been associated with impairments in verbal fluency,[27] as well as memory encoding and retrieval.[53]

Attention and executive function impairment profiles present a challenge because they are nonspecific findings without unique PNES links. Consequently, these findings may simply represent network disruption common to many psychiatric and neurological conditions. Nevertheless, the presence of attention and executive functioning difficulties is accounted for by conceptual models of PNES,[6,54] and the neurocognitive profile then provides evidence for overlapping network involvement between cognitive, motor, and psychopathological symptoms. The neuropsychology literature in PNES does not report focal findings or evidence for lateralized profiles, and demonstrating such findings on clinical neuropsychological evaluation would suggest the presence of a comorbid condition.

4.2. Psychopathological Heterogeneity and PNES Subgroups

A number of psychopathological mechanisms, such as conversion/dissociation, somatization, and PTSD, co-occur in PNES (for a review, see Baslet, 2010 [6]) and require examination in the context of a comprehensive neuropsychological evaluation. Self-report personality inventories, including the Minnesota Multiphasic Personality Inventory (MMPI-2/MMPI2-RF) and the Personality Assessment Inventory (PAI), have demonstrated good sensitivity to identifying conversion and somatization in PNES.[53,55] However, these inventories are lengthy and may lead to inconsistent responses. Inconsistent responses can invalidate profiles and are problematic in patient populations with dysregulated attention.

A number of studies have investigated subgroups within PNES.[2,56-63] These studies examine topics closely related to psychopathology, but focus on mechanisms that may be particularly informative to understand the development of PNES. They suggest that PNES patients have difficulty regulating emotion, and at least two types of maladaptive emotional regulation styles have emerged: "undermodulators" and "overmodulators."[57] The "undermodulator" group is characterized by emotional reactivity, poor arousal tolerance, and difficulties controlling affect. The "overmodulator" group is characterized by relatively normal personality profiles, minimal psychiatric comorbidity, emotional avoidance, excessively controlled behavior, and a tendency toward somatization.

Ultimately, the presence of subgroups will likely refine multiple aspects of the PNES literature and lead to improved treatment recommendations. The current challenge for neuropsychology is to determine how best to characterize these symptoms in a clinical evaluation. Self-report inventories and personality measures offer a number of options (see Table 9.4), although a measure specific to PNES subgroups, as they

Table 9.4. Self-Report Measures to Characterize Psychopathological and Emotion Regulation Subgroups

Psychopathology	
Somatoform dissociation	Somatoform Dissociation Questionnaire (SDQ-20)[64]
Psychoform dissociation	Dissociative Experiences Scale (DES)[43]
Emotion Processing and Coping Styles	
Subjective cognitive concerns	Everyday Problems Checklist (EPCL)[65]
	Memory Complaints Inventory[66]
	QOLIE-31[67]
Alexithymia	Toronto Alexithymia Scale-20 (TAS-20)[68]
	Berkeley Expressivity Questionnaire (BEQ)[69]
Emotion regulation	Affective Style Questionnaire [70]
	Difficulties in Emotion Regulation Scale (DERS)[71]
	Emotion Regulation Questionnaire (ERQ)[72]
Emotional intelligence	Trait Meta-Mood Scale (TMMS)[73]
Experiential avoidance	Multidimensional Experiential Avoidance Questionnaire (MEAQ)[74]
	Acceptance and Action Questionnaire-II[75]
Coping strategies	Brief COPE[76]
Perceived level of stress	Perceived Stress Scale[77]
	Depression Anxiety and Stress Scale[78]
Perceived capacity to tolerate distress	Distress tolerance Scale[79]

are currently defined, has not been developed. The addition of a personality instrument and a number of self-report inventories can significantly increase the duration of an already lengthy comprehensive evaluation. Treatment outcome research according to PNES subtype is also limited, thus some would argue that the characterization of subtypes on clinical neuropsychological evaluation has limited value. While this may be true, the information derived from these characterizations may be helpful to therapists who do not have particular expertise in treating PNES but are able to utilize information regarding personality constructs, emotion regulation styles, and coping strategies.

5. THERAPEUTIC GOALS OF NEUROPSYCHOLOGICAL EVALUATION IN PNES

Three therapeutic goals of the clinical neuropsychological evaluation in PNES include efforts to (1) improve a patient's understanding of cognitive symptoms (and correct misperceptions), (2) promote cognitive self-efficacy, and (3) direct patients to the most effective treatments. We discuss these goals in more detail in the next sections.

5.1. Improving Insight into Cognitive Symptoms

PNES patients often present with cognitive complaints that significantly contribute to functional impairment. While multiple studies demonstrate PNES patients overestimate cognitive impairment,[80,81] others found no such differences between PNES and epilepsy patients.[82,83] Specific patterns in PNES patients include a bias toward underestimating memory functioning and overestimating language functioning, but accurately assessing attention and concentration.[80] This suggests some misinterpretation of abilities, similar to somatization as a misinterpretation of bodily symptoms. Providing patients with psychoeducation regarding their cognitive profile and offering explanations for how these findings relate to their everyday difficulties has been shown to improve insight in both psychiatric and neurologic populations.[9,84,85] This is particularly true in patient groups with limited insight.[86,87] Improving insight has been shown to have downstream effects on treatment motivation[88] and improving insight into cognitive difficulties in PNES may have important implications for treatment.

The delivery of the PNES diagnosis is one opportunity for providing a patient with psychoeducation regarding their cognitive profile and how this profile fits within the diagnosis of PNES. It creates an opportunity to highlight the overlap in mechanisms underlying somatic and cognitive symptoms. This integrative understanding of the vulnerable cognitive-emotional system in PNES is described in more detail in an earlier chapter (Chapter 5). In brief, this model proposes that a stimulus (internal or external) that has emotional valence can "destabilize" or desynchronize the components of the cognitive-emotional system, and interfere with the coordination of attentional resources, resulting in aberrant behavioral, cognitive, and/or sensorimotor responses.[6] This model predicts the presence of cognitive symptoms in PNES and provides an integrated explanation for the coexistence of these symptoms. Therefore, one goal of integrating neuropsychological profiles into the presentation of the PNES diagnosis is to improve patient motivation to follow through with the recommended treatment plan by providing a more comprehensive explanation that involves various symptoms.

Specific psychoeducationally oriented cognitive interventions have not been reported in the PNES research literature. However, research in psychiatric populations that commonly present with cognitive deficits has demonstrated improved outcomes with the addition of psychoeducational interventions focused on cognition.[9,84] Therefore, the inclusion of neuropsychological data at the time of PNES diagnosis provides an opportunity to educate patients regarding their cognitive profile and potentially correct misperceptions regarding subjective concerns which can be held onto steadfastly by this population.

5.2. Promoting Cognitive Self-Efficacy

Cognitive self-efficacy describes the relationship between confidence and perceptions regarding effectiveness of cognitive functioning.[89,90] Among individuals with physical or medical illness, functional disability has been more strongly predicted by perceived self-efficacy than by level of impairment or duration of illness.[91,92] This finding is mirrored when specifically looking at cognitive dysfunction, such that studies have found cognitive self-efficacy and cognitive complaints to be more closely related than cognitive self-efficacy and cognitive capacity.[93-95] It has been suggested that cognitive self-efficacy may mediate the degree of improvement during cognitive training programs, such that an increase in cognitive self-efficacy facilitates more positive outcomes.[91]

For some patients, cognitive self-efficacy may be facilitated by providing psychoeducation at the time of PNES diagnosis (described in the previous section). However, other patients may benefit from engaging in longer-term work to improve insight, understand their cognitive abilities, and develop skills to compensate for their cognitive difficulties. *Compensatory skills training* describes the process of establishing new patterns of activity or behavior through external compensatory strategies or internal metacognitive strategies. The most frequently reported external compensatory strategies in the literature are written memory notebooks or daily planners.[96] *Internal metacognitive strategies* refer to interventions that develop patients' awareness and an approach to various cognitive tasks, such as sustaining attention, time/task management, and problem-solving. There are currently no treatment studies of cognitive rehabilitation in the PNES research literature, but this treatment modality has been successfully applied to a range of other psychiatric disorders, including depression,[8-10] bipolar disorder,[11] anorexia nervosa,[12] and obsessive–compulsive disorder.[13] There exists a need for more formal research on cognitive rehabilitation interventions as stand-alone treatments or a component of similar skills-based treatments (e.g., cognitive behavioral therapy) in PNES.

5.3. Informing Treatments Plans and Directing Patients to Specific Treatments

As more information is gathered to further characterize the heterogeneity of the PNES population, neuropsychologists will play an ever more important role in informing treatment plans and directing patients to the most effective treatments. To illustrate this, we describe how the neuropsychological evaluation accomplishes this in patients with low IQ or developmental disorders. We also highlight the potential for PNES subtyping as a means to inform treatment.

5.3.1. Treatment Planning in Developmental and Intellectual Disorders with PNES

Full Scale IQs (FSIQs), ranging from extremely low (intellectual disability range) to superior, have been reported in PNES.[49,52,80,97,98] However, many studies have found mean FSIQ in PNES groups to be significantly below the normative mean of 100.[7] Some authors argue that attention and working memory weaknesses may be influencing these findings[52]; however, detailed investigations of individual FSIQ constructs have not been reported in PNES.

Individuals with intellectual or learning disabilities may represent a unique subtype of PNES. Events in this group are thought to result from reinforced behavior as opposed to psychopathological mechanisms.[98,99] That is, in individuals with low IQ, events may be unconsciously learned behaviors that allow patients to control the environment and are reinforced by caregivers.[98] Immediate circumstantial triggers are also more common in PNES patients with learning disabilities,[98] suggesting that events are perhaps manifestations of reinforced behaviors. IQ has also been shown to correlate with the availability of psychological resources (e.g., frustration tolerance, self-esteem) and ability to cope effectively with stress.[100]

When a developmental or intellectual disorder is demonstrated as part of an individual's neuropsychological profile, this should prompt the neuropsychologist and the team to further examine the patient's history to determine if there are environmental or behavioral triggers that immediately precede PNES events. A functional behavioral assessment, where antecedents, behaviors, and consequences are defined, may be particularly helpful to understand the development of PNES in these patients.

Several studies have demonstrated that people with learning disabilities have the necessary prerequisite skills to engage in a range of cognitive-behavioral therapy (CBT) interventions,[101-103] including the ability to link situations to emotions,[101] the capacity to differentiate between thoughts, feelings, and behavior,[103] and the ability to correctly identify emotions.[102] However, CBT often has to be adapted for use in the treatment of individuals with developmental and intellectual disorders. For example, adaptions have improved outcomes in people with mild to moderate learning disabilities who suffer from a range of symptoms, including anger,[104,105] psychosis,[106] obsessive-compulsive disorder,[107] and depression.[108,109] Examples of adaptations include being more specific and didactic, presenting key concepts in extremely concrete ways, and providing extra support in the form of visual aids such as pictures, drawings, and signs for certain tasks.[110] Therefore, the neuropsychological evaluation can provide an understanding of the degree of developmental or intellectual impairment in order to recommend when adaptations to psychotherapeutic interventions for PNES are necessary.

5.3.2. Treatment Planning for PNES Subgroups

While treatment outcome research on PNES subtypes is limited, subtype classification has the potential to identify differential response to treatment variables that in turn have the potential to improve outcomes in this population. As mentioned earlier, at least two types of maladaptive emotional regulation styles have emerged in the PNES literature: "undermodulators" and "overmodulators."[57] "Undermodulators" are characterized by emotional reactivity and may align with PNES groups that employ emotion-focused coping strategies.[111] "Overmodulators," by contrast, are characterized by emotional avoidance and excessively controlled behavior and may utilize more task-oriented and avoidant coping strategies.[111] Therefore, it may be that "undermodulators" will have a greater treatment response to focusing on improving distress tolerance often described in the context of dialectical behavioral therapy,[112] whereas "overmodulators" may show a greater treatment effect for CBT strategies that build insight into one's emotional responses through monitoring and mindfulness.[113] Of course, these hypotheses require formal examination through treatment outcome research, but they illustrate the point that more nuanced characterization of PNES patients on neuropsychological evaluation has great potential to inform treatment and improve outcomes by tailoring treatment approaches to patients' psychological and behavioral profiles.

6. SUMMARY

The objective of this chapter was to present practical and diagnostic challenges in the clinical neuropsychological assessment of PNES patients in order to guide neuropsychologists in refining their approach to this patient population. These challenges were formulated from the perspective of a neuropsychologist functioning as a member of an interdisciplinary epilepsy team. As such, we recommend that neuropsychologists develop an integrated team-based plan (with input from other epilepsy team members) to inform neuropsychological decision-making. The final focus of the chapter was on therapeutic goals of the neuropsychological evaluation. PNES patients often present with subjective cognitive concerns, and the neuropsychological evaluation presents an opportunity to promote a patient's understanding of cognitive symptoms and identify cognitive, psychological, and personality characteristics that may ultimately be helpful for directing patients to the most effective treatments. The neuropsychological challenges and therapeutic goals addressed in this chapter are summarized as follows.

6.1. Practical Challenges for the Neuropsychologist

- Responding to PVT failures
- Different clinical environments (inpatient versus outpatient)
- Medications with cognitive sequelae
- Acute psychological distress
- Comprehensive evaluations versus abbreviated screening batteries

6.2. Diagnostic Challenges for the Neuropsychologist

- *Lack of specificity of cognitive profiles*—The presence of attention and executive functioning difficulties is accounted for by conceptual models of PNES, but these difficulties also represent network disruption common to many psychiatric and neurological conditions.
- *Psychopathological heterogeneity*—PNES subtyping may be a promising way to break down the population heterogeneity, but it requires further research to effectively inform treatment planning.

6.3. Therapeutic Goals of the Neuropsychological Evaluation

- Promote understanding of cognitive symptoms (and correct misperceptions)
- Promote cognitive self-efficacy through cognitive interventions
- Inform treatment planning and direct patients to the most effective treatments

REFERENCES

1. Binder LM, Kindermann SS, Heaton RK, Salinsky MC. Neuropsychologic impairment in patients with nonepileptic seizures. *Arch Clin Neuropsychol.* 1998;13(6):513–522.
2. Drane DL, Williamson DJ, Stroup ES, et al. Cognitive impairment is not equal in patients with epileptic and psychogenic nonepileptic seizures. *Epilepsia.* 2006;47(11):1879–1886.
3. LaFrance WC, Jr., Barry JJ. Update on treatments of psychological nonepileptic seizures. *Epilepsy Behav.* 2005;7(3):364–374.
4. van der Kruijs SJ, Bodde NM, Vaessen MJ, et al. Functional connectivity of dissociation in patients with psychogenic non-epileptic seizures. *J Neurol Neurosurg Psychiatry.* 2012;83(3):239–247.
5. Ding J, An D, Liao W, et al. Abnormal functional connectivity density in psychogenic non-epileptic seizures. *Epilepsy Res.* 2014;108(7):1184–1194.
6. Baslet G. Psychogenic non-epileptic seizures: a model of their pathogenic mechanism. *Seizure.* 2011;20(1):1–13.
7. Cragar DE, Berry DT, Fakhoury TA, Cibula JE, Schmitt FA. A review of diagnostic techniques in the differential diagnosis of epileptic and nonepileptic seizures. *Neuropsychol Rev.* 2002;12(1):31–64.
8. Elgamal S, McKinnon MC, Ramakrishnan K, Joffe RT, MacQueen G. Successful computer-assisted cognitive remediation therapy in patients with unipolar depression: a proof of principle study. *Psychol Med.* 2007;37(9):1229–1238.
9. Naismith SL, Diamond K, Carter PE, et al. Enhancing memory in late-life depression: the effects of a combined psychoeducation and cognitive training program. *Am J Geriatr Psychiatry.* 2011;19(3):240–248.
10. Naismith SL, Redoblado-Hodge MA, Lewis SJ, Scott EM, Hickie IB. Cognitive training in affective disorders improves memory: a preliminary study using the NEAR approach. *J Affect Disord.* 2010;121(3):258–262.
11. Deckersbach T, Nierenberg AA, Kessler R, et al. RESEARCH: cognitive rehabilitation for bipolar disorder: an open trial for employed patients with residual depressive symptoms. *CNS Neurosci. Therap.* 2010;16(5):298–307.
12. Wood L, Al-Khairulla H, Lask B. Group cognitive remediation therapy for adolescents with anorexia nervosa. *Clinical Child Psychol Psychiatry.* 2011;16(2):225–231.
13. Buhlmann U, Deckersbach T, Engelhard I, et al. Cognitive retraining for organizational impairment in obsessive-compulsive disorder. *Psychiatry Res.* 2006;144(2-3):109–116.
14. Larrabee GJ. Performance validity and symptom validity in neuropsychological assessment. *J Int Neuropsychol Soc.* 2012;18(4):625–630.
15. Bilder RM, Sugar CA, Hellemann GS. Cumulative false positive rates given multiple performance validity tests: commentary on Davis and Millis (2014) and Larrabee (2014). *Clin Neuropsychol.* 2014;28(8):1212–1223.
16. Mittenberg W, Patton C, Canyock EM, Condit DC. Base rates of malingering and symptom exaggeration. *J Clin Exp Neuropsychol.* 2002;24(8):1094–1102.
17. Williamson DJ, Drane DL, Stroup ES, Holmes MD, Wilensky AJ, Miller JW. Recent seizures may distort the validity of neurocognitive test scores in patients with epilepsy. *Epilepsia.* 2005;46(Suppl 8).
18. Orbach D, Ritaccio A, Devinsky O. Psychogenic, nonepileptic seizures associated with video-EEG-verified sleep. *Epilepsia.* 2003;44(1):64–68.
19. Bigler ED. Symptom validity testing, effort, and neuropsychological assessment. *J Int Neuropsychol Soc.* 2012;18(4):632–640.

20. Bigler ED. Effort, symptom validity testing, performance validity testing and traumatic brain injury. *Brain Injury.* 2014;28(13-14):1623–1638.
21. Dickson A, Toft A, O'Carroll RE. Neuropsychological functioning, illness perception, mood and quality of life in chronic fatigue syndrome, autoimmune thyroid disease and healthy participants. *Psychol Med.* 2009;39(9):1567–1576.
22. Ogden P, Pain C, Fisher J. *Trauma and the Body: A Sensorimotor Approach to Psychotherapy.* New York: W. W. Norton & Company; 2006.
23. Dandachi-FitzGerald B, Ponds RW, Merten T. Symptom validity and neuropsychological assessment: a survey of practices and beliefs of neuropsychologists in six European countries. *Arch Clin Neuropsychol.* 2013;28(8):771–783.
24. Marcopulos BA, Caillouet BA, Bailey CM, Tussey C, Kent JA, Frederick R. Clinical decision making in response to performance validity test failure in a psychiatric setting. *Clin Neuropsychol.* 2014;28(4):633–652.
25. Reuber M, Fernandez G, Bauer J, Helmstaedter C, Elger CE. Diagnostic delay in psychogenic nonepileptic seizures. *Neurology.* 2002;58(3):493–495.
26. Stulemeijer M, Andriessen TM, Brauer JM, Vos PE, Van Der Werf S. Cognitive performance after mild traumatic brain injury: the impact of poor effort on test results and its relation to distress, personality and litigation. *Brain Injury.* 2007;21(3):309–318.
27. Black LC, Schefft BK, Howe SR, Szaflarski JP, Yeh HS, Privitera MD. The effect of seizures on working memory and executive functioning performance. *Epilepsy Behav.* 2010;17(3):412–419.
28. Wechsler D. *Wechsler Adult Intelligence Scale*-Fourth Edition. San Antonio, TX: Pearson; 2008.
29. Conners CK. *Conners' Continuous Performance Test.* Toronto, Canada: Multi-Health System; 2002.
30. Schretlen D. *The Brief Test of Attention.* Lutz, FL: Psychological Assessment Resources; 1989.
31. Lezak MD, Howieson DB, Loring DW. *Neuropsychological Evaluation.* New York: Oxford University Press; 2004.
32. Golden C, Freshwater SM. *The Stroop Color and Word Test.* Wood Dale, IL: Stoelting Co.; 1994.
33. Heaton RK, Miller SW, Taylor MJ, Grant I. *Revised Comprehensive Norms for the Expanded Halstead-Reitan Battery: Demographically Adjusted Neuropsychological Norms for African American and Caucasion Adults.* Lutz, FL: Psychological Assessment Resources; 2004.
34. Strauss E, Sherman EMS, Spreen O. *Compendium of Neuropsychological Test.* Vol. 776-807. New York: Oxford University Press; 2006.
35. Wechsler D. *Wechsler Memory Scale*-Fourth Edition. San Antonio, TX: Pearson; 2009.
36. Benedict R. *Brief Visuospatial Memory Test-Revised Professional Manual.* Odessa, FL: Psychological Assessment Resources; 1997.
37. Goodglass H, Kaplan E. *The Assessment of Aphasia and Related Disorders*, 2nd ed. Philadelphia: Lea & Febiger; 1983.
38. Instrument L. *Grooved Pegboard Test User Instructions.* Layayette, IN; 2002.
39. Beck AT, Steer RA, Brown GK. *Manual for the Beck Depression Inventory Second Edition (BDI-II).* San Antonio, TX: Psychological Corporation; 1996.
40. Beck AT. An inventory for measuring clinical anxiety:psychometric properties. *Journal of Consulting and Clinical Psychology.* 1988;56(6):893–897.
41. Spitzer RL, Kroenke K, Williams JB, Lowe B. A brief measure for assessing generalized anxiety disorder: the GAD-7. *Archives of Internal Medicine.* 2006;166(10):1092–1097.

42. Zimmerman M, Mattia JI. The psychiatric diagnostic screening questionnaire: development, reliability and validity. *Compr Psychiatry.* 2001;42(3):175–189.
43. Bernstein EM, Putnam FW. Development, reliability, and validity of a dissociation scale. *J Nerv Ment Dis.* 1986;174(12):727–735.
44. Morey LC. *Personality Assessment Inventory–Professional Manual.* Odessa, FL: Psychological Assessment Resources, Inc.; 1991.
45. Heilbronner RL, Sweet JJ, Morgan JE, Larrabee GJ, Millis SR, Conference P. American Academy of Clinical Neuropsychology Consensus Conference Statement on the neuropsychological assessment of effort, response bias, and malingering. *Clin Neuropsychol.* 2009;23(7):1093–1129.
46. Tombaugh T. *Test of Memory Malingering (TOMM).* New York: Multi-Health Systems; 1996.
47. Axelrod BN, Fichtenberg NL, Millis SR, Wertheimer JC. Detecting incomplete effort with Digit Span from the Wechsler Adult Intelligence Scale-Third Edition. *Clin Neuropsychol.* 2006;20(3):513–523.
48. Randolph C, Tierney MC, Mohr E, Chase TN. The Repeatable Battery for the Assessment of Neuropsychological Status (RBANS): preliminary clinical validity. *J Clin Exp Neuropsychol.* 1998;20(3):310–319.
49. Kalogjera-Sackellaris D, Sackellares JC. Intellectual and neuropsychological features of patients with psychogenic pseudoseizures. *Psychiatry Res.* 1999;86(1):73–84.
50. Swanson SJ, Springer JA, Benbadis SR, Morris GL. Cognitive and psychological functioning in patients with nonepileptic seizures. In: Gates JR, Rowan AJ, eds. *Non-epileptic Seizures.* Boston: Butterworth-Heinemann; 2000:124–137.
51. Gene-Cos N, Pottinger R, Barrett G, Trimble MR, Ring HA. A comparative study of mismatch negativity (MMN) in epilepsy and non-epileptic seizures. *Epileptic Disord.* 2005;7(4):363–372.
52. Strutt AM, Hill SW, Scott BM, Uber-Zak L, Fogel TG. A comprehensive neuropsychological profile of women with psychogenic nonepileptic seizures. *Epilepsy Behav.* 2011;20(1):24–28.
53. Wagner MT, Wymer JH, Topping KB, Pritchard PB. Use of the Personality Assessment Inventory as an efficacious and cost-effective diagnostic tool for nonepileptic seizures. *Epilepsy Behav.* 2005;7(2):301–304.
54. LaFrance WC, Jr., Devinsky O. The treatment of nonepileptic seizures: historical perspectives and future directions. *Epilepsia.* 2004;45(Suppl 2):15–21.
55. Cragar DE, Schmitt FA, Berry DT, Cibula JE, Dearth CM, Fakhoury TA. A comparison of MMPI-2 decision rules in the diagnosis of nonepileptic seizures. *J Clin Exp Neuropsychol.* 2003;25(6):793–804.
56. Cragar DE, Berry DT, Schmitt FA, Fakhoury TA. Cluster analysis of normal personality traits in patients with psychogenic nonepileptic seizures. *Epilepsy Behav.* 2005;6(4):593–600.
57. Brown RJ, Bouska JF, Frow A, et al. Emotional dysregulation, alexithymia, and attachment in psychogenic nonepileptic seizures. *Epilepsy Behav.* 2013;29(1):178–183.
58. Duncan R, Oto M. Predictors of antecedent factors in psychogenic nonepileptic attacks: multivariate analysis. *Neurology.* 2008;71(13):1000–1005.
59. Kuyk J, Swinkels WA, Spinhoven P. Psychopathologies in patients with nonepileptic seizures with and without comorbid epilepsy: how different are they? *Epilepsy Behav.* 2003;4(1):13–18.

60. Holmes MD, Dodrill CB, Bachtler S, Wilensky AJ, Ojemann LM, Miller JW. Evidence that emotional maladjustment is worse in men than in women with psychogenic nonepileptic seizures. *Epilepsy Behav.* 2001;2(6):568–573.
61. Uliaszek AA, Prensky E, Baslet G. Emotion regulation profiles in psychogenic non-epileptic seizures. *Epilepsy Behav.* 2012;23(3):364–369.
62. Selkirk M, Duncan R, Oto M, Pelosi A. Clinical differences between patients with non-epileptic seizures who report antecedent sexual abuse and those who do not. *Epilepsia.* 2008;49(8):1446–1450.
63. Reuber M, Pukrop R, Bauer J, Derfuss R, Elger CE. Multidimensional assessment of personality in patients with psychogenic non-epileptic seizures. *J Neurol Neurosurg Psychiatry.* 2004;75(5):743–748.
64. Nijenhuis ER, Spinhoven P, Van Dyck R, Van der Hart O, Vanderlinden J. The development and psychometric characteristics of the Somatoform Dissociation Questionnaire (SDQ-20). *J Nerv Ment Dis.* 1996;184(11):688–694.
65. Vingerhoets AJ, Van Tilburg MA. *The Everyday Problems Checklist.* Lisse: Swets and Zeitlinger; 1994.
66. Green P, Gervais R, Merten T. The memory complaints inventory (MCI): memory impairment, symptom presentation, and test effort. *Neurologie Rehabilitation.* 2005;11(3):139–144.
67. Vickrey BG, Perrine K, Hays RD, et al. *Quality of Life in Epilepsy QOLIE-31 (Version 1.0) Scoring Manual.* Santa Monica, CA: RAND; 1993.
68. Bagby RM, Parker JD, Taylor GJ. The Twenty-item Toronto Alexithymia Scale-I. Item selection and cross-validation of the factor structure. *J Psychosom Res.* 1994;38:23–32.
69. Gross JJ, John OP. Facets of emotional expressivity: three self-report factors and their correlates. *Pers Individ Dif.* 1995;19:555–568.
70. Hofmann SG, Kashdan TB. The Affective Style Questionnaire: development and psychometric properties. *J Psychopathol Behav Assess.* 2010;32(2):255–263.
71. Gratz KL, Roemer L. Multidimensional assessment of emotion regulation and dysregulation: development, factor structure, and initial validtion of the difficulties in emotional regulation scale. *J Psychopathol Behav Assess.* 2004;26(1):141–154.
72. Gross JJ, John OP. Individual differences in two emotion regulation processes: implications for affect, relationships, and well-being. *J Pers Soc Psychol.* 2003;85(2):348–362.
73. Salovey P, Mayer JD, Goldman SL, Turvey C, Palfai TP. Emotional attention, clarity, and repair: exploring emotional intelligence using the Trait Meta-Mood Scale. In: Pennebaker JW, ed. *Emotion, Disclosure, and Health.* Washington, DC: American Psychological Association; 1995:125–154.
74. Gamez W, Kotov R, Watson D. The validity of self-report assessment of avoidance and distress. *Anxiety Stress Coping.* 2010;23(1):87–99.
75. Bond FW, Hayes SC, Baer RA, et al. Preliminary psychometric properties of the Acceptance and Action Questionnaire-II: a revised measure of psychological inflexibility and experiential avoidance. *Behav Ther.* 2011;42(4):676–688.
76. Carver CS. You want to measure coping but your protocol's too long: consider the brief COPE. *Int J Behav Med.* 1997;4(1):92–100.
77. Cohen S, Kamarck T, Mermelstein R. A global measure of perceived stress. *J Health Soc Behav.* 1983;24(4):385–396.
78. Lovibond SH, Lovibond PF. *Manual for the Depression Anxiety Stress Scales*, 2nd ed. Sydney: Psychology Foundation; 1995.

79. Simons JS, Gaher RM, Oliver MN, Bush JA, Palmer MA. An experience sampling study of associations between affect and alcohol use and problems among college students. *J Stud Alcohol.* 2005;66(4):459–469.
80. Fargo JD, Schefft BK, Szaflarski JP, et al. Accuracy of self-reported neuropsychological functioning in individuals with epileptic or psychogenic nonepileptic seizures. *Epilepsy Behav.* 2004;5(2):143–150.
81. Szaflarski JP, Hughes C, Szaflarski M, et al. Quality of life in psychogenic nonepileptic seizures. *Epilepsia.* 2003;44(2):236–242.
82. Breier JI, Fuchs KL, Brookshire BL, et al. Quality of life perception in patients with intractable epilepsy or pseudoseizures. *Arch Neurol.* 1998;55(5):660–665.
83. Loring DW, Meador KJ, King DW, Hermann BP. Relationship between quality of life variables and personality factors in patients with epilepsy and non-epileptic seizures. In: Rowan AJ, Gates J, eds. *Non-Epileptic Seizures*, 2nd ed. Boston: Butterworth-Heinemann; 2000:159–168.
84. Ruzanna Z, Marhani M, Parveen K, Cheah YC. Does psychoeducation improve insight of patients with schizophrenia? *Malays J Psychiatry.* 2010;9:27–40.
85. Hughes AJ, Beier M, Hartoonian N, Turner AP, Amtmann D, Ehde DM. Self-efficacy as a longitudinal predictor of perceived cognitive impairment in individuals with multiple sclerosis. *Arch Phys Med Rehabil.* 2015;96(5):913–919.
86. Yen CF, Chen CC, Lee Y, Tang TC, Ko CH, Yen JY. Insight and correlates among outpatients with depressive disorders. *Compr Psychiatry.* 2005;46(5):384–389.
87. Medalia A, Thysen J. Insight into neurocognitive dysfunction in schizophrenia. *Schizophren Bull.* 2008;34(6):1221–1230.
88. Markland D, Ryan RM, Tobin VJ, Rollnick S. Motivational interviewing and self-determination theory. *J Soc Clin Psychol.* 2005;24:811–831.
89. Cavanaugh JC, Green EE. I believe, therefore I can: self-efficacy beliefs in memory aging. In: Lovelace E, ed. *Aging and Cognition: Mental Processes, Self-Awareness, and Interventions.* Amsterdam: Elsevier; 1990:189–230.
90. McDougall GJ, Jr. A framework for cognitive interventions targeting everyday memory performance and memory self-efficacy. *Fam Community Health.* 2009;32(1 Suppl):S15–S26.
91. Cicerone KD, Mott T, Azulay J, Friel JC. Community integration and satisfaction with functioning after intensive cognitive rehabilitation for traumatic brain injury. *Arch Phys Med Rehabil.* 2004;85(6):943–950.
92. Kohler CL, Fish L, Greene PG. The relationship of perceived self-efficacy to quality of life in chronic obstructive pulmonary disease. *Health Psychol* 2002;21(6):610–614.
93. Aben L, Ponds RW, Heijenbrok-Kal MH, Visser MM, Busschbach JJ, Ribbers GM. Memory complaints in chronic stroke patients are predicted by memory self-efficacy rather than memory capacity. *Cerebrovasc Dis.* 2011;31(6):566–572.
94. Comijs HC, Deeg DJ, Dik MG, Twisk JW, Jonker C. Memory complaints; the association with psycho-affective and health problems and the role of personality characteristics. A 6-year follow-up study. *J Affect Disord.* 2002;72(2):157–165.
95. Reid LM, Maclullich AM. Subjective memory complaints and cognitive impairment in older people. *Dement Geriatr Cogn Disord.* 2006;22(5-6):471–485.
96. Cicerone KD, Langenbahn DM, Braden C, et al. Evidence-based cognitive rehabilitation: updated review of the literature from 2003 through 2008. *Arch Phys Med Rehabil.* 2011;92(4):519–530.

97. Bortz JJ, Prigatano GP, Blum D, Fisher RS. Differential response characteristics in nonepileptic and epileptic seizure patients on a test of verbal learning and memory. *Neurology*. 1995;45(11):2029–2034.
98. Duncan R, Oto M. Psychogenic nonepileptic seizures in patients with learning disability: comparison with patients with no learning disability. *Epilepsy Behav*. 2008;12(1):183–186.
99. Magaudda A, Gugliotta SC, Tallarico R, Buccheri T, Alfa R, Lagana A. Identification of three distinct groups of patients with both epilepsy and psychogenic nonepileptic seizures. *Epilepsy Behav*. 2011;22(2):318–323.
100. van den Hout M, Arntz A, Merckelbach H. Contributions of psychology to the understanding of psychiatric disorders. In: Gelder MG, Lopez-Ibor JLJr., Andreasen NC, eds. *New Oxford Textbook of Psychiatry*. Oxford, UK: Oxford University Press; 2000:277–292.
101. Dagnan D, Chadwick P, Proudlove J. Towards an assessment of the suitability of people with mental retardation for cognitive therapy. *Cogn Ther Res*. 2000;24(6):627–636.
102. Joyce T, Globe A, Moody C. Assessment of component skills for cognitive therapy in adults with intellectual disability. *J Appl Res Intellect Disabil*. 2006;19:17–23.
103. Sams S, Collins S, Reynolds S. Cognitive therapy abilities in people with learning disabilities. *J Appl Res Intellect Disabil*. 2006;19(1):25–33.
104. Rose J, West C, Clifford D. Group interventions for anger in people with intellectual disabilities. *Res Dev Disabil*. 2000;21(3):171–181.
105. Gulbenjoglu H, Hagiliassis N. *Anger Management: An Anger Management Training Package for Individuals with Disabilities*. London: Jessica Kingsley Publishers; 2006.
106. Kirkland J. Cognitive-behaviour formulation for three men with learning disabilities who experience psychosis: how do we make it make sense? *Br J Learn Disabil*. 2005;33:160–165.
107. Willner P, Goody R. Interaction of cognitive distortions and cognitive deficits in the formulation and treatment of obsessive-compulsive behaviors in a woman with an intellectual disability. *J Appl Res Intellect Disabil*. 2006;19(67–73).
108. McCabe MP, McGillivray JA, Newton DC. Effectiveness of treatment programmes for depression among adults with mild/moderate intellectual disability. *J Intellect Disabil Res*. 2006;50(Pt 4):239–247.
109. McGillivray JA, McCabe MP, Kershaw MM. Depression in people with intellectual disability: an evaluation of a staff-administered treatment program. *Res Dev Disabil*. 2008;29(6):524–536.
110. Hassiotis A, Serfaty M, Azam K, Martin S, Strydom A, King M. *A Manual of Cognitive Behaviour Therapy for People with Mild Learning Disabilities and Common Mental Disorders*. Camden & Islington NHS Foundation Trust and University College London; 2012.
111. Myers L, Fleming M, Lancman M, Perrine K, Lancman M. Stress coping strategies in patients with psychogenic non-epileptic seizures and how they relate to trauma symptoms, alexithymia, anger and mood. *Seizure*. 2013;22(8):634–639.
112. Linehan MM. *Cognitive Behavioral Treatment of Borderline Personality Disorder*. New York: Guilford Press; 1993.
113. Baslet G, Dworetzky B, Perez DL, Oser M. Treatment of psychogenic nonepileptic seizures: updated review and findings from a mindfulness-based intervention case series. *Clin EEG and Neurosci*. 2015;46(1):54–64.

Section IV
Principles of Treatment

10

Communicating the Diagnosis

Markus Reuber, MD, PhD

1. INTRODUCTION

A poor explanation of the diagnosis of PNES can seriously undermine a patient's confidence in the clinician and reduce the patient's ability to learn how to stop the seizures or to engage in further treatment. The conversation in which the clinician communicates the diagnosis of PNES is the greatest single opportunity in patients' illness trajectory to gain an understanding of the nature of their problem, which may allow them to find ways of controlling seizures or start them off on a longer process of recovery. This conversation is often complicated by the fact that patients are not only given the new diagnosis of PNES but also told that the previous diagnosis of epilepsy was incorrect.[1] What is more, a doctor with sufficient expertise to explain the diagnosis of PNES is usually not the first health professional to talk to patients about their seizures. Many patients have encountered clinicians with very negative attitudes toward PNES before speaking to an expert.[2,3] A previous experience of being considered a "faker" by a health professional is likely to make subsequent doctor–patient communications more difficult. While the studies discussed in this chapter leave no doubt about the therapeutic potential of the communication of the diagnosis, there is no compelling evidence base informing us how best to tell patients and their families about PNES. This chapter refers to what evidence there is regarding such communication, and because it is intended to be useful to practicing clinicians, it also draws on my personal experience in this area.

2. CHALLENGES INVOLVED IN COMMUNICATING THE DIAGNOSIS OF PNES

Clinicians with experience in this field are likely to be aware of the stark contrast between interactions after which patients stop having PNES when the diagnosis has been explained to them, and clinic conversations that extend well beyond the allocated appointment time and still leave patients feeling angry and with continued PNES—and that leave the physician feeling frustrated. Perhaps it is for this reason that clinicians tend to approach this conversation in a very cautious manner.[4] A qualitative study using conversation analysis to examine doctor–patient communication in depth has also provided objective evidence documenting that this conversation is often difficult and that almost all patients exhibit interactional resistance to a "psychological" explanation of their disorder.[5]

PNES are usually conceptualized as a dissociative response to threatening internal or external stimuli likely to have been caused by the interaction of predisposing, precipitating, and perpetuating factors.[6-8] However, most patients initially feel that their seizures could not possibly be related to "stress" or to how their brain deals with difficult emotions, difficult memories, or adverse life events. While patients with PNES are more likely to acknowledge that they have experienced more negative life events before developing seizures than those who have just developed epilepsy, they find it much more difficult to accept that these experiences could be relevant to the etiology of their seizure disorder.[9,10] What is more, the relationship between the development of PNES and adverse life events may be complicated. One study found no increased number of adverse experiences in a group of patients with PNES, but suggested that patients with this disorder had less effective ways of coping with their problems when compared to epilepsy controls.[11] Patients' coping skills may well be shaped by experiences in earlier life, which they may not be able to recall or find difficult to link to symptoms that developed many years later. Adverse experiences in early life may also be linked to alexithymia, a feature in many patients with PNES, which may make it harder for them to perceive or acknowledge any link between PNES and emotions.[12-16] An understanding of the personal relevance of experiences that are "objectively" only modestly traumatic may also be hindered by behavioral and cognitive avoidance tendencies which characterize the preferred coping strategies of many patients with PNES.[17] The combination of alexithymia and avoidance may explain why caregivers of patients with PNES usually have greater insight into the link between PNES and emotions than patients themselves.[18,19] These personal characteristics may also affect how patients experience their PNES. For instance, one study showed that patients are more aware of seizure-associated physical symptoms of emotional arousal than they are of mental anxiety symptoms. They may, therefore, report symptoms characteristic of a physiological stress response without recognizing the possible subjective emotional valence of these symptoms.[6]

In marked contrast to patients, neurologists tend to perceive PNES as a largely or entirely "psychological" problem.[20] In keeping with this, they think of psychotherapy as the treatment of choice for the disorder, whereas patients may fail to understand how psychological treatment could help address a physical problem.[21,22]

3. CHOOSING THE BEST SETTING FOR COMMUNICATING THE DIAGNOSIS

In this section I will discuss the best time and place of the conversation in which the diagnosis of PNES is explained, and who should be present during this encounter.

The experience of any episode of transient impairment of consciousness or self-control is likely to be frightening and may have social consequences (such as work or driving restrictions). Thus it is likely that patients would like to know as quickly possible what caused the paroxysmal symptoms. An accurate diagnosis at the earliest point possible is also important because the choice of treatment will depend on it.

Last but not least, outcome may be better in patients diagnosed early on in their illness trajectory (within a small number of weeks) rather than when they have adjusted to a chronic condition (after several months or even years).[23] Having said that, treatment (with, e.g., antiepileptic drugs [AEDs] or psychotherapy) is only likely to work if a correct diagnosis is made, and it may take time to collect enough information about seizures from the patient, witnesses, and investigations to make a clear diagnosis. Starting inappropriate treatment (e.g., AEDs for patients with PNES) is likely to make the disorder more chronic and intractable[24,25] and increases the challenge the clinician will ultimately face, for instance when the diagnosis of PNES is explained, and the previous diagnosis of epilepsy has to be "taken away."[1] There is no evidence about the relative merits of watchful waiting as opposed to early treatment based on an uncertain diagnosis. Both choices are associated with risks and benefits. There is also no evidence demonstrating whether it is easier or more effective to communicate the diagnosis of PNES after it has been confirmed by video-EEG. However, clinical experience suggests that clinicians are more comfortable and certain explaining PNES when the diagnosis is supported by the recording of a typical attack with video-EEG. The level of certainty of the diagnosis may also impact the patient and family's acceptance of the diagnosis. While studies examining the outcome of communicating the diagnosis are not directly comparable, studies in which almost all patients had video-EEG-supported diagnoses have reported higher rates of PNES cessation than those in which the diagnosis was based on clinical grounds alone in many patients.[23,26,27]

Given that there is evidence that experts are more likely to make correct diagnoses,[28] patients with seizure-like episodes should have access to an expert in this field within weeks of the initial manifestation of the disorder. An expert will also have a better understanding of when it is possible to make a diagnosis and when the diagnosis is sufficiently clear for treatment to be started.

In reality, the setting of the communication of the diagnosis of PNES is likely to be determined by local circumstances. However, the following issues may be considered: as stated earlier, doctors and patients hold markedly different views about PNES. The recommendation of psychotherapy is unlikely to make sense to patients who feel that they have a "physical" problem. It is likely to take time for patients to understand that they do not have epilepsy or another "physical" problem and that psychological treatment may help them. The situation is even more challenging when the clinician also has to explain that the previous diagnosis of epilepsy was erroneous and the treatment for it inappropriate.[1] What is more, in some cases the explanation that seizures could be linked to previous adverse experiences may cause patients to reveal serious traumas. If they are able to plan the conversation about the PNES diagnosis, clinicians should ensure that there is enough time to address the patient's doubts, questions or revelations. If a patient is admitted for video-EEG because of diagnostic doubt, the reason for admission should be discussed with the patient so that the potential diagnosis of PNES is not sprung on the person all of a sudden just before going home. Clinicians may consider offering two appointments 1 week apart to address any questions that have arisen after the explanation of the diagnosis or providing additional support from another member of their healthcare team after the diagnosis.[3,29] It may also be helpful if the explanation of the PNES diagnosis is followed by a brief psychoeducational intervention. Both one-to-one and group approaches have been described, aiming to give patients a better understanding of how stress or emotions can affect the body, recognizing stress factors in their own lives and learning basic grounding or relaxation techniques.[30-32]

Most neurologists in Western countries accept that explanation of PNES is part of their role.[21,22] It has been suggested that the additional early involvement of mental health professionals may be helpful, not only to address comorbid mental health problems but also to enable patients to make better sense of PNES and to facilitate engagement in further treatment.[33] Notwithstanding the particular specialisation of the person communicating the diagnosis, it is likely to be helpful if this person has a thorough understanding of both epilepsy and PNES, has made the diagnosis themselves or understands clearly why it was made, and is able to communicate the diagnosis with conviction. They should also be able to answer any questions the patient has about the condition or the diagnostic process.

Given how important caregivers or family members can be for support during seizures and for patients' acceptance of psychotherapeutic intervention, it makes a lot of sense to involve family members when the diagnosis is explained. While the input provided by some caregivers may contribute to patients' level of disability (for instance, when caregivers are overprotective), studies show that caregivers are likely to have more insight into links between stress or emotional problems and PNES than do the patients themselves, and that they are less reluctant than patients to accept psychological accounts of the disorder.[18,19] Caregivers may therefore support the explanation of the diagnosis and help the clinician convey a psychological account of PNES, not just by helping the patient remember what the clinician said. If caregivers are hostile to the diagnosis, their involvement in the conversation in which the diagnosis is explained provides the clinician with an opportunity to tackle their concerns.

4. HOW TO EXPLAIN THE DIAGNOSIS OF PNES

While a number of communication strategies have been provided to clinicians with advice on *what* to say when they explain the diagnosis of PNES, the question of *how* to talk about this diagnosis has been relatively neglected. Two studies based on one data set of video or audio recordings of 20 conversations in which neurologists explained their diagnosis and treatment recommendations to patients with functional neurological problems have provided some relevant insights (patients with PNES made up 17 of 20 cases). One of these publications provided objective evidence that almost all patients display resistance to the doctor's attempts to link their apparently physical problem to emotional causes or adverse life events.[5] The other publication demonstrated that the experienced neurologists whose activities were observed in this study seemed to anticipate these interactional difficulties, treating the upcoming diagnosis of PNES as problematic from the very start of the encounter (and at a point at which the patient had not demonstrated any resistance to their conversational objective). For instance, clinicians initially retook the history in almost all cases, even though they had done this previously and had already formulated their diagnosis and treatment plan. Most patients were initially told what was not wrong with them before they were given the diagnosis. These interactional maneuvers would be unexpected prior to the communication of a less problematic diagnosis and could conceivably provoke patients' resistance.[4] During the more difficult phases of the conversation, in which psychological causes for the disorder were discussed, doctors' talk was characterized by increased formulation effort (mid-sentence silences, repetitions, self-corrections, syllable stretching, self-interruptions, cutoffs, etc.) and accounting activities (doctors defending their conclusions). The resulting complex talk may well have contributed to the confusion that many patients report after the diagnosis of PNES has been explained to them.[3,34]

Based on these studies, there is considerable scope for clinicians to improve the effectiveness of their explanation of the PNES diagnosis. If the clinician wants to communicate that PNES are a relatively common problem that is neither more nor less "legitimate" or "real" than other causes of temporary impairment of self-control, they should find an explanation they can deliver fluently and with conviction. They should announce their diagnosis before discussing what the condition is not.

5. WHAT TO SAY ABOUT PNES

Four detailed communication strategies have been published advising clinicians what they may want to tell patients newly diagnosed with PNES (Table 10.1).[35-38] These strategies should not be seen as scripts suitable for all patients with PNES. The group of patients with PNES is very heterogeneous, with subpopulations that are distinctly different from the majority of patients presenting to neurologists (such as older people or patients with intellectual disabilities).[39,40] Communication of the diagnosis is likely to be most effective if it is adapted to the patients' particular circumstances. For instance, a study based on interviews with patients after communication of the PNES diagnosis suggested that patients with a history of significant trauma found it helpful if the neurologist mentioned that development of PNES may be linked to trauma, whereas those unaware of a history of trauma found it difficult to accept the diagnosis after the neurologist had strongly linked PNES with previous trauma.[3]

One key question is what to call the attacks and the disorder. The label "PNES" has dominated the scientific literature over the last 20 years, whereas "nonepileptic attack disorder" has been the preferred label in the UK. While "psychogenic" makes a clear statement about the presumed etiology of the attacks, this word does not reflect patients' own experience of their disorder as "physical."[20] What is more in a study of lay people's ratings of different terms, "psychogenic seizures" was perceived as only slightly less offensive than "pseudoseizures" or "hysterical seizures," suggesting that its use may raise doubts in the patient's mind that the doctor understands their problem as "real."[41] The term "nonepileptic" is also problematic: some patients never thought they had epilepsy, for instance, when PNES superficially resemble syncope rather than epilepsy.[42] Psychiatric labels ("conversion" or "dissociative" seizures) are not commonly used in publications or clinical practice, at least in English-speaking countries.[21,22] Seizure experts may not feel comfortable applying labels referring to particular intrapsychic mechanisms, which they do not feel able to identify. However, given that "dissociative" has the distinct advantage of being a "positive" term (not limited to stating what the seizures are not) and is the label

Table 10.1. Published Strategies for Communicating the Diagnosis of PNES

	Shen et al. (1990)[38]	Mellers (2005)[37]	Duncan (2010)[35]	Hall-Patch et al. (2010)[36]
Framing	• Good news—the seizures are not caused by epilepsy; explain video-EEG findings. • Bad news—we do not know the precise cause of the seizures but they are nonepileptic; antiepileptic drugs do not work. • Antiepileptic drugs may cause serious side effects.	• Cover reasons for concluding that the patient does not have epilepsy. • Convey what the patient does have (explain "switching off"; describe dissociation). • Emphasize that the patient is not suspected of "putting on" the events. • Reassure patient that he or she is not "mad"; the problem is common, and seizures are disabling.	• Explain how video-EEG works and how it has helped with the diagnosis.	• Genuine symptoms, real events can be frightening or disabling. • Label. Give a name for the condition. Give alternative names the patient may hear. • Reassure patient that this is a common and recognized condition.
Etiology	• Communicate to patient that we may never know what these seizures are but can work together on the problems. • In most cases seizures are eventually related to upsetting emotions of which patients are unaware. • Patients should be told that they are not crazy, that the seizures occur at a subconscious level. • A history of sexual abuse is discovered in many cases.	• Events are stress related but stresses may be difficult to identify. • Triggering "stresses" may not be immediately apparent. • Convey relevance of etiological factors in each patient's case. • Address maintaining factors. Worry about seizures may make them worse or more frequent. • Avoidant behavior may make seizures worse.	• Seizures are related to emotional and psychological factors, are due to past or present issues, and are not a medical condition. • List possible predisposing factors as "specimen causes" not directly linked to the patient. • Seizures are not under conscious control, but patients can learn to control them with help from a therapist. • Patients may have anxiety or low mood but are otherwise not mentally ill or "mad."	• Convey cause and maintaining factors: not epilepsy; predisposing factors are difficult to identify, can be related to stress; perpetuating factors are important (vicious cycle: worry or stress → events get worse → more worry). • Provide a model for the events—e.g., the brain becomes overloaded and shuts down.

Treatment	• This may be best addressed by a psychiatrist, psychologist, or counselor. • Neurological follow-up will continue.	• Caution that AED withdrawal should be gradual. • Describe psychological treatment.	• Describe psychological intervention. • Ask whether patients want psychological intervention.	• Talk about referral to a treatment specialist. • AEDs are not effective. • There is evidence that psychological treatment is effective.
Prognosis	• The seizures may stop spontaneously. • Seizures are subconscious but conscious effort can stop them. • Counseling may not control seizures immediately, but seizures can improve as treatment progresses.	• Symptoms may improve after correct diagnosis.	• Drug treatment does not work, psychological treatment can work, no other treatment is available.	• Seizures can resolve, the patient can expect improvement.

AED, antiepileptic drug.

suggested for the condition in ICD-10, this is currently my preferred description of the episodes.

It is also debatable whether the terms "attack" or "seizure" are most suitable.[43] "Attack" would differentiate PNES more clearly from epileptic seizures but suggests that PNES are caused by an external agent doing something to the patient. This is not how PNES are experienced by most patients.[44] "Seizure" is associated with the same problem; one linguistic study suggests that patients with PNES treat both terms as problematic.[45] The use of the words "turn," "do," "event," or "episode" may be acceptable to patients and doctors and help to demedicalize the problem. A "spell" would also imply causation by an outside force and may be something associated with witchcraft or evil spirits in the minds of some English speakers.

While reflecting on these issues may help doctors understand some of the difficulties patients face when the diagnosis is explained, it is likely to be more important that the diagnosis is presented empathetically than which label is employed (or whether a label is used at all). It is also important to ensure that the words used are supported by concordant nonverbal communication, supporting the messages that the clinician is trying to get across.

If PNES have been captured by video-EEG, all proposed strategies should be preceded by a search for confirmation that the recorded events are typical of the patient's habitual events. The strategy proposed by Shen also involves clinicians showing patients and caregivers a video recording of the PNES before delivering the diagnosis.[38] The benefits and drawbacks of looking at seizure recordings with patients and caregivers have not been studied. Patients may not be keen to watch videos of their seizures, but experience suggests that this can be helpful in a number of ways. Sharing the video may help to normalize the patient's seizure experience. The clinician's objective commentary on what is happening in the seizure may enable patients (and any caregivers present) to feel and think about their seizures differently. For instance, seeing a seizure in the presence of a clinician may help desensitize patients who may want to avoid looking at what happens in a seizure. What is more, patients may be more likely to think that the doctor understands the seriousness of their problem and less likely to think that their PNES are not being taken seriously if they know that the doctor has seen a seizure. Some patients look anxious or sad during their PNES, providing the clinician with an additional argument to convince the patient of the emotional etiology of their seizures. Last but not least, the video may allow the clinician to give more specific advice to caregivers about the acute management of PNES. Watching videos of a patient's PNES (and their epileptic seizures) together with caregivers is particularly important in the 10% (or so) of patients who have PNES and concurrent epilepsy.[46] In such cases, healthcare professionals need to invest time and effort to educate patients (and caregivers) about the differences between their PNES and other symptoms.

Unfortunately, there are no comparative studies to tell us which strategy works best in those areas in which the strategies diverge. Only one of these strategies has been tested in a prospective (but uncontrolled) study. This study concluded that the strategy (consisting of a crib sheet for neurologists and a booklet for patients) was acceptable and effective at communicating the possibility of a psychological etiology of PNES.[36] One in six patients who received the diagnosis in this way reported being PNES-free 6 months later.[26]

In contrast to the four strategies summarized in Table 10.1, I currently explain PNES as a reflex with which the brain has learned to deal with internal triggers (such as memories or feelings) or external triggers (such as perceived threats in the current environment). The trigger may be so fleeting (and the response so rapid) that the patient never becomes aware of it. By causing the brain to go into a kind of "freeze" mode, the reflex stops people from being aware of the threatening trigger. This means that each PNES moves the patient from a moment of perceived serious threat to a place after the seizure, when they may feel exhausted or upset but not acutely distressed. In this sense PNES work well. The fact that each PNES "works" means that the brain is more likely to use this reflex again to deal with similar triggers in the future. Unfortunately, many people also become unaware of their environment during their PNES and are unable to control their body. They may find the symptoms associated with their PNES unpleasant and become anxious about having PNES and the risks associated with PNES. PNES may help the brain deal with a problem in the moment, but they tend to cause problems in the longer term. Framing PNES as a reflex communicates that seizures are not willfully produced, although they may be suppressed. Reflexes are generally understood to be rapid, making it more acceptable that PNES could have been triggered by emotional reactions that the patient was not aware of. The reflex model also allows clinicians to explain how reflexes can be unlearned and replaced by other reflexes, providing a rationale for psychotherapeutic interventions.

Last but not least, the reflex model breaks away from traditional dualism, the separation of psychological and physical problems, that can become a major obstacle to patients engaging with psychological treatment for a problem they perceive as physical. In clinical situations in which PNES are associated with other functional neurological symptoms, this explanation can be extended by explaining that reflex action is taken in parts of the brain that process sensory inputs to the brain outside people's awareness. Symptoms such as sensory loss, abnormal posturing, tremor, and even weakness can be explained by slightly different things going wrong in the same parts of the brain.

6. OUTCOME AFTER EXPLANATION OF THE DIAGNOSIS OF PNES

Communication of the diagnosis is a potentially effective and highly important therapeutic step in the management pathway of patients with PNES. A study conducted in a video-EEG unit showed that the number of PNES was reduced in the 24 hours after the diagnosis had been explained.[47] Several retrospective studies suggest that about one third of patients will report that PNES have stopped when asked 3 to 6 months after diagnosis and with no further intervention.[48–50] Outcomes are even better when patients receive the diagnosis within a few weeks of seizure onset and from the first expert they see.[23,27] One prospective multicenter study with 6 months follow-up also demonstrated that PNES can cease with the explanation of the diagnosis alone, although in this study only 16% of patients were PNES-free at follow-up.[26,51]

Different studies have identified a range of (sometimes diverging) features predicting the likelihood of PNES cessation after communication of the diagnosis alone. Predictors of persistence of seizures include depression, personality disorder, and abuse history.[50]

Proposed predictors of PNES cessation include recent onset; acceptance of the clinician's explanation of the diagnosis; absence of comorbid anxiety, depression, personality disorder, or abuse history; access to friends; and continued employment at the time of diagnosis or lack of reliance on state financial benefits.[27,52,53]

The communication of the diagnosis, however, seems to have more significant effects on healthcare utilization than on seizure control. Reductions in healthcare expenditure overall, and in the use of emergency services more specifically, have been observed in several studies—even in those patients whose PNES failed to stop.[27,54,55] One large prospective study showed that the risk of patients developing other somatoform problems when PNES have ceased is small (at least in the short term).[56]

Having said that, it is important to highlight that explanation of the diagnosis has little impact on self-report measures of psychological distress, functioning, or health-related quality of life. The biggest prospective study of this issue showed no significant change in relevant measures after 6 months even when PNES had improved or stopped.[26] Furthermore, the encouraging short-term outcomes after explanations of the PNES diagnosis are not matched by those seen over the longer term.[51,53] Some early relapses after initial seizure cessation have been described in the short term.[23] These observations suggest that it is a minority of patients whose PNES stop in the long term with the explanation of the diagnosis alone. Most need more intensive and longer-term treatment.

Even with the clinician's best efforts, a substantial proportion of patients will fail to accept the diagnosis of PNES. Long-term outcome studies demonstrate that over 30% of patients with PNES and no additional epilepsy diagnosed at epilepsy centers continue to take AEDs several years after the diagnosis has been explained to them.[34,53] While there is no evidence for this, the risk of diagnostic drift from PNES (back) to epilepsy can perhaps be reduced and the effect of the conversation about the diagnosis enhanced if the patient is given written material about the diagnosis such as a leaflet, if the diagnosis is re-explained to the patient in a letter from the clinician, and if all relevant healthcare practitioners involved in the patient's care are informed about the diagnosis. It may also be helpful to offer patients a follow-up appointment, provide them with an opportunity to present any questions that emerge after the initial encounter, and ensure that they do not feel abandoned after the diagnosis of PNES has been made.[3] A website such as www.nonepilepticattackdisorders.info may enable patients to gain a better understanding of their problem on their own time.

7. SUMMARY

Communication of the diagnosis is a key moment in the course of a PNES disorder. Disabling PNES that have persisted for years may stop if the patient's thoughts and feelings about the problem have changed as a result of interaction with the clinician. PNES disorders, in contrast, may become more entrenched and future attempts to enable patients to gain control of their seizures less likely to succeed. While this chapter has provided some guidance regarding this conversation, it is important to note that explanation of the PNES diagnosis is likely to be most effective if it is adapted to the individual circumstances of the patient; one size will not fit all. The way in which the diagnosis is

Table 10.2. Do's and Don'ts in Communicating the Diagnosis of PNES

Do's	Don'ts
Do establish an alliance with the patient even before EMU diagnosis and mention the possibility of PNES.	Don't just spring the diagnosis on the patient.
Do ask what the patient's understanding of the problem is before embarking on an explanation.	Don't follow the same explanatory script for all patients.
Do demonstrate that you believe the patient (that the events are real and serious); show empathy verbally and nonverbally.	Don't imply that the patient is faking by contrasting PNES with "real" seizures or by telling the patient that the diagnosis is "good news."
Do name it: PNES, nonepileptic attack disorder, dissociative attacks	Don't just say what it is NOT (i.e., not epilepsy).
Do consider using a "reflex model" to provide an acceptable explanation in terms your patient can understand.	Don't just say the seizures are caused by stress.
Do reflect back with the patient and family to see what they understand and what they don't understand.	Don't rush the conversation.
Do assure patients that you will be part of their care as they transition to a mental health provider.	Don't say "I'm sorry, I can't help you. This isn't neurological."
Do use additional resources to back up your explanation (letter to patient, leaflets, Internet resources, e.g., www.nonepilepticattacks.info).	Don't continue AEDs "just in case."
Do communicate the diagnosis clearly to care givers and other health professionals involved.	Don't use ambiguous terms for PNES that can be misinterpreted.

AEDs, antiepileptic drugs; EMU, epilepsy monitoring unit; PNES, psychogenic nonepileptic seizures.

communicated is likely to be as important as the words that are used. Table 10.2 summarizes some thoughts about this important interaction between clinician, patient, and caregivers, in the form of do's and don'ts.

- The manner in which the diagnosis of PNES is communicated affects the prognosis of the disorder.
- The communication style has to be adapted to the individual patient's circumstances and must take into account the level of certainty of the diagnosis.
- How the diagnosis is communicated is as important as the words that are used.
- It is advisable to support the conversation in which the diagnosis is communicated with written information or reference to Internet-based resources.

REFERENCES

1. Karterud HN, Knizek BL, Nakken KO. Changing the diagnosis from epilepsy to PNES: patients' experiences and understanding of their new diagnosis. *Seizure*. 2010;19:40–46.
2. Worsley C, Whitehead K, Kandler R, Reuber M. Illness perceptions of health care workers in relation to epileptic and psychogenic nonepileptic seizures. *Epilepsy Behav*. 2011;20:668–673.
3. Thompson R, Isaac CL, Rowse G, Tooth CL, Reuber M. What is it like to receive the diagnosis of non-epileptic seizures? *Epilepsy Behav*. 2009;14:508–515.
4. Monzoni CD, Grunewald R, Reuber M. How do neurologists talk about medically unexplained symptoms? A conversation analytic study. *J Psychosom Res*. 2011;71:377–383.
5. Monzoni CM, Duncan R, Grunewald R, Reuber M. Are there interactional reasons why doctors may find it hard to tell patients that their physical symptoms may have emotional causes? A conversation analytic study in neurology outpatients. *Patient Educ Couns*. 2011;85:e189–e200.
6. Goldstein LH, Mellers JD. Ictal symptoms of anxiety, avoidance behaviour, and dissociation in patients with dissociative seizures. *J Neurol Neurosurg Psychiatry*. 2006;77:616–621.
7. Roberts NA, Reuber M. Alterations of consciousness in psychogenic nonepileptic seizures: emotion, emotion regulation and dissociation. *Epilepsy Behav*. 2014;30:43–49.
8. Reuber M. The etiology of psychogenic non-epileptic seizures: toward a biopsychosocial model. *Neurol Clin*. 2009;27:909–924.
9. Binzer M, Stone J, Sharpe M. Recent onset pseudoseizures—clues to aetiology. *Seizure*. 2004;13:146–155.
10. Stone J, Binzer M, Sharpe M. Illness beliefs and locus of control: a comparison of patients with pseudoseizures and epilepsy. *J Psychosom Res*. 2004;57:541–547.
11. Testa SM, Krauss GL, Lesser RP, Brandt J. Stressful life event appraisal and coping in patients with psychogenic seizures and those with epilepsy. *Seizure*. 2012;21:282–287.
12. Kooiman CG, van Rees Vellinga S, Spinhoven P, Draijer N, Trijsburg RW, Rooijmans HG. Childhood adversities as risk factors for alexithymia and other aspects of affect dysregulation in adulthood. *Psychother Psychosom*. 2004;73:107–116.
13. Brown RJ, Bouska JF, Frow A, et al. Emotional dysregulation, alexithymia, and attachment in psychogenic nonepileptic seizures. *Epilepsy Behav*. 2013;29:178–183.
14. Novakova B, Howlett S, Barker R, Reuber, M. Emotion processing and psychogenic nonepileptic seizures: a cross-sectional comparison of patients and healthy controls. *Seizure*. 2015;29:4–10.
15. Bewley J, Murphy PN, Mallows J, Baker GA. Does alexithymia differentiate between patients with nonepileptic seizures, patients with epilepsy and nonpatient controls. *Epilepsy Behav*. 2005;7:1165–1173.
16. Tojek TM, Lumley M, Barkley G, Mahr G, Thomas A. Stress and other psychosocial characteristics of patients with psychogenic nonepileptic seizures. *Psychosomatics*. 2000;41:221–226.
17. Dimaro LV, Dawson DL, Roberts NA, Brown I, Moghaddam NG, Reuber M. Anxiety and avoidance in psychogenic nonepileptic seizures: the role of implicit and explicit anxiety. *Epilepsy Behav*. 2014;33C:77–86.
18. Whitehead K, Stone J, Norman P, Sharpe M, Reuber M. Differences in relatives' and patients' illness perceptions in functional neurological symptom disorders compared with neurological diseases. *Epilepsy Behav*. 2015;42:159–164.

19. Reuber M, Jamnadas-Khoda J, Broadhurst M, et al. Psychogenic non-epileptic seizures: seizure manifestations reported by patients and witnesses. *Epilepsia.* 2011;52:2028–2035.
20. Whitehead K, Kandler R, Reuber M. Patients' and neurologists' perception of epilepsy and psychogenic nonepileptic seizures. *Epilepsia.* 2013;54:708–717.
21. LaFrance WC, Jr., Rusch MD, Machan JT. What is "treatment as usual" for nonepileptic seizures? *Epilepsy Behav.* 2008;12:388–394.
22. Mayor R, Smith P, Reuber, M. Management of patients with nonepileptic attack disorder in the United Kingdom: a survey of healthcare professionals. *Epilepsy Behav.* 2011;21:402–406.
23. Duncan R, Razvi S, Mulhern S. Newly presenting psychogenic nonepileptic seizures: Incidence, population characteristics, and early outcome from a prospective audit of a first seizure clinic. *Epilepsy Behav.* 2011;20:308–311.
24. Oto M, Espie CA, Duncan R. An exploratory randomized controlled trial of immediate versus delayed withdrawal of antiepileptic drugs in patients with psychogenic nonepileptic attacks (PNEAs). *Epilepsia.* 2010;51:1994–1999.
25. Oto M, Russell AJ, McGonigal A, Duncan R. Misdiagnosis of epilepsy in patients prescribed anticonvulsant drugs for other reasons. *BMJ.* 2003;326:326–327.
26. Mayor R, Brown RJ, Cock H, et al. Short-term outcome of psychogenic nonepileptic seizures after communcation of the diagnosis. *Epilepsy Behav.* 2012;25:676–681.
27. McKenzie P, Oto M, Russell A, Pelosi A, Duncan, R. Early outcomes and predictors in 260 patients with psychogenic nonepileptic attacks. *Neurology.* 2010;74:64–69.
28. Leach JP, Lauder R, Nicolson A, Smith DF. Epilepsy in the UK: misdiagnosis, mistreatment and undertreatment. *Seizure.* 2005;14:514–520.
29. Thompson NC, Osorio I, Hunter EE. Nonepileptic seizures: reframing the diagnosis. *Perspect Psych Care.* 2005;41:71–78.
30. Mayor R, Brown RJ, Cock H, et al. A feasibility study of a brief psycho-educational intervention for psychogenic nonepileptic seizures. *Seizure.* 2013;22:760–765.
31. Zaroff CM, Myers L, Barr WB, Luciano D, Devinsky O. Group psychoeducation as treatment for psychological nonepileptic seizures. *Epilepsy Behav.* 2004;5:587–592.
32. Myers L, Zaroff C. The successful treatment of psychogenic nonepileptic seizure using a disorder-specific treatment modality. *Brief Treat Crisis Interv.* 2004;4:343–352.
33. Harden CL, Ferrando S. Controversies in epilepsy and behavior: delivering the diagnosis of psychogenic pseudoseizures, should the neurologist or psychiatrist be responsible. *Epilepsy Behav.* 2001;2:519–523.
34. Carton S, Thompson PJ, Duncan JS. Non-epileptic seizures: patients' understanding and reaction to the diagnosis and impact on outcome. *Seizure.* 2003;12:287–294.
35. Duncan R. Psychogenic non-epileptic seizures: diagnosis and initial management. *Expert Rev Neurother.* 2010;10:1803–1809.
36. Hall-Patch L, Brown R, House A, et al. Acceptability and effectiveness of a communication strategy for the diagnosis of non-epileptic attacks. *Epilepsia.* 2010;51:70–78.
37. Mellers JDC. The approach to patients with "non-epileptic seizures." *Postgrad Med J.* 2005;81:498–504.
38. Shen W, Bowman ES, Markand ON. Presenting the diagnosis of pseudoseizure. *Neurology.* 1990;40:756–759.
39. Duncan R, Oto M, Martin E, Pelosi A. Late onset psychogenic nonepileptic attacks. *Neurology.* 2006;66:1644–1647.

40. Duncan R, Oto M. Psychogenic non-epileptic seizures in patients with learning difficulties: comparison with patients with no learning difficulties. *Epilepsy Behav.* 2008;12:183–186.
41. Stone J, Campbell K, Sharma N, Carson A, Warlow CP, Sharpe M. What should we call pseudoseizures? The patient's perspective. *Seizure.* 2003;12:568–572.
42. Benbadis SR, Chichkova R. Psychogenic pseudosyncope: an underestimated and provable diagnosis. *Epilepsy Behav.* 2006;9:106–110.
43. LaFrance WC, Jr. Psychogenic nonepileptic "seizures" or "attacks"? It's not just semantics: seizures. *Neurology.* 2010;75:87–88.
44. Plug L, Sharrack B, Reuber M. Seizure metaphors differ in patients' accounts of epileptic and psychogenic non-epileptic seizures. *Epilepsia.* 2009;50:994–1000.
45. Plug L, Sharrack B, Reuber M. Seizure, fit or attack? The use of diagnostic labels by patients with epileptic and non-epileptic seizures. *Appl Linguistics.* 2009;31:94–114.
46. Lesser RP, Lueders H, Dinner DS. Evidence for epilepsy is rare in patients with psychogenic seizures. *Neurology.* 1983;33:502–504.
47. Farias ST, Thieman C, Alsaadi TM. Psychogenic nonepileptic seizures: acute change in event frequency after presentation of diagnosis. *Epilepsy Behav.* 2003;4:424–429.
48. Aboukasm A, Mahr G, Gahry BR, Thomas A, Barkley GL. Retrospective analysis of the effects of psychotherapeutic interventions on outcomes of psychogenic nonepileptic seizures. *Epilepsia.* 1998;39:470–473.
49. Arain AM, Hamadani AM, Islam S, Abou-Khalil BW. Predictors of early seizure remission after diagnosis of psychogenic nonepileptic seizures. *Epilepsy Behav.* 2007;11:409–412.
50. Kanner AM, Parra J, Frey M, Stebbins G, Pierre-Louis S, Iriarte J. Psychiatric and neurologic predictors of psychogenic pseudoseizure outcome. *Neurology.* 1999;53:933–938.
51. Wilder C, Marquez AV, Farias ST, et al. Long-term follow-up study of patients with PNES. *Epilepsia.* 2004;45(Supp. 7):349.
52. Ettinger AB, Dhoon A, Weisbrot DM, Devinsky O. Predictive factors for outcome of non-epileptic seizures after diagnosis. *J Neuropsychiatry Clin Neurosci.* 1999;11:458–463.
53. Reuber M, Pukrop R, Bauer J, Helmstaedter C, Tessendorf N, Elger CE. Outcome in psychogenic nonepileptic seizures: 1 to 10 year follow-up in 164 patients. *Ann Neurol.* 2003;53:305–311.
54. Martin RC, Gilliam FG, Kilgore M, Faught E, Kuzniecky R. Improved health care resource utilization following video-EEG-confirmed diagnosis of nonepileptic psychogenic seizures. *Seizure.* 1998;7:385–390.
55. Razvi S, Mulhern S, Duncan R. Newly diagnosed psychogenic nonepileptic seizures: health care demand prior to and following diagnosis at a first seizure clinic. *Epilepsy Behav.* 2012;23:7–9.
56. McKenzie PS, Oto M, Graham CD, Duncan R. Do patients whose psychogenic non-epileptic seizures resolve, 'replace' them with other medically unexplained symptoms? Medically unexplained symptoms arising after a diagnosis of psychogenic non-epileptic seizures. *J Neurol Neurosurg Psychiatry.* 2011;82:967–969.

11

Clinicians' Response to the Diagnosis

Sigita Plioplys, MD, Shan Abbas, MD, and Brien Smith, MD

1. INTRODUCTION

A clinician's response to medically unexplained symptoms (MUS), such as psychogenic nonepileptic seizures (PNES), is a complex psychological process influenced by the dynamic interactions between clinician, patient, and medical and social systems–related factors. Patients with MUS comprise up to 30% of neurology outpatients[1] and they often experience physical and mental suffering as well as poor quality of life.[2,3] Although clinicians accept management of these patients as an important part of their daily clinical responsibilities,[4] the overwhelming majority find them difficult to deal with.

Patients with MUS often feel discounted and misunderstood by their physicians because of difficulties finding a medical explanation for their symptoms.[5] Lingering MUS and worries about undiagnosed "true" illness motivate patients to seek more medical services, use more time during doctors' appointments, and often dismiss the clinician's recommendations. A combination of patients' underlying personality and mood disorders further complicate patient–clinician interactions and communication. Excessive demands for personal attention, requests for disability to cover sick-leave or out-of-school time, and dissatisfaction with received care are additional variables associated with clinicians' perception of these patients as difficult.[6]

As a result, patients with MUS often carry a negative label of being "emotionally difficult, frustrating." Furthermore, the burden of excessive time commitment, consumption of medical and financial resources, coping with diagnostic uncertainties, and feeling professionally challenged, as well as doubts and frustration toward the patient's demands and symptoms, contribute to the clinician's negative attitudes.[4,7–11]

The therapeutic relationship between the patient and clinician is based on mutual trust and commitment to help. It is also influenced by the traditionally defined doctor's and patient's roles with socially accepted privileges and obligations. The patient assumes the "sick role," which carries the privilege of not being responsible for the illness, requiring care and support, and being exempted from daily responsibilities.[12,13] The obligations of the sick role include that the patient perceives the illness as "undesirable" and cooperates with others to achieve health.[12,13] The clinician's professional obligation is to decide which person is ill and therefore who can take on the sick role with the associated privileges. In cases of PNES, this obligation may be highly uncomfortable for the clinician and can be perceived as a "social cheating," particularly if the clinician doubts the diagnosis, believes that the presenting symptoms are under the patient's control, or perceives that the patient refuses to follow the clinician's recommendations to resolve the illness.[7] A clinician's personal discomfort with this diagnosis and its management may lead to difficulties reaching common ground with the patient, resulting in mutual frustration, premature termination of treatment, and further doctor shopping.

2. CLINICIANS' ATTITUDES TOWARD PNES DIAGNOSIS

More recent studies show that clinicians' attitudes toward the PNES diagnosis have been changing and becoming more positive. Two recent surveys of neurology clinicians in the United Kingdom and United States show that clinicians report having sufficient knowledge about PNES, with the majority of them accepting PNES's psychological model and feeling that they can diagnose PNES with confidence.[14,15] However, attitudes vary according to medical specialty.

Clinicians, including mental health providers, report conceptual and clinical misperceptions about PNES. Despite increased interest in and research on PNES, clinicians overwhelmingly report a better understanding of epilepsy than of PNES.[15] Several studies demonstrate that a large proportion of emergency and 35% of primary care clinicians do not accept PNES as a valid diagnosis, feel that video-EEG (vEEG) is not needed to make this diagnosis, and believe that patients use the PNES symptoms as voluntary attention-seeking behaviors.[16-18] A survey of 85 neurologists and psychiatrists in the United Kingdom revealed that both groups of clinicians think that PNES patients have greater personal control over their illness than those with epilepsy.[15] Further, 48% of nurses feel that PNES are "fake" and that patients have voluntary control over the symptoms.[16] Psychiatrists also report skepticism about the value of the vEEG in diagnosing PNES.[19]

Among the clinician-related factors, limited understanding and education about PNES can contribute to the sense of professional incompetency and anxiety about making diagnostic and treatment mistakes. As a result, a clinician may develop a negative attitude toward the disorder, which can further impact the therapeutic relationship with the patient, influence premature termination and affect treatment outcome, increase health care utilization, and contribute to stigma.[10,20,21]

Pridmore et al.[7] proposed that clinicians' attitudes toward any illness can range from protective and paternalistic to mistrustful and avoidant. A clinician who is doubtful about the accuracy of the diagnosis may develop a protective and paternalistic approach and recommend continuing the search for a "true" diagnosis, leading to additional testing, consultations, and continuation of treatment with antiepileptic drugs (AEDs). On the other hand, a clinician who feels skeptical about the nature and validity of this diagnosis or feels that the patient is "faking it" may develop a mistrustful and avoidant attitude. Negative illness-related attitudes affect how clinicians present the diagnosis and explain its development and treatment to the patients. A clinician's communication impacts how the patient perceives his or her condition.[7] A clinician's negative attitude may trigger patients' anger at and mistrust in the doctor, resulting in demands for further testing to prove the "real" nature of the illness.[7]

2.1. Case Vignettes

Cases	Comments
A 37-year-old veteran of the Iraq war with a history of mild traumatic brain injury (TBI) and post-traumatic stress disorder (PTSD) is referred to a university medical center by his neurologist in the community for drug-resistant seizures. He undergoes vEEG and is diagnosed with PNES. He is counseled about his diagnosis at the epilepsy center but is unable to attend psychotherapy as an outpatient because of the lack of available resources around his rural home. Three months later, he returns to see his neurologist for the first time since the PNES diagnosis. He has continued to experience seizures. The neurologist is frustrated and demands that the patient "just stop having these things."	This all-too-common scenario could have been avoided had the neurologist had a better understanding of PNES. Some neurologists have difficulty relating to the concept of dissociation or an altered conscious state that does not correlate with a specific neuroanatomical or neurophysiological abnormality and think that there may be a conscious or volitional component in symptom development and maintenance. The first opportunity for getting mentoring and education about PNES and having supervised engagement with PNES patients takes place during residency training; this opportunity can be pivotal in the development of empathy for the patient with PNES.
A 16-year-old female with a diagnosis of a drug-resistant seizure disorder for 3 years undergoes vEEG monitoring. The study records multiple habitual seizures and a diagnosis of PNES is made. Upon discharge, she is asked to follow up with her psychiatrist, who has been treating the patient for attention-deficit/hyperactivity and anxiety disorders for the past 4 years. The psychiatrist expresses uncertainty when the patient's parents ask how accurate the vEEG results are. The possibility that certain patients may have a mixed seizure disorder with epileptic and nonepileptic events is raised. The patient's parents subsequently ask her pediatrician to refer her for a second opinion. A repeat vEEG reaffirms PNES, with no data to support epileptic seizures.	In this case, reinforcement of the vEEG results and the PNES diagnosis by the psychiatrist may have saved thousands of healthcare dollars. It is important to acknowledge that some clinicians, including psychiatrists, feel that vEEG is accurate only some of the time. Collegial discussions about the strengths and weaknesses of vEEG should occur between mental health and neurology clinicians to achieve a common understanding of shared patients.

3. CLINICIANS' ATTITUDES TOWARD PNES TREATMENT

Despite the lack of evidence-based PNES treatment guidelines and confusion and skepticism about the diagnosis, clinicians show a positive attitude toward providing treatment for PNES patients. In a recent survey of academic neurology clinicians, 68% reported having sufficient knowledge about PNES treatment and 96% were very or moderately likely to discontinue AEDs for patients with PNES only.[14] Ongoing treatment by a mental health professional was a factor influencing the strength of decision to discontinue AEDs in about 35% of responders.[14] Also, responders with sufficient knowledge about the PNES diagnosis and treatment were less concerned about the potential for medical errors and were less influenced by requests made by patients or parents to continue prescribing AEDs.[14] Neurology clinicians report stronger confidence than primary care clinicians in managing PNES patients,[16] with 69% of neurologists continuing to follow the patients after the PNES diagnosis.[22] Fifty-two percent of primary care physicians felt comfortable following patients with PNES either with or without neurology back-up,[17] although up to 71% of primary care physicians said they would not adjust antiepileptic medications before a neurology consultation.[16]

Neurologists find patients whose symptoms are not explained by organic disease more difficult to help than those with well-explained neurological problems.[6] Thus, even though many clinicians are willing to treat PNES, frustration is still a common theme. In an attitudinal survey of primary care clinicians in the United Kingdom, 72% of responders perceived patients with MUS as causing considerable stress.[23] Clinicians may decrease their focus on and attention to the patient who presents with the same symptoms over and over again despite all of the interventions provided; clinicians may feel "stuck" with the same diagnostic and treatment dilemmas in chronic cases or as new somatic symptoms emerge. They may feel frustrated that they are unable to help the patient, despite their best efforts.[8]

A significant barrier in effective PNES management is difficulty arranging multidisciplinary collaboration between the mental health clinicians, neurologists, and primary care staff. Some neurologists understand their primary role as strictly providing a diagnostic evaluation and then referring patients to psychiatry for outpatient care. Yet the psychiatrists may resist treating new patients with PNES, especially if they are still taking AEDs, leaving patients with a sense of medical abandonment and a need to search for new clinicians who would "understand better."

Although it is generally agreed upon that mental health clinicians should take the primary role in PNES management,[16,24] the transition to psychiatry is often challenged by patients' resistance and limited referral sources, especially in child psychiatry.

Table 11.1. Clinicians' Attitude Problems toward PNES and Subsequent Consequences

Attitudes	Consequences
• The majority of clinicians find that patients with MUS, including PNES, are difficult to understand and manage.	• Clinicians experience feelings of professional incompetency, anxiety, stress, and frustration working with PNES patients.
• Clinicians often receive little formal training related to PNES.	• Many clinicians do not accept the diagnosis as valid and believe that the symptoms are voluntary, under the patient's control, and used to gain attention. • Clinicians' negative attitudes regarding PNES impact their relationship with the patient and the treatment outcome.
• Many patients with PNES also experience their own negative attitudes surrounding PNES and report feeling discounted and misunderstood by their clinicians.	• The patients' own desire for a medical explanation for their symptoms, along with the clinician's ambivalence about the PNES diagnosis, lead patients to seek additional medical services and ongoing treatment with AEDs.
• Many clinicians do not feel comfortable managing PNES, and the transition to psychiatric care can be viewed as ineffective and challenging.	• Difficulties with PNES treatment, including patient-related factors and difficulty with multidisciplinary collaboration, can lead to frustration among clinicians and avoidance of clinical involvement.

AEDs, antiepileptic drugs; MUS, medically unexplained symptoms; PNES, psychogenic nonepileptic seizures.

Furthermore, some primary care physicians and neurologists perceive psychiatric treatment as ineffective and mental health clinicians as not so skillful in treating patients with somatoform or conversion disorders.[4,24,25]

Clinicians' attitudes toward PNES patients and the consequences of such attitudes are summarized in Table 11.1.

3.1. Case Vignettes

Cases	Comments
A 35-year-old female with a long-standing history of physical, emotional, and sexual abuse is evaluated in the epilepsy monitoring unit. Her typical events are consistent with PNES. She is counseled about the diagnosis by a neurologist and starts a cognitive-behavioral therapy program with a therapist. She is also co-managed by a psychiatrist for depression, anxiety, and PTSD. Her primary care physician is given frequent management updates by her neurologist, psychiatrist, and therapist. Overall, the patient is very satisfied with her management plan; however, she continues to have PNES intermittently. She also develops multiple gastrointestinal symptoms with normal examination despite extensive testing.	PNES can be a chronic condition and its management is often prolonged. Transition from PNES to some other constellation of MUS is common. Multidisciplinary management strategies are key in successful PNES management. Primary care physicians' involvement is important, as often they will take the responsibility of coordinating and orchestrating care for the patient's somatoform symptoms and contain the amount of medical testing done.
A 15-year-old female with a history of seizures, juvenile-onset diabetes, and gastroparesis undergoes vEEG monitoring and PNES are captured. During the evaluation the treating neurologist also feels that the patient has a bipolar disorder and the neurologist is comfortable providing all care independent of a psychiatric consultation. The patient is placed on lithium, which worsens her gastric emptying, and she develops malnutrition. She presents to the emergency department with visual changes, unsteady gait, and sixth nerve abnormalities, leading to a diagnosis of Wernicke's encephalopathy.	Certain healthcare providers are overconfident in their understanding of the psychological underpinnings and psychiatric comorbidities associated with PNES and choose to manage complex patients independently. Not only may that lead to significant iatrogenic morbidity, it frequently creates an uncomfortable work environment where healthcare providers (nursing staff, medical assistants) are fielding phone calls and directing patients, with very little baseline psychiatric training.

4. POTENTIAL SOLUTIONS AND RECOMMENDATIONS

1) Knowledge about the developmental PNES models, clinical PNES features, differential diagnosis, classification, and practical management clinical skills help clinicians develop professional confidence and foster a more positive attitude toward patients with PNES and perceive them as "interesting" rather than "difficult."[6] Comprehensive

education and training about PNES should start early, in medical school or in residency training.

2) "Stepping into the patient's shoes" helps clinicians to better understand each unique patient's experience related to PNES and his or her personal suffering. For the patient, experiencing a clinician's empathy can promote bonding and aid in developing trust, cooperation, and compliance.[26] The perception that a clinician is available to understand and address the patient's emotional needs may reduce the patient's use of somatic symptoms to communicate psychological distress. For the clinician, experiencing empathy helps with building and strengthening rapport with the patient and contributes to better data collection and more effective care because the patient's communication will be clearer and will be predominantly verbal rather than "somatic."[26] Improved outcome and a trustworthy therapeutic relationship with the patient will increase professional satisfaction despite the challenging ambiguity of the disorder and the excessive time and effort spent on these patients.

3) When building a clinician–patient therapeutic relationship, "patient-centered" rather than "physician-centered" communication may be helpful.[5] A patient-centered, partnering approach includes and validates patients' illness-related experiences, acknowledges ambiguity, and seeks patients' input regarding the diagnostic testing and treatment. In contrast, in the "physician-centered" model, ambiguity is denied and termination of involvement is sought.[5] A partnering approach helps clinicians to develop more trustworthy relationships, guide patients to use appropriate health care services, and lower malpractice litigations.[5,27,28]

4) To better cope with frustration when dealing with PNES, clinicians can self-reflect to recognize their own anxiety, negative attitudes, disbelief, and reduced empathy toward PNES patients. Self-reflection can be facilitated through consultations with colleagues about difficult cases, seeking mentorship by an expert in the field, or through individual psychotherapy.

5) Active collaboration and communication with the multidisciplinary treatment team members can help clinicians feel more confident about the PNES diagnosis and less frustrated and more supported in providing care for patients with PNES. Mental health clinicians must become a central figure in the multidisciplinary treatment team, to provide necessary resources for the other clinicians and education about conversion disorder and comorbid psychopathology.

5. SUMMARY

- Many clinicians perceive patients with PNES as difficult to understand and manage and may experience professional anxiety, frustration, and a negative attitude toward providing care for these patients.
- Clinicians' negative attitude toward PNES patients can impact the therapeutic relationship with the patient, influence premature termination of treatment, increase health care utilization, and contribute to stigma.

- Education about PNES will help clinicians to develop clinical confidence and foster a more positive attitude toward patients with PNES.
- A patient-centered and partnering approach is critical to the successful therapeutic relationship and delivery of healthcare services to PNES patients.
- Mental health clinicians must become a central resource for the multidisciplinary care team members in coordinating services and communication between all parties involved.

REFERENCES

1. Carson AJ, Ringbauer B, Stone J, McKenzie L, Warlow C, Sharpe M. Do medically unexplained symptoms matter? A prospective cohort study of 300 new referrals to neurology outpatient clinics. *J Neurol Neurosurg Psychiatry*. 2000;68(2):207–210.
2. Reilly C, Menlove L, Fenton V, Das KB. Psychogenic nonepileptic seizures in children: a review. *Epilepsia*. 2013;54(10):1715–1724.
3. Barsky AJ, Ettner SL, Horsky J, Bates DW. Resource utilization of patients with hypochondriacal health anxiety and somatization. *Med Care*. 2001;39(7):705–715.
4. Reid S, Whooley D, Crayford T, Hotopf M. Medically unexplained symptoms—GPs' attitudes towards their cause and management. *Fam Pract*. 2001;18(5):519–523.
5. Epstein RM, Shields CG, Meldrum SC, et al. Physicians' responses to medically unexplained symptoms. *Psychosom Med*. 2006;68(2):269–276.
6. Carson AJ, Stone J, Warlow C, Sharpe M. Patients whom neurologists find difficult to help. *J Neurol Neurosurg Psychiatry*. 2004;75(12):1776–1778.
7. Pridmore S, Skerritt P, Ahmadi J. Why do doctors dislike treating people with somatoform disorder? *Australas Psychiatry*. 2004:12(2);134–138.
8. Ringsberg KC, Krantz G. Coping with patients with medically unexplained symptoms: work-related strategies of physicians in primary health care. *J Health Psychol*. 2006;11(1):107–116.
9. Salmon P. Conflict, collusion or collaboration in consultations about medically unexplained symptoms: the need for a curriculum of medical explanation. *Patient Educ Couns*. 2007;67:246–254.
10. Salmon P, Wissow L, Carroll J, et al. Doctors' responses to patients with medically unexplained symptoms who seek emotional support: criticism or confrontation? *Gen Hosp Psychiatry*. 2007;29(5):454–460.
11. Salmon P, Ring A, Dowrick CF, Humphris GM. What do general practice patients want when they present medically unexplained symptoms, and why do their doctors feel pressurized? *J Psychosom Res*. 2005;59(4):255–260.
12. Pilowsky I. *Abnormal Illness Behaviour*. Chichester, UK: John Wiley & Sons; 1997.
13. Parsons T. *The Social System*. Glencoe, IL: The Free Press; 1951.
14. Plioplys S, Siddarth P, Asato MR, Caplan R. Clinicians' views on antiepileptic medication management in nonepileptic seizures. *J Child Neurol*. 2013;29(6):746–750.
15. Whitehead K, Reuber M. Illness perceptions of neurologists and psychiatrists in relation to epilepsy and nonepileptic attack disorder. *Seizure*. 2012;21(2):104–109.
16. Sahaya K, Dholakia SA, Lardizabal D, Sahota PK. Opinion survey of health care providers towards psychogenic nonepileptic seizures. *Clin Neurol Neurosurg*. 2012;114(10):1304–1307.

17. O'Sullivan SS, Sweeney BJ, McNamara B. The opinion of the general practitioner toward clinical management of patients with psychogenic nonepileptic seizures. *Epilepsy Behav.* 2006;8(1):256–260.
18. Shneker BF, Elliott JO. Primary care and emergency physician attitudes and beliefs related to patients with psychogenic nonepileptic spells. *Epilepsy Behav.* 2008;13(1):243–247.
19. Harden CL, Ferrando SJ. Delivering the diagnosis of psychogenic pseudoseizures: should the neurologist or the psychiatrist be responsible? *Epilepsy Behav.* 2001;2(6):519–523.
20. Heijmans MJ. Coping and adaptive outcome in chronic fatigue syndrome: importance of illness cognitions. *J Psychosom Res.* 1998;45(1):39–51.
21. Morris A, Ogden, J. Making sense of children's medically unexplained symptoms: managing ambiguity, authenticity and responsibility. *Psychol Health Med.* 2012;17(3):285–294.
22. LaFrance WC Jr, Rusch MD, Machan JT. What is "treatment as usual" for nonepileptic seizures? *Epilepsy Behav.* 2008;12(3):388–394.
23. Dowrick C, Gask L, Hughes JG, et al. General practitioners' views on reattributions for patients with medically unexplained symptoms: a questionnaire and qualitative study. *BMC Fam Prac.* 2008;9:46.
24. McMillan KK, Pugh MJ, Hamid H, et al. Providers' perspectives on treating psychogenic nonepileptic seizures: frustration and hope. *Epilepsy Behav.* 2014;37:276–281.
25. Benbadis SR. The problem of psychogenic symptoms: is the psychiatric community in denial? *Epilepsy Behav.* 2005;6(1):9–14.
26. Klyman CM, Browne M, Austad C, Spindler EJ, Spindler AC. A workshop model for educating medical practitioners about optimal treatment of difficult-to-manage patients: utilization of transference-countertransference. *J Am Acad Psychoanal Dyn Psychiatry.* 2008;36(4):661–676.
27. Dugdale DC, Epstein R, Pantilat SZ. Time and the patient-physician relationship. *J Gen Intern Med.* 1999;14(Suppl 1):S34–S40.
28. Levinson W, Roter DL, Mullooly JP, Dull VT, Frankel RM. Physician-patient communication. The relationship with malpractice claims among primary care physicians and surgeons. *JAMA.* 1997;277(7):553–559.

12

Models of Care

Tyson Sawchuk, MSc, RPsych, Joan K. Austin, PhD, RN, FAAN
and Debbie Terry, MS CNP

1. INTRODUCTION

Diagnosis of psychogenic nonepileptic seizures (PNES) can pose challenges to medical and healthcare systems, as described earlier in this book, in Chapters 7–9 (Section III). Managing care in PNES is no exception and must be approached with careful thought to achieve maximum likelihood of success from both the patient's and caregiver's point of view. Once identified, the diagnosis of PNES must be adequately described to patients and their families. Additional care providers, including primary care physicians and mental health professionals, must also be given clear direction and rationale for the diagnosis. Treatment requires formulation and presentation to the patient in a manner that informs consent for treatment as well as expectations regarding outcome.

There are effective interventions available for PNES (see Part V of this book). Clinicians who are able to administer these treatments while monitoring results and managing difficulties along the way will maximize likelihood of success. Emerging evidence has begun to inform which treatments may be effective in managing PNES; however, there is an increasing need to translate theoretical knowledge into practice. Common setbacks in this process include nonresponse or nonadherence to recommended treatment due to factors including disbelief of the diagnosis. Reinvestigation by healthcare providers unfamiliar with PNES may also occur. The literature does not tell us what to do when these approaches fail, what to try next, or how to combine approaches. Despite frequent presentation of patients with PNES to epilepsy centers, no overarching models of care exist to guide providers through the many pitfalls encountered toward potential solutions.

Models of care for PNES are sorely lacking. Furthermore, a survey of healthcare providers within the United States Veterans Affairs (VA) healthcare system recently revealed substantial variation in care. Frustration was expressed by providers in regard to low patient acceptance, uncertainty about treatment approaches, lack of evidence-based treatment, complexity of care, and lack of collaboration between neurologists and mental health care providers.[1] Among patients themselves, there is uncertainty about the diagnosis and how best to proceed in managing their condition.[2] This uncertainty presents additional barriers, as patient perceptions profoundly impact PNES adjustment, acceptance, and compliance with treatment recommendations.[3,4] Clinicians and their patients, as well as healthcare systems, require models encompassing the necessary components of care while providing guidance on how to initiate, support, and fund treatments to manage this complex and challenging condition.[5,6]

2. BARRIERS TO CARE

2.1. A PNES Narrative

Consider the following example of a new PNES diagnosis. A patient is diagnosed with PNES by a neurologist. Unfortunately, because PNES is not considered a neurological disorder, the neurologist may not feel he or she needs to be involved in the patient's care after the diagnosis is communicated. The neurologist may not be entirely comfortable with the PNES diagnosis and therefore not provide an explanation of treatment that is understandable to the patient. This patient is referred to a mental health provider, but because of the lack of access, the person may not be seen for weeks or months, and even when seen may not be effectively treated because of the provider's lack of knowledge about evidence-based treatments for PNES. While waiting for appropriate treatment, the patient may continue to seek out opinions from other providers. As a result of poor communication among the different healthcare systems, further unnecessary evaluations are performed. The patient may be seen in multiple emergency departments and, owing to inadequate communication of the diagnosis and insufficient professional knowledge, may be treated inappropriately and even stigmatized, being told directly or indirectly that he or she is "faking it." Because the patient is interacting with several healthcare providers with varying degrees of knowledge about the diagnosis, he or she may become less and less confident the diagnosis is correct.

This narrative will resonate with most clinicians who have worked with PNES patients. Even when an accurate diagnosis is achieved, patients are often discharged from medical care. What happens next is poorly understood. Will the patient get better "on their own?" While this appears to be the case for a minority of patients,[7] it is unclear how long short-term improvements are sustained beyond follow-up periods.

2.2. Barriers Related to Clinician Knowledge

There are several factors that interfere with optimal and appropriate care for persons with PNES. These relate to inadequate knowledge of PNES care and negative attitudes toward the patient suffering the symptoms. Neurology providers recognize the importance of psychiatry in the treatment of PNES, but lack of access to psychiatric care can negatively impact outcomes.[8,9] Although in many areas access to mental health services can be limited, it may be particularly difficult for patients with PNES to access care from a provider who is knowledgeable about the diagnosis and confident in overseeing treatment. Many neurologists also believe that mental health providers are not interested in treating PNES, a belief that may be reinforced by prior negative experiences of treatment failure.[1]

Knowledge of PNES is limited among practitioners across several disciplines, including neurologists, psychiatrists, emergency department physicians, primary care physicians

(PCPs), EEG technologists, emergency medical technicians, and nurses.[9-13] Surprisingly, psychiatrists report a better understanding of epilepsy than of PNES.[11] Another study found that 35% of PCPs demonstrated disagreement with diagnoses of PNES despite lack of epileptiform correlation upon capturing an event.[13] Neurology providers report negative attitudes and frustration toward patients with a PNES diagnosis.[1] In another study, Worsley et al.[12] found that healthcare staff viewed PNES as a less chronic or serious condition than epilepsy, while 38% of general practitioners believed that PNES events are voluntarily induced![10] In another survey, 39% of healthcare professionals, 38% of PCPs, 25% of neurologists, and 48% of nurses endorsed that PNES patients should, in fact, have volitional control over their events.[14]

These studies demonstrate the prominence of erroneous beliefs among those most likely to come into contact with a PNES patient. The resulting attitudes may limit the empathy shown by healthcare workers toward persons with PNES while limiting the urgency they feel to diagnose and treat the condition. Being misunderstood and even blamed for their condition undermines patients' acceptance of a PNES diagnosis and will discourage follow-up with treatment.

2.3. Lack of Empirical Argument

The evidence for treatment in PNES has rapidly increased in recent years (see Parts IV and V of this book). The accumulation of studies to date is promising, and a number of educational, psychotherapeutic (group and individual), and psychopharmacology interventions have been described. What remains to be demonstrated are sufficiently powered randomized controlled trials establishing the impact of individual and combined treatments for PNES. The majority of studies to date are also limited by relatively short follow-up periods, rarely exceeding a year. Mental health comorbidity is the norm rather than the exception in PNES, and in fact typical diagnoses are likely to be relatively long term and chronic (e.g., depression, anxiety, dissociation). Another limitation of PNES studies lies in the definition of treatment "success." Although event frequency is the most common outcome variable in PNES studies, it is well established that productivity and quality of life are also severely affected and likely persist beyond resolution of PNES events themselves.[15] Adaptive functions, usually measured in the form of work or school days missed and disability status, are also negatively impacted in PNES populations and likely persist beyond typical treatment periods.[7,15]

2.4. Barriers Related to Diagnosis

Communication among health providers caring for a person with PNES is lacking. Patients often refuse to accept the diagnosis of PNES[16,17] and have lingering doubts,[18] leading patients and families to seek multiple opinions from different providers.[19] They often do not disclose the results of previous evaluations indicating diagnosis of PNES to avoid being dismissed by the provider. Persons with PNES and their families also do not share their diagnosis with coworkers or school personnel, resulting in unnecessary calls to emergency medical services.[20] An integrated medical record that can be accessed by healthcare providers in multiple systems could enhance communication and avoid repeated evaluations, but is unfortunately a luxury, not the norm, in most healthcare systems.

2.5. Barriers Related to Treatment

Once a diagnosis has been made, it is imperative that follow-up is made to ensure that the patient does not continue to seek out multiple opinions leading to unnecessary medical investigations. If care or follow-up is needed, who should be responsible? While 60% of healthcare practitioners in a recent U.S. survey thought it should be psychiatrists, 25% also thought it should be primary care physicians.[13] Patients are usually diagnosed by a neurologist and then referred to a mental health provider for treatment. The handoff between providers is often poorly coordinated. Patients may feel abandoned by the neurology provider. Often there is a time gap between the diagnosis and initiation of treatment due to a lack of mental health resources or refusal of the patient (and sometimes mental health providers) to believe the diagnosis.[18] Many neurologists do not continue to follow the patient after diagnosis and patients may become "lost in the system."[21] Patients may not follow through with the mental health provider and "fall through the cracks."[22] Communication and collaboration between the neurology and mental health care systems is needed; fortunately, there is increasing evidence of this collaboration. For example, McMillan et al.[1] found that some American VA facilities were developing cross-disciplinary teams with a neurology and mental health provider to treat somatoform disorders. Thompson et al.[18] have also shown that an educational intervention by a mental health provider at the time of diagnosis can improve follow-through with mental health appointments.

PNES events often occur in the community, including at work and in school environments. Without adequate communication between patient, family, healthcare providers, and staff at the school/work setting, bystanders may respond inappropriately, resulting in unnecessary hospital visits which only delay treatment and recovery. Children with PNES are often transported from school to the emergency department (ED) according to school policies for the treatment of epileptic seizures.[20,23] A consistent message that the events are not epileptic and do not require emergency intervention or rescue medication is needed in order to prevent ongoing doubts about the correct diagnosis. Anyone who interacts with the person should respond consistently to events so as to build the person's skill in aborting them. Care plans can be developed for school and emergency medical services to facilitate these types of responses, while first responders can also be taught to recognize signs of a PNES event.[24]

2.6. Barriers Related to Healthcare Systems

Additional barriers are posed by the structure of healthcare systems. In publically funded healthcare (Canada, for example), care may be undermined by a lack of co-ordination among clinics with separate and finite operating budgets. In the absence of a collaborative care model, administrators across medical and mental health departments often find it difficult to achieve common resource allocation in the service of PNES patients. Similar barriers exist in the United States, where communication between medical and mental health care systems is often fragmented. Care coordination challenges may also be observed among rurally located EDs and PCPs, where a diagnosis of PNES in one geographic region may not be communicated or known in another. In another example, sufferers of PNES in Japan have benefitted historically from continuity of care by psychiatrists able to diagnose and manage both epilepsy as well as PNES, thereby preventing lost follow-up due to care "handover" among providers.[25]

2.7. Lack of Integrated Care Models

Finally, while many factors are at play in achieving effective management in PNES, there is also a paucity of information and resources available to medical administrators on how best to provide these services. Healthcare systems require effective models for managing patients with PNES according to age, chronicity, comorbidity, and level of impairment. Effective care for PNES does occur, in our opinion, when provided by clinicians who have taken the time to understand PNES symptoms. Those who have done so have usually developed specific strategies for treating a population characterized by high levels of alexithymia and lack of emotional insight. They have developed successful collaborations among neurology specialists, primary care providers, and mental health providers in their communities. They also understand the strengths and weaknesses of the system within which they deliver their services and how this impacts patients. Determination of effective care in the case of PNES can be feasibly achieved by incorporating these components in clinically relevant and cost-effective deployments. Once developed, these models can be tested for positive outcomes independent of individual skill levels and personal characteristics. A summary of barriers to care in PNES is provided in Table 12.1.

3. PNES CARE MODELS: THEORETICAL CONSIDERATIONS

A model of care provides a conceptual representation of the relationships among health care personnel, resources, and services that are needed to provide patient-centered,

Table 12.1. Barriers to Care

Patient-Related Barriers
1. Lack of patient acceptance of PNES diagnosis
2. Lack of patient disclosure at work or school settings

Clinician-Related Barriers
1. Lack of knowledge and understanding
2. Lack of empathy and negative attitudes
3. Lack of ownership for management of treatment (i.e., mental health vs. neurology)

Healthcare System–Related Barriers
1. Lack of access to neurology and mental health services
2. Lack of care coordination and communication among different healthcare systems and providers

comprehensive care for patients. An ideal model of care for PNES should provide clear direction for making treatment decisions that are based on evidence-based interventions. Care models also need to take into consideration patient and family preferences and clearly identify resources needed for optimal treatment outcomes. It is important to distinguish that while treatment models often focus on evidence-based treatments in a specific, sequential manner, care models provide an overview of care components from an overarching healthcare system perspective. For example, while optimal treatment for PNES may include multidisciplinary diagnosis and treatment delivery within an integrated epilepsy clinic, such services may not be readily available given finite resources and logistical limitations within healthcare systems.

An example of a well-established model that has been found to be effective in improving outcomes in patients with a range of chronic illnesses is the chronic care model (CCM).[26,27] The CCM is an approach to improving ambulatory care for patients with chronic illness. The CCM contains six elements recommended for quality outcomes: a health system to provide structure and goals, links to community resources, support for patient self-management, provider access to evidence-based guidelines, clinical information systems that provide timely patient information, and a structure that supports team care. These six elements have been incorporated by health care systems to provide ambulatory care for a number of different health conditions.[28–31] In the CCM model, care is patient centered, and patients and families are informed and actively engaged with health care providers in making care decisions.[28] Another important element in care models is evaluation of treatment outcomes, or how well patients meet the goals of care.[32,33] The CCM has also been identified as relevant for treatment of epilepsy by the Institute of Medicine report on epilepsy.[34]

Care models require an understanding of patient perception, desires, and expectations. The patient perspective may be represented by identity, causes, consequences, timeline, and controllability of symptoms. Green and colleagues showed illness identity to be the most confusing aspect of care among PNES patients.[35] As a result, they proposed a self-regulation model in PNES care, primarily based on the belief that patient illness perceptions are key to recovery. Their model assumes people are active problem-solvers and motivated to treat illness according to their understanding of the problem. Any adequate model of care requires integration, not just of healthcare provider needs but of the patients themselves, who may then understand and take responsibility for their care.

It is recommended that, where possible, mental health care providers be located within the epilepsy center or neurology unit, as this facilitates overcoming many of the barriers to achieving effective care in PNES. The effectiveness of "co-locating" mental health care within an epilepsy monitoring unit (EMU) has been demonstrated to improve outcomes.[36] Benefits potentially include enhancing delivery of diagnosis (team approach by medical and psychiatric staff), avoiding care providers unfamiliar with PNES, avoiding premature discharge from medical care (which has been shown to reduce acceptance of diagnosis by patients and families), and provide buy-in of treatment by lessening stigma.

In an optimal model of care, patients would receive an early diagnosis, as neurology and ED staff/providers would have current knowledge of the diagnosis and how it is treated. The diagnosis would be explained clearly by both a neurology and mental health provider to help the patient and family understand it. The patient would then be connected with appropriate mental health services in a timely manner. The patient, family, and all members of the patient's healthcare team would understand the diagnosis and the plan for treatment and management of the events. Staff at school and work environments would also be educated about how to respond to new events. All of these care elements would help to ensure follow-through with evidence-based treatments for PNES as a result of participants having good understanding of 1) where to start, 2) where to go, and 3) when treatment may end.

4. PNES CARE MODELS: PRACTICAL CONSIDERATIONS

4.1. Stepped-Care

A stepped-care approach offers a strategy for efficiently managing health care resources.[37] This approach to treatment is based on the following assumptions: that minimal interventions (i.e., basic-level care, Level 1 care) are beneficial to PNES, that a stepped approach uses resources more efficiently than traditional care, and that incremental care is acceptable to both patients and providers.[38] Treatment provided in stepped-care models begins with the lowest intensity interventions and services and builds with each step, where greater intensity interventions and more services are offered. If patients respond to the lowest level of care, they are not offered higher, more intensive levels of care. By contrast, only those patients who do not respond are offered more intensive services involving greater cost and use of resources.

Stepped-care models have promise in treatment of PNES, and there is evidence that brief interventions may be effective in helping some patients with PNES. For example, an informational leaflet with 14 points describing patients' representations of their health condition was given to 50 patients newly diagnosed with PNES. A guide was also provided to their physicians with a communication strategy for providing information to patients. In follow-up interviews, 94% of patients who recalled receiving the leaflet found it easy to understand, with only 11% desiring additional information that was not included. At 11 weeks following diagnosis, seizure frequency had reduced in 63% of patients.[39] In another study, Mayor and colleagues[7] demonstrated that education alone led to 16% of adult PNES sufferers being seizure-free at 6-month follow-up, with an additional 23% showing 50% or greater reduction in seizure frequency. Very little change was observed however, on measures of impairment, including physical health, work/social adjustment, and activities of daily living, underscoring need for further intervention in these areas.

Use of a stepped-care model is also appropriate for PNES, as 1) patients differ in event severity and extent of comorbidities and 2) their relationships and families vary in level of dysfunction as well as in their ability to provide supportive and healthy environments. In our pediatric experience for example, desire for service may also vary according to a family's perceived ability to manage PNES symptoms on their own. These differences suggest that some patients might benefit from less treatment than others. Finally, Bower and Gilbody[38] suggest that for models to be successfully implemented, it is critical that providers are committed to following a stepped-care approach and that patients are willing to participate in care that involves initially receiving minimal level care, where indicated. For families to actively participate in a stepped-care approach, it is critical that they become knowledgeable about PNES and the outcomes associated with a stepped-care model.

4.2. Patient-Centered Care

Patient-centered care, a general approach to providing health care services in a manner that takes into consideration the patients' expressed needs, desires, and preferences, is recognized as an important element of high-quality care.[40] Historically, the roots for patient-centered care occurred in the 1970s when there was a shift from traditional disease-oriented approaches to care to more holistic healthcare that focuses on the whole person.[40] A patient-centered approach to care for PNES places the patient at the center of care, rather than the PNES symptoms being the primary focus. When the patient is a child, it is the child and the family who are at the center of care. Sidani et al.[41] describe three components of patient-centered care: 1) holistic care that addresses all domains of health; 2) healthcare professional and patient and family work together in a partnership; and 3) the care that the patient and family receive is consistent with their needs, desires, and preferences. This approach is also consistent with recommendations for optimal epilepsy care outcomes by Gruman et al.,[42] who emphasize the importance of productive interactions between healthcare providers and patients at key points of care, beginning at initial screening/assessment and continuing throughout treatment and follow-up.

4.3. The Care Manager

Care coordination has been defined by the Agency for Healthcare Research and Quality (AHRQ) as the deliberate organization of patient care activities and sharing of information among all participants concerned with a patient's care to achieve safer and more effective care. Ideally, one person should be tasked with managing the care coordination. The particular person who fills this role may vary from one setting to another. As an example, the Institute for Healthcare Improvement (IHI) has suggested social workers may have an ideal skill set for coordinating care among persons with mental health disorders.[43]

Examples of care coordination activities include the following: 1) establishing accountability and agreeing on responsibilities; 2) communicating/sharing knowledge; 3) helping with transitions in care; 4) assessing patient needs and goals; 5) creating a proactive care plan; 6) monitoring; and 7) follow-up, including responding to changes in the patients' needs, supporting patients' self-management goals, linking to community resources, and working to align resources with patient and population needs (AHRQ).

Persons with PNES are often seen by a number of different providers in different facilities. Once a diagnosis of PNES is suspected or diagnosed, clear communication is needed among all providers regarding the diagnosis, treatment plan, and response plan for events. This may reduce unnecessary investigations and potentially harmful interventions for assumed epileptic seizures, while optimizing appropriate treatment for the diagnosis. A summary of these recommendations is provided in Table 12.2.

Table 12.2. Recommended Components of Care Models in PNES

Psychogenic Nonepileptic Seizures (PNES)
Care Model Recommendations
1. A stepped-care approach that recognizes
    a. PNES symptoms may respond to time-limited intervention (education, brief psychotherapy).
    b. Where non-response occurs, increased intensity and resources may be required.
2. A patient-centered approach is used that addresses patients' expressed needs, desires, and preferences.
3. Ideally, a mental health clinician familiar with PNES is embedded or co-located within the neurology clinic or epilepsy monitoring unit (EMU).
4. Treat PNES under the respectful assumption that patients and their families are active problem-solvers and motivated to treat their illness according to their understanding of the problem.
5. A care manager is designated in the model:
    a. May be clinic nurse, psychologist, physician, or social worker
    b. Designated professional must have timely access to care provider team as well as decision-making capacity
    c. Patient and family agree to access the care manager, who is available to respond to concerns in a timely manner.
6. Regular and timely follow-up (preferably by care manager or clinic nurse) occurs, to maintain continuity of care and identification of deviations from care model.
7. Neurology and medical services maintain involvement until discharge from PNES treatment.

5. CARE MODEL EXAMPLES

5.1. Pediatrics

The PNES Care Model implemented at Alberta Children's Hospital (ACH) is a systematic approach to the treatment of PNES in children and their families.[44] The model uses a stepped-care approach involving evaluation of responses to treatment and interactions with the family at each level of care. The ACH model (Figure 12.1) describes the care process at the immediate point paroxysmal events are suspected as having a psychogenic origin. All patients and their families receive base level of care, identified as initial presentation of diagnosis and reassurance by the neurologist. This is followed by education and first aid instructions for PNES events by the clinic nurse. Initiation of antiepileptic drug (AED) reduction follows where indicated. At the base level of care, families are offered psychological consultation but may also choose a self-help approach to facilitating recovery (e.g., removing an environmental trigger, arranging for private third-party services) or decline treatment in favor of a "wait and see" approach. Families accepting psychological consultation or experiencing remission failure at base-level care are expedited to Level 1, consisting of formal psychological assessment/consultation and feedback around psychological functioning as it relates to PNES symptoms.

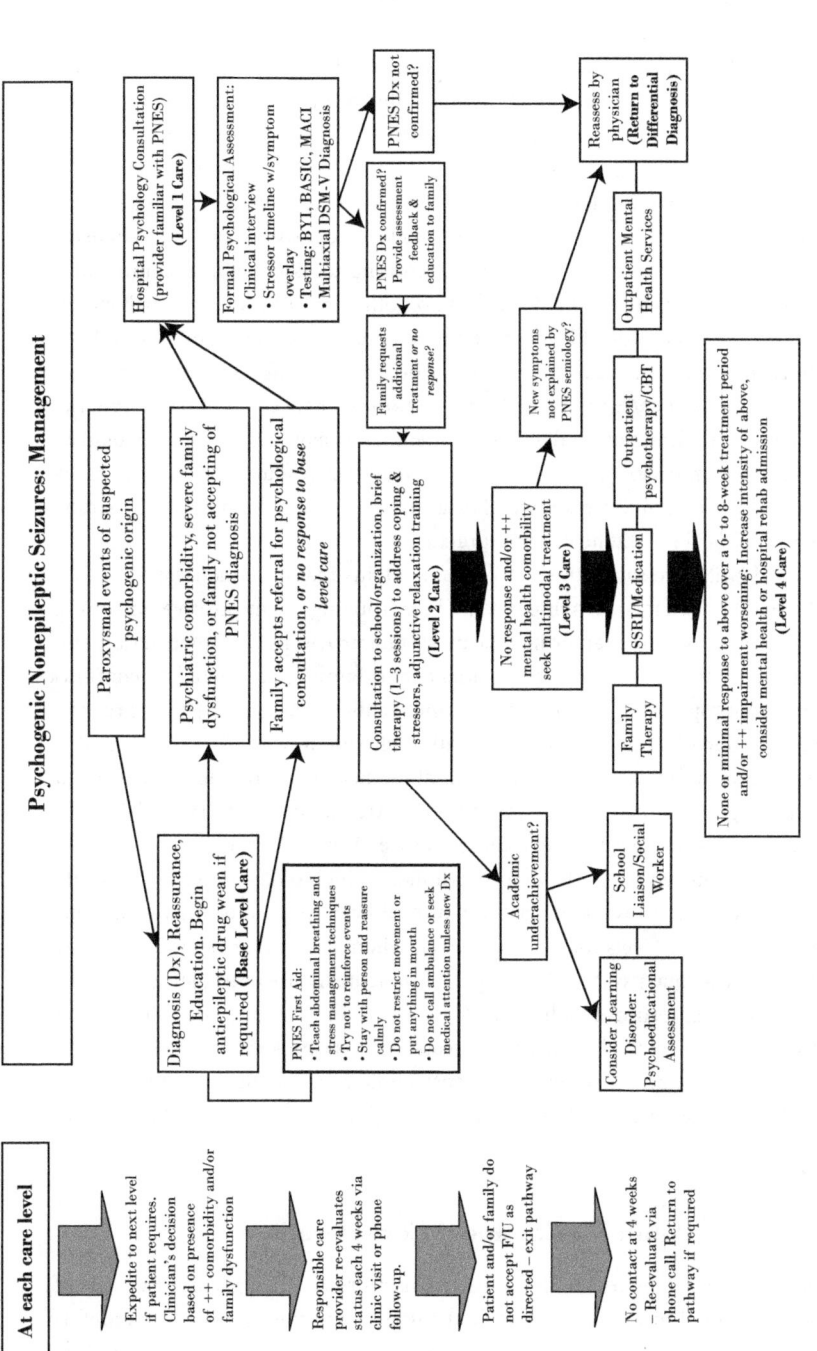

Figure 12.1 Alberta Children's Hospital (ACH) pediatric psychogenic nonepileptic seizures (PNES) care model. CBT, cognitive-behavioral therapy; DSM-IV, *Diagnostic & Statistical Manual of Mental Disorders*, fourth edition; F/U, follow-up; SSRI, serotonin selective reuptake inhibitor; BASC, Behavior Assessment System for Children; BYI, Beck Youth Inventories; MACI, Millon Adolescent Clinical Inventory.

At any stage, if the PNES diagnosis is not confirmed by psychological assessment, the child and family may be referred back to their neurologist for reassessment. Cross-disciplinary collaboration may occur in favor of a working diagnosis while ruling out other possible psychological or physiological causes of paroxysmal events (e.g., panic attack, migraine, vasovagal response). Lack of response to Level 1 care leads to the child and family receiving Level 2 care, consisting of increased involvement by a clinical psychologist specializing in PNES, consultation to outside agencies (e.g., school personnel, social services), and initiation of psychotherapy in the context of PNES symptom management (e.g., address acute stressors, teach coping strategies). In accordance with a stepped-care approach, lack of response to Level 2 care leads to Level 3, consisting of comprehensive outpatient mental health services (determined according to assessment recommendations) and may include psychiatric medication, psychotherapy (i.e., cognitive behavioral therapy), family therapy, and social work (as required for parent support and resourcing). Lack of response to Level 3 over a 6- to 8-week period, prompts efforts to increase intensity of treatment at Level 4 care. In this highest and most intensive level of treatment, the child is considered for admission to daily or inpatient treatment, usually in a hospital or rehabilitation setting, in order to receive intensive treatment resources.[44] Level 4 care is intended to represent maximum resource allocation, followed by maintenance therapy consistent with standard mental health care practice.

The pediatric PNES care model just described contains many characteristics similar to those in the CCM described as being essential for bringing about positive outcomes. Treatment is delivered within a larger healthcare system providing for organization and support for implementation of team care; patients and families are linked to community resources as appropriate (or preferred) by family; children and their parents receive self-management education and support; evaluation of patient response to treatment is assessed at each level of care; and children and families meet with providers to engage in decision making regarding their future care. Another strength of the ACH model lies in provision of an infrastructure for patient-centered care. At each level of care, the family engages in conversations with healthcare professionals, which offers ample opportunity for families and providers to work as partners in healthcare decisions. This is demonstrated primarily at earlier levels (base, 1, or 2 level) where parents (or neurologist) may be hesitant to initiate formal psychiatric care given the acute nature of triggers (e.g., transient family crises or "exposure" of a hidden stressor) or out of respect for autonomy of the child and family to elect for less intensive treatment. As care level increases, so does more specialized support provided by the epilepsy clinic psychologist and allied health team, in collaboration with other hospital areas (psychiatry, pediatrics, rehabilitation services, etc.).

5.2. Adult PNES Model Considerations

An adult PNES model is depicted in Figure 12.2. This representation includes aspects of the pediatric care model just described while demonstrating the necessity for redefining stepped-care decisions based on type of impairment (e.g., work versus school). The adult model also incorporates family members and recognizes adult PNES may be more chronic and requiring longer-term follow-up than in children. As a result, the adult care

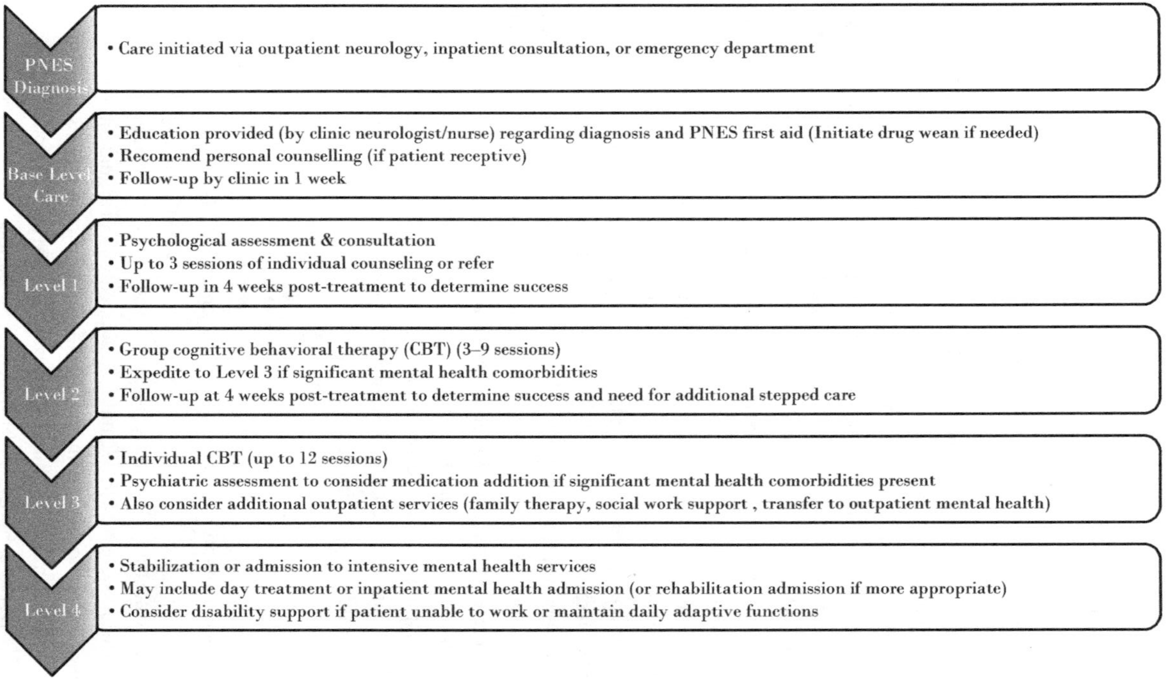

PNES Diagnosis
- Care initiated via outpatient neurology, inpatient consultation, or emergency department

Base Level Care
- Education provided (by clinic neurologist/nurse) regarding diagnosis and PNES first aid (Initiate drug wean if needed)
- Recomend personal counselling (if patient receptive)
- Follow-up by clinic in 1 week

Level 1
- Psychological assessment & consultation
- Up to 3 sessions of individual counseling or refer
- Follow-up in 4 weeks post-treatment to determine success

Level 2
- Group cognitive behavioral therapy (CBT) (3–9 sessions)
- Expedite to Level 3 if significant mental health comorbidities
- Follow-up at 4 weeks post-treatment to determine success and need for additional stepped care

Level 3
- Individual CBT (up to 12 sessions)
- Psychiatric assessment to consider medication addition if significant mental health comorbidities present
- Also consider additional outpatient services (family therapy, social work support , transfer to outpatient mental health)

Level 4
- Stabilization or admission to intensive mental health services
- May include day treatment or inpatient mental health admission (or rehabilitation admission if more appropriate)
- Consider disability support if patient unable to work or maintain daily adaptive functions

Figure 12.2 Care model example—adult PNES care.

model also includes identification of community supports and considerations for coverage by disability insurance.

6. FUTURE DIRECTIONS

Significant barriers to care exist in the diagnosis and management of PNES in children and adults. Although empirically supported treatments have begun to emerge, care models are lacking. We have suggested several theoretical and practical issues in the development of care models for PNES in both children and adults. These include consideration of stepped-care approaches that are patient-centered and include a "care manager" taking on responsibility for coordination of resources. A full list of recommendations is depicted in Table 12.2. Two PNES care model examples are further provided (one in current use and another theoretical). We acknowledge cultural, regional and professional biases in these models, requiring refinement and empirical validation of outcomes as well as patient/care-provider satisfaction. It is recommended that PNES care models include identification of appropriate resources required at each level of care as well as time points for making care level decisions. Further study and measurement is also required to compare care approaches that integrate various components. Given multiple etiologies for PNES and corresponding psychological subtypes,[45-48] further study should also seek to determine flexible decision rules regarding treatment and initial level of care.

We expect models of care for PNES to vary across divergent healthcare systems in response to resource availability and allocation. In addition to improving the lives of patients and families with PNES, care models can be used to demonstrate individual clinic and societal cost-savings stemming from reduced disability and increased productivity. Subsequent economic evaluation of care models may help to establish cost-effectiveness and thereby increase acceptance of specialized treatment and services for PNES. Studies of various PNES cohorts have begun to identify economic savings as a result of reduced medical visits, diagnostic tests, AED and ED/EMS utilization. Demonstrating reduced demand on fiscal budgets and reimbursement systems will in turn lead to acceptance of care models by healthcare administrators.

7. SUMMARY

- Despite advancements in diagnosis and management of PNES, significant barriers to care exist.
- These barriers relate to: 1) diagnostic barriers, 2) clinician knowledge, 3) treatment barriers, 4) healthcare system barriers, and 5) lack of empirical argument.
- Theoretical and practical issues in the development of care models for PNES can be informed by existing models within chronic care, stepped care, and patient-centered care.
- Examples of PNES care models are provided and described.
- Significant barriers to care in PNES exist and may be addressed by development of care models that take into account clinician, patient, and healthcare system factors and are adapted according to resource availability and cultural context.
- Once developed, PNES care models can be used to demonstrate improved patient outcome, healthcare utilization, and societal benefit.

REFERENCES

1. McMillan KK, Pugh MJ, Hamid H, et al., Providers' perspectives on treating psychogenic nonepileptic seizures: frustration and hope. *Epilepsy Behav.* 2014;37:276–281.
2. Baxter S, Mayor R, Baird W, et al., Understanding patient perceptions following a psycho-educational intervention for psychogenic non-epileptic seizures. *Epilepsy Behav.* 2012;23(4):487–493.
3. Sharpe M, Walker J, Williams C, et al. Guided self-help for functional (psychogenic) symptoms: a randomized controlled efficacy trial. *Neurology.* 2011;77:564–572.
4. Stone J, Campbell K, Sharm N, Carson A, Warlow CP, Sharpe M. What should we call pseudoseizures? The patient's perspective. *Seizure.* 2003;12(8):568–572.
5. Magee JA, Burke T, Delanty N, Pender N, Fortune GM. The economic cost of nonepileptic attack disorder in Ireland. *Epilepsy Behav.* 2014;33:45–48.
6. Razvi S, Mulhern S, Duncan R. Newly diagnosed psychogenic nonepileptic seizures: health care demand prior to and following diagnosis at a first seizure clinic. *Epilepsy Behav.* 2012;23(1):7–9.
7. Mayor R, Brown RJ, Cock H, et al. Short-term outcome of psychogenic non-epileptic seizures after communication of the diagnosis. *Epilepsy Behav.* 2012;25(4):676–681.
8. Plioplys S, Siddarth P, Asato MR, Caplan R. Clinicians' views on antiepileptic medication management in nonepileptic seizures. *J Child Neurol.* 2014;29(6):746–750.
9. Benbadis SR. The problem of psychogenic symptoms: is the psychiatric community in denial? *Epilepsy Behav.* 2005;6:9–14.
10. Shneker BF, Elliott JO. Primary care and emergency physician attitudes and beliefs related to patients with psychogenic nonepileptic spells. *Epilepsy Behav.* 2008;13(1):243–247.
11. Whitehead K, Reuber M. Illness perceptions of neurologists and psychiatrists in relation to epilepsy and nonepileptic attack disorder. *Seizure.* 2012;21(2):104–109.
12. Worsley C, Whitehead K, Kandler R, Reuber M. Illness perceptions of health care workers in relation to epileptic and psychogenic nonepileptic seizures. *Epilepsy Behav.* 2011;20(4):668–673.
13. O'Sullivan SS, Sweeney BJ, McNamara B. The opinion of the general practitioner toward clinical management of patients with psychogenic nonepileptic seizures. *Epilepsy Behav.* 2006;8(1):256–260.
14. Sahaya K, Dholakia SA, Lardizabal D, Sahota PK. Opinion survey of health care providers towards psychogenic non epileptic seizures. *Clin Neurol Neurosurg.* 2012;114(10):1304–1307.
15. LaFrance WC Jr, Ranieri R, Bamps Y, et al. Comparison of common data elements from the Managing Epilepsy Well (MEW) Network integrated database and a well-characterized sample with nonepileptic seizures. *Epilepsy Behav.* 2015;45:136–141.
16. LaFrance WC Jr, Alper K, Babcock D, Vert C. Nonepileptic seizures treatment workshop summary. *Epilepsy Behav.* 2006;8(3):451–461.
17. LaFrance WC Jr, Reuber M, Goldstein LH. Management of psychogenic nonepileptic seizures. *Epilepsia.* 2013;54(Suppl 1):53–67.
18. Thompson R, Isaac CL, Rowse G, Tooth CL, Reuber M. What is it like to receive a diagnosis of nonepileptic seizures? *Epilepsy Behav.* 2009;14(3):508–515.
19. Dickinson P, Looper KJ. Psychogenic nonepileptic seizures: a current overview. *Epilepsia.* 2012;53(10):1679–1689.
20. Cole CM, Falcone T, Caplan R, Timmon-Mitchell J, Jares K, Ford PJ. Ethical dilemmas in pediatric and adolescent psychogenic nonepileptic seizures. *Epilepsy Behav.* 2014;37:145–150.

21. Plioplys S, Asato MR, Bursch B, Salpekar JA, Shaw R, Caplan R. Multidisciplinary management of pediatric nonepileptic seizures. *J Am Acad Child Adolesc Psychiatry.* 2007;46(11):1491–1495.
22. Howlett S, Grünewald RA, Khan A, Reuber M. Engagement in psychological treatment for functional neurological symptoms—barriers and solutions. *Psychotherapy (Chic).* 2007;44(3):354–360.
23. Plioplys S, Laux LC. Pediatric psychogenic nonepileptic seizures in the emergency department: recognition and interventions. *Clin Ped Emerg Med.* 2008;9:101–105.
24. De Paola L, Terra VC, Silvado CE, et al. Improving first responders' psychogenic nonepileptic seizures diagnosis accuracy: development and validation of a 6-item bedside diagnostic tool. *Epilepsy Behav.* 2016;54:40–46.
25. Yamauchi T, Epilepsy and psychiatry: how can psychiatry contribute to the care of patients with epilepsy? *Seishin Igaku (Clinical Psychiatry).* 2011;53:423–435.
26. Coleman K, Austin BT, Brach C, Wagner EH. Evidence on the chronic care model in the new millennium. *Health Aff (Millwood).* 2009;28(1):75–85.
27. Tsai AC, Morton SC, Mangione CM, Keeler EB. A meta-analysis of interventions to improve care for chronic illnesses. *Am J Manag Care.* 2005;11(8):478–488.
28. Wagner EH, Bennett SM, Austin BT, Greene SM, Schaefer JK, Vonkorff M. Finding common ground: patient-centeredness and evidence-based chronic illness care. *J Altern Complement Med.* 2005;11(Suppl 1):S7–S15.
29. Siminerio LM, Piatt GA, Emerson S, et al. Deploying the chronic care model to implement and sustain diabetes self-management training programs. *Diabetes Educ.* 2006;32(2):253–260.
30. Stroebel RJ, Gloor B, Freytag S, et al. Adapting the chronic care model to treat chronic illness at a free medical clinic. *J Health Care Poor Underserved.* 2005;16(2):286–296.
31. Dancer S, Courtney M. Improving diabetes patient outcomes: framing research into the chronic care model. *J Am Acad Nurse Pract.* 2010;22(11):580–585.
32. Meyer RM, Wang S, Li X, Thomsen D, O'Brien-Pallas S. Evaluation of a patient care delivery model: patient outcomes in acute cardiac care. *J Nurs Scholarsh.* 2009;41(4):399–410.
33. Yu GC, Beresford R. Implementation of a chronic illness model for diabetes care in a family medicine residency program. *J Gen Intern Med.* 2010;25(Suppl 4):S615–S619.
34. (Institute of Medicine), *Epilepsy across the Spectrum: Promoting Health and Understanding.* 2012; Washington, DC: National Academies Press.
35. Green A, Payne S, Barnitt R. Illness representations among people with non-epileptic seizures attending a neuropsychiatry clinic: a qualitative study based on the self-regulation model. *Seizure.* 2004;13:331–339.
36. Chen JJ, Caller TA, Mecchella JN, et al. Reducing severity of comorbid psychiatric symptoms in an epilepsy clinic using a colocation model: results of a pilot intervention. *Epilepsy Behav.* 2014;39:92–96.
37. Haaga DA. Introduction to the special section on stepped care models in psychotherapy. *J Consult Clin Psychol.* 2000;68(4):547–548.
38. Bower P, Gilbody S. Stepped care in psychological therapies: access, effectiveness and efficiency. Narrative literature review. *Br J Psychiatry.* 2005;186:11–17.
39. Hall-Patch L, Brown R, House A, et al.; NEST collaborators. Acceptability and effectiveness of a strategy for the communication of the diagnosis of psychogenic nonepileptic seizures. *Epilepsia.* 2010;51(1):70–78.

40. Robinson JH, Callister LC, Berry JA, Dearing KA. Patient-centered care and adherence: definitions and applications to improve outcomes. *J Am Acad Nurse Pract.* 2008;20(12):600–607.
41. Sidani S, Collins L, Harbman P, et al. Development of a measure to assess healthcare providers' implementation of patient-centered care. *Worldviews Evid Based Nurs.* 2014;11(4):248–257.
42. Gruman J, VonKorff M, Reynolds J, Wagner EH, Organizing health care for people with seizures and epilepsy. *J Ambul Care Manage.* 1998;21(2):1–13; discussion 14–17.
43. Craig C, Eby D, Whittington J. *Care Coordination Model: Better Care at Lower Cost for People with Multiple Health and Social Needs.* IHI Innovation Series white paper. Cambridge, MA: Institute for Healthcare Improvement; 2011.
44. Sawchuk T, Buchhalter J. Psychogenic nonepileptic seizures in children—psychological presentation, treatment, and short-term outcomes. *Epilepsy Behav.* 2015;52(Pt A):49–56.
45. Brown RJ, Bouska JF, Frow A, et al. Emotional dysregulation, alexithymia, and attachment in psychogenic nonepileptic seizures. *Epilepsy Behav.* 2013;29(1):178–183.
46. Uliaszek AA, Prensky E, Baslet G. Emotion regulation profiles in psychogenic nonepileptic seizures. *Epilepsy Behav.* 2012;23(3):364–369.
47. Baslet G, Roiko A, Prensky E. Heterogeneity in psychogenic nonepileptic seizures: understanding the role of psychiatric and neurological factors. *Epilepsy Behav.* 2010;17(2):236–241.
48. Hingray C, Maillard L, Hubsch C, et al. Psychogenic nonepileptic seizures: characterization of two distinct patient profiles on the basis of trauma history. *Epilepsy Behav.* 2011;22(3):532–536.

13

Readiness to Start Treatment and Obstacles to Adherence

Benjamin Tolchin, MD and Gaston Baslet, MD

1. INTRODUCTION

Effective evidence-based treatments for psychogenic nonepileptic seizures (PNES) are increasingly available. Nevertheless, difficulties in engaging and keeping patients in treatment remain major obstacles, and these are probably major contributors to patients' poor long-term outcomes. We will review a number of patient- and provider-related factors that contribute to poor adherence to treatment. Several potential strategies for improving adherence are currently under development. This is a key area for ongoing research to improve treatment and outcomes for patients with PNES.

2. THE PROBLEM: POOR ADHERENCE TO TREATMENT

While effective treatments for PNES have historically been limited, psychiatrists and neurologists are establishing strong evidence for the efficacy of specific treatments (see Chapter 14). Multiple studies, including two randomized clinical trials, have demonstrated the short-term effectiveness of cognitive-behavioral therapy (CBT)–based regimens in decreasing seizure frequency and improving quality of life for patients with PNES.[1-4] Uncontrolled studies have suggested the effectiveness of other psychotherapeutic modalities, including psychodynamic and group therapy regimens.[5-8]

Long-term outcomes are not favorable in PNES (see Chapter 17). The majority of patients do not receive effective treatment, and up to 75% of patients continue to have psychogenic seizures and associated disability over the long term.[9-12] These studies were conducted prior to the availability of proven effective therapies. As evidence-based treatments become more widely available, it remains unknown if these treatments will have a positive *long-term* impact. One issue that appears to undermine their long-term effectiveness is patients' poor adherence to therapy regimens. As we will discuss, the same randomized trials and observational studies that show that CBT-based regimens and other psychotherapeutic modalities are effective for patients who fully participate also show that the majority of patients do not complete these treatments, even when offered within the structure and support of a clinical trial setting.[4,13–16]

In clinical practice, there are at least three time points at which poor adherence with treatment is known to arise, typically resulting in treatment failure, ongoing symptoms, and disability (see Figure 13.1).

1) Diagnostic confirmation usually takes places during an elective admission to an epilepsy monitoring unit (EMU). Immediately following this admission, many patients fail to follow up with their neurologist and the diagnostic team, even before they are referred to a mental health provider for treatment. Observational studies document approximately 30% of patients being lost to follow-up after first receiving the diagnosis of PNES.[13,14] It is important to note that these studies were performed without the involvement of mental health providers at the time of diagnosis or at first follow-up, and with first follow-up occurring a full 6 months after diagnosis. These features are by no means unusual among comprehensive epilepsy centers diagnosing PNES but are different from the model of integrated care we are currently piloting, as we will discuss later in this chapter.
2) A second time point at which dropout is known to occur is in the referral from the diagnosing neurology team to the treating mental health provider or team. Approximately 30% of patients refuse referral by their neurologist to a psychiatrist or psychotherapist.[15]
3) Finally, among those patients who begin treatment with a mental health provider, at least 50% drop out of treatment before completing a psychotherapeutic regimen.

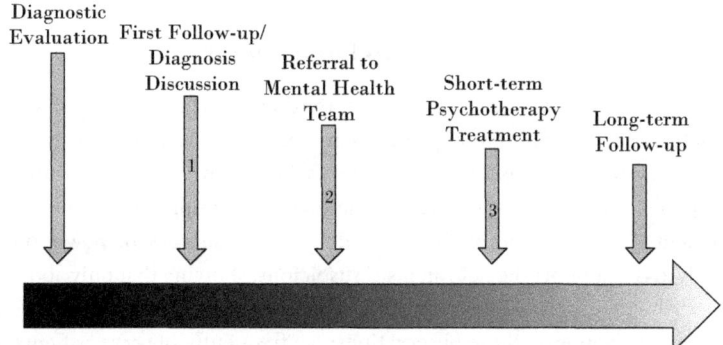

Time point		Rate of adherence
1	Immediate follow-up with neurological team following PNES diagnosis	71–72% (13–14)
2	Initial referral to behavioral health team	66% (15)
3	Completion of psychotherapy	31–54% (4,16)
1-3	Composite Adherence Rate (time points 1–3 considered in series)	15–26%

Figure 13.1 Stages during the evaluation and treatment of patients with psychogenic nonepileptic seizures (PNES). Time points 1, 2, and 3 highlight the specific time points at which PNES patients have a risk of not engaging in or dropping out of treatment.

This high rate of noncompletion is observed in study conditions as well as in conventional clinic settings and increases to approximately 70% when the therapist is based at a different institution from the referring physician.[4,16] These results are consistent with studies of adherence rates with psychotherapy in other psychiatric conditions, which also show astounding dropout rates of approximately 50%.[17,18] Clinical experience suggests that a further fraction of those patients who do attend an entire psychotherapeutic regimen do not engage with the treatment program and do not implement changes to their behavior as recommended in most behavioral-based interventions. This subset of patients is considered "adherent to treatment" in only the most superficial sense.

When the three time points of potential nonadherence are considered in series, we can calculate that, on average, less than 25% of patients diagnosed with PNES in an EMU actually follow through with their diagnosing neurologist, accept a referral to a mental health provider, and then fully participate in a behavioral health treatment regimen. As effective as modern psychotherapy regimens may be for the treatment of PNES, care for these patients will remain inadequate so long as the large majority of diagnosed patients do not fully and meaningfully participate in treatment.

3. UNDERLYING CAUSES OF THE ADHERENCE PROBLEM IN PNES

The causes for the difficulty in engaging patients in treatment can be divided into patient-related and provider- and systems-related factors (Table 13.1).

3.1. Patient-Related Factors

To begin with, acceptance and understanding of the diagnosis of PNES, especially its psychogenic nature, is often poor among patients and particularly among newly diagnosed patients. Surveys of neurologists show that they believe only about 40% of their newly diagnosed patients understand and accept the diagnosis, improving to approximately 60% of patients by 6–12 months following diagnosis.[13] Surveys of newly diagnosed patients with PNES support the neurologists' suspicions, showing that only about 30% of patients describe their problems as "mainly or entirely psychological" in etiology.[19] Our clinical experience supports these observations: we frequently observe patients returning to clinic after being diagnosed in the EMU, reporting that they were never given a specific diagnosis or never told that their seizure-like events were psychological in etiology, even when the same team members who delivered the diagnosis of PNES in the EMU are sitting in the clinic room with them. In our experience, it often takes time and gentle, repeated explanations for patients to hear and process this complex and—for many—distressing explanation for their symptoms. In other psychiatric disorders, such as depression or anxiety, emotional distress motivates the clinical evaluation, and a psychological explanation therefore accords with the patients' experiences and expectations. In contrast, patients with PNES perceive their distress as primarily physical, and a psychological explanation is therefore often unexpected and contrary to their experience.

Table 13.1. Patient-Related, Provider-Related, and Systemic Factors that Interfere with PNES Treatment Adherence

Patient-Related Factors	Potential Interventions
Failure to accept or understand the diagnosis	Rapid and streamlined initiation of psychotherapy. Joint delivery of diagnosis by neurology/behavioral health teams.
Additional psychiatric comorbidities	Early psychiatric assessment (prior to or at time of diagnosis). Rapid and streamlined initiation of psychotherapy/psychiatric treatment.
Ambivalence	Motivational interviewing. Values clarification therapy.
Alexithymia, avoidant personality	Values clarification therapy. Nonthreatening presentation of the diagnosis, emphasis on concrete and achievable goals. Emotion recognition training.
Social isolation	Include family or close friends with patient's permission. Encourage patients to participate in support groups and clinic-based wellness activities.
Low socioeconomic status	Social worker/case manager as part of integrated healthcare team.

Provider- or System-Related Factors	Potential Interventions
Shortage of mental health providers	Increased training by professional organizations. Establishing an integrated healthcare team including neurologist, psychiatrist, psychotherapist, primary care provider.
Gaps in care between diagnosing neurologists and treating mental health providers	Integrated healthcare team, single primary care provider/gatekeeper, early psychiatric assessment, open communication between neurologist and mental health professionals.
Lack of familiarity with diagnosing and treating PNES among psychiatrists and neurologists	Increased training efforts by professional organizations. Open communication within integrated healthcare team.
Stigmatization of patients	Early psychiatric assessment, open communication regarding differential diagnosis prior to final diagnosis, joint delivery of diagnosis by neurology/behavioral health teams.
Liability concerns	Establish emergency care protocol in advance. Open communication within integrated healthcare team. Option for re-evaluation by primary care provider or neurologist if new symptoms develop.

It is understandable that many patients who have difficulty accepting a psychological basis for their symptoms will not be motivated to begin or complete a psychotherapeutic treatment.

Approximately 50–70% of patients with PNES suffer from an additional psychiatric comorbid disorder, such as depression, post-traumatic stress disorder (PTSD), generalized anxiety disorder, and/or a personality disorder (most often a cluster B personality disorder).[20,21] Some, but not all, studies have found that the presence of psychiatric comorbidities are a poor prognostic indicator and may contribute to poor adherence to treatment.[11,14,16] The presence of subjective cognitive complaints in PNES, generally thought to be the result of variable motivation and/or emotionally driven factors on cognitive function rather than neuropathology (see Chapter 5), strongly correlates with poor adherence.[16] The majority of patients with PNES have additional somatic symptoms (also known as "medically unexplained symptoms"), and these symptoms may become more common as seizure-like events become less frequent, in some sense "replacing" PNES.[22] These new somatic symptoms can interfere with engagement with treatment, as patients become focused on the new somatic symptom, seeking new medical explanations, and lose interest in their ongoing psychotherapy regimen.

While most patients with PNES clearly long for freedom from seizures and can easily describe the many ways in which their work, family, and social lives would be better without PNES, they often simultaneously exhibit behaviors that perpetuate their seizure-like events and interfere with therapy. Therapy-interfering behaviors among patients include using small difficulties—a missed appointment, a minor conflict with a healthcare provider or staff, a temporary conflict between work and treatment, the presence of minor symptoms—as a justification for stopping participation in treatment altogether. We surmise that these behaviors indicate an unconscious tendency to continue experiencing symptoms and to continue inhabiting the sick role, with the increased attention from family members and care providers and the diminished responsibility that this role entails. We believe this tendency exists simultaneously with a conflicting desire to achieve seizure-freedom, creating a vacillating ambivalence toward remaining symptomatic with PNES and toward treatment. In addition, we believe that several of the patient-related factors detailed here, including difficulty accepting the diagnosis of PNES, subjective cognitive symptoms, and newly emerging somatic symptoms, are at least in part manifestations of this ambivalence. We note that desire for treatment and freedom from seizures often peaks during periods of crisis and increased seizure frequency, but that ambivalence grows when the crisis has passed and seizure frequency is more manageable, making it difficult for patients to sustain long-term interest in treatment.

In addition to ambivalence, other psychological factors may contribute to poor adherence among patients with PNES. *Alexithymia* is defined as difficulty with identifying and especially verbally expressing one's own emotions. Patients with PNES rank highly on scales of alexithymia, and patients with related somatic symptom disorders score particularly low on scales of emotional awareness, even in comparison to other psychiatric patients.[23] Similarly, patients with PNES rate higher on measures of avoidant behavior than matched patients with epilepsy, indicating a greater tendency to avoid unpleasant thoughts and internal stimuli.[24] Indeed, alexithymia and avoidant behavior may play causal roles in PNES as patients experience intense affect without the ability to address, resolve, express, or even recognize such emotions, potentially contributing to seizure events as involuntary, explosive reactions to intense unconscious affect. Regardless, the difficulty with recognition and verbal expression of emotions and the tendency to avoid unpleasant thoughts and emotions are clear obstacles to active participation in psychotherapy, which may be experienced as exceptionally unpleasant and difficult for some patients with PNES.

Social isolation is another personal factor that is strongly associated with poor adherence to treatment among patients with PNES. In one observational study, the best predictor of follow-up after the diagnosis of PNES was the presence of a caretaker—either a spouse, family member, or friend—at the delivery of the diagnosis. Initial acceptance of the diagnosis of PNES by the caretaker (but not the patient) predicted decreased use of healthcare resources for treatment of PNES at 5–10 years.[13] In another study, marriage or domestic partnership was the best predictor of adherence to psychotherapy over 3 months.[16] The active engagement of close social contacts in the management and treatment of PNES appears to be a key factor in treatment adherence and a successful outcome.

Patients with PNES are disproportionately economically dependent, and we have observed that low socioeconomic status, including limited healthcare insurance, is another factor that raises barriers to treatment.[9] Patients who are economically disadvantaged often have less flexibility in arranging their work schedule to accommodate participation in treatment and have more difficulty in arranging the childcare and transportation that is necessary for adherence to regular weekly or biweekly appointments. Driving restrictions or concerns over experiencing an event in public add to the logistical limitations that impact treatment participation. These very real obstacles to care can sometimes be amplified further by the ambivalent feelings that patients may have toward their treatment, leading them to give up treatment over what might otherwise be temporary or workable difficulties. Additionally, in the United States, low-cost and low-quality medical insurance often provides very limited mental health benefits, which exacerbates the systemic shortage of healthcare providers—the first of many provider-related and systemic barriers to treatment.

3.2. Provider-Related and Systemic Factors

Perhaps the most fundamental systemic difficulty in initiating treatment for PNES is obtaining an initial appointment with a mental health provider. Regardless of one's insurance or even nationality, behavioral health specialists are often in short supply, with long wait times for an initial appointment. In the United Kingdom's National Health Service, standard wait times of more than 12 months have been repeatedly documented for patients newly diagnosed with PNES to see a mental health provider.[14,19] While access to mental health services is more variable in the United States, depending on an individual's insurance, wait times of 6 months are not uncommon in our experience. In a national survey of U.S. primary care physicians (PCPs), two-thirds reported that their patients could not access adequate outpatient mental health services, primarily because of a lack of behavioral health professionals.[25] Partly as a result, it is estimated that only one third of U.S. patients with mental health problems receive adequate treatment.[26] It is therefore not surprising that one third of our patients with PNES cite difficulty in finding a mental health provider who accepts their insurance as an important obstacle to treatment (unpublished data).

Patients with PNES face additional systemic obstacles above and beyond those encountered by other patients with mental illness, in part because PNES falls between two medical specialties: neurologists who make the diagnosis, and psychiatrists and other mental health professionals who provide treatment.[27-29] Patients often experience the referral from neurology to psychiatry with surprise and may interpret it as a dismissal and abandonment—sometimes mixed with stigmatization as a "faker" or even "lunatic." Additionally, as a result of the division of labor, many psychiatrists and psychotherapists are unfamiliar with the diagnosis of PNES and are in the uncomfortable position of depending on other specialists to confirm the diagnosis and rule out alternatives, such as epileptic seizures or other physiological paroxysms. Less than 20% of psychiatrists feel that video-EEG (vEEG)—the gold standard for diagnosis of PNES—is reliable in making the diagnosis.[29] This disconnect suggests an important lack of formal and informal communication between neurologists and psychiatrists regarding this condition. Limited collaboration between disciplines creates gaps in the care of these patients across multiple settings, including emergency departments, neurology clinics, and eventually outpatient mental health clinics. These gaps allow miscommunication, erratic follow-up patterns, and the emergence of patient behaviors that interfere with therapy.

Within both the neurology and psychiatry literature, PNES receives scant attention in comparison to its clinical frequency and its associated disability.[30] Training programs in each specialty devote limited time and attention to functional neurological symptom disorders (FNSD) such as PNES. As a result, providers diagnosing and treating PNES often have to learn about the disorder on their own, without clear guidelines or role models to follow. Even when patients do receive proper referrals to behavioral health professionals with clear communication of the diagnosis by the neurologist, many mental health professionals are simply unfamiliar with the evidence-based treatments for PNES.[30]

The relative lack of communication around the topic of PNES, both within the specialties of neurology and psychiatry and especially between the specialties, may be due in part to the significant frustration with which healthcare providers view PNES.[30,31] Specific areas of frustration include difficulty in treating the illness, concerns that patients are seeking primary or secondary gain, the stigma that patients face, the complexity of the illness, and the lack of clear evidence-based guidelines.[31] Many healthcare providers deal with these frustrations through dark humor and the disparaging of patients, unfortunately reinforcing the stigma that patients experience.[32,33] In our experience, most patients are very much aware of the frustration and disdain directed at them by healthcare providers (see Chapter 11). This frustration and stigmatization are additional substantive obstacles to patients initiating and continuing treatment.

Neurologists frequently demonstrate a "dualist" perspective in their views of PNES, categorizing it as an "entirely psychological" rather than physical problem.[34] In contrast, they view epilepsy as a "mainly or entirely physical" problem (despite the fact that depression, anxiety, and other psychiatric comorbidities are more common among patients with epilepsy than in the general population). In making this distinction, neurologists often disregard the presumably cortically based neurological underpinnings of PNES and other psychiatric disorders. This is an issue for adherence because most patients understand PNES as a "partly psychological and partly physical" problem, and a significant minority view the disorder as mainly or entirely physical.[19,34] The discrepancy in conceptualization may contribute to patients' difficulty in accepting and understanding PNES as a psychiatric diagnosis.[13] Furthermore, neurologists' categorization of PNES as purely psychological without any physical basis may contribute to the frustration and stigma that some direct toward patients with the disorder.

Finally, liability concerns represent another provider-dependent barrier to treatment. The nature of this disease involves episodes during which patients can become transiently confused and injure themselves. Psychiatrists who are unfamiliar with or skeptical of the diagnostic process may fear that epileptic seizures misdiagnosed as PNES will cause permanent injury or death. Unfamiliarity with the disorder and limited planning may leave many practitioners fearful of potential liability while treating PNES patients.[35]

Table 13.1 lists all the patient-related, provider-related, and systemic factors that interfere with engagement in treatment. The table also summarizes some of the potential interventions to target these problems, which are described in detail in the next section.

4. POTENTIAL SOLUTIONS TO PROMOTE ADHERENCE TO TREATMENT AMONG PATIENTS WITH PNES

The array of impediments to treatment facing patients with PNES can appear overwhelming to patients and providers alike. There are steps that clinicians can take to facilitate patients engaging and participating in treatment. These interventions can be directed toward both patient-related and provider-related causes of nonadherence, though there is a certain amount of overlap, as some interventions are helpful in addressing multiple obstacles (see Table 13.1).

4.1. Interventions Targeting Patient-Related Factors

Creating an efficient and well-organized transition from the moment the diagnosis is made until the patient is engaged in treatment minimizes the opportunity for second-guessing and dropout by ambivalent patients. Rapid transition decreases the immediate post-diagnosis dropout rate from 30% to 20%.[13,14,36] It is very useful for neurologists to have pre-established referral relationships with mental health professionals who are skilled, interested, and available to treat PNES. If practical, this referral should take place within a single institution or network, recalling that adherence deteriorates when referrals are made to behavioral health providers in different institutions.[16] Ideally, the behavioral health team should be involved in evaluating patients with probable PNES even before the diagnosis is confirmed with vEEG in the EMU. This allows the behavioral health team to evaluate for risk factors for PNES (a history of trauma, psychosocial reinforcing factors, personality factors, etc.) as well as psychiatric comorbidities and suicidal or parasuicidal behaviors. An early mental health evaluation also allows patients to familiarize themselves with a mental health provider (if they have had not mental health treatment before) and may help them consider PNES as a possible diagnosis even before the vEEG confirmation, decreasing their surprise and rejection of the diagnosis. Finally, it is also beneficial for a unified healthcare team including both a neurologist and a behavioral health specialist to jointly present the diagnosis to the patient once confirmed. This approach helps patients to better understand and accept the psychological etiology of PNES and can alleviate the stigma associated with a psychiatric diagnosis and the sense of abandonment that patients may experience with the transition to behavioral health treatment.

In our practice, a psychiatrist evaluates all patients with suspected PNES during the EMU admission and then joins the neurology team to deliver and discuss the diagnosis together with the patient prior to discharge. PNES is presented as a disorder on the differential diagnosis throughout the admission, rather than as a secret or a "bombshell" surprise revealed right before discharge. Patients then follow up within 2–3 weeks in our post–long-term monitoring (LTM) clinic, where they meet simultaneously with a neurologist, a psychiatrist, and a social worker to review the diagnosis again, discuss the treatment plan, and initiate psychiatric treatment. At least one member of the EMU team is always present in the post-LTM clinic to ensure continuity of care. We are currently studying the effects of this integrated process on patient adherence to treatment and long-term outcomes; preliminary data suggest that adherence is improved by about 10%.[36]

Given the ambivalence demonstrated by patients with PNES toward the diagnosis and treatment, the technique of motivational interviewing may be valuable in improving their adherence to treatment. Motivational interviewing (MI) is "a person-centered counseling style for addressing the common problem of ambivalence about change."[37] It de-emphasizes confronting or persuading patients and focuses instead on evoking patients' own reasons for change, thereby minimizing resistance.[37] MI was originally developed to decrease risky alcohol consumption but has since been successfully used for such varied purposes as promoting weight loss among obese patients and increasing adherence to antiretroviral therapy among those with HIV.[38–40] MI has been learned and successfully employed by physicians, nurses, psychotherapists, and social workers, among others.[41] It has been shown to produce durable effects up to 1 year post-treatment.[42] We are currently studying the effect of MI on adherence to treatment among patients with PNES in a randomized controlled trial (unpublished data).

Values clarification therapy may also play an important role in helping ambivalent patients who do not actively engage with treatment. As noted, some patients with PNES may attend therapy sessions and yet not meaningfully engage or make significant changes in their lives. Values clarification techniques are designed to help individuals increase awareness of the core values or behavioral standards that they hold and to assess the desirability of behavioral options with respect to the identified values.[43] Some studies have shown that values clarification exercises can improve the decision-making process for individuals facing new and complex decisions.[43] These techniques may be especially helpful for patients with PNES who are focused on their somatic symptoms and thus have particular difficulty redirecting their attention toward their core life values.

There are additional strategies for ameliorating the effects of alexithymia and avoidant personality traits among patients with PNES. In particular, presenting the diagnosis in a nonthreatening, nonaccusatory manner needs to be a priority (see Chapter 10). It may be helpful to normalize the diagnosis by comparing it to more common and better known phenomena such as panic attacks or physiological tachycardia and diaphoresis during a stressful encounter. In discussing treatment, providers should not focus on simple "symptom resolution" but should instead address the underlying difficulties that led to PNES, while concentrating on goals that are concrete, achievable, and not overwhelming. It can be helpful for patients to write out clear goals, the specific methods they will use to achieve these goals, problems they anticipate, and strategies they will use to address anticipated problems. Specific training in emotion recognition, acceptance, and regulation, as part of the psychotherapy program, can help patients overcome the underlying vulnerabilities leading to somatic expressions of distress.

Social isolation is another patient-related factor that strongly predicts nonadherence among patients with PNES. It is therefore essential to recruit partners, family, and/or close friends to participate in patient care. Provided that the patient is amenable, healthcare providers should actively engage close social contacts in the diagnostic and treatment process. Patients who are willing should be encouraged to invite a loved one to meetings in which the diagnosis and treatment plan are discussed and to share their treatment goals and plans with trusted social contacts. Patients who "publicize" their treatment plans in this manner have been shown to be more likely to adhere to those plans.[36] Additionally, patients should be encouraged to form new social contacts through support groups and, if available, through clinic-based wellness activities (e.g., gentle exercise, meditation, etc.).

Low socioeconomic status, which disproportionately affects patients with PNES, is another key obstacle to treatment adherence, bridging the gap between patient-related and systemic issues. If available, a case manager or social worker can be especially helpful to patients dealing with the many difficulties associated with low socioeconomic status. They can help to coordinate appointments and address logistical obstacles, such as transportation, childcare, and disruptions to medical insurance. A case manager can often assist patients in rescheduling missed appointments if not avoiding them altogether. The case manager also monitors patients' overall health and functioning, provides guidelines on how to cope with newly presenting or deteriorating symptoms, and keeps all members of the treatment team informed. Such a contact can help prevent unnecessary medical utilization and reorient patients and their families when new symptoms emerge and the diagnosis is questioned again.

4.2. Interventions Targeting Provider-Related and Systemic Factors

Some systemic obstacles to adherence, such as the shortages of mental health providers and the general lack of training in the diagnosis and treatment of PNES, will need to be addressed by professional organizations and training programs, rather than by individual clinics or providers. Professional organizations such as the American Academy of Neurology, the American Psychiatric Association, and the American Psychological Association can play key roles in developing and promulgating guidelines and educational programs on the evidence-based diagnosis and treatment for PNES and other functional neurological disorders.[35] Continuing educational programs for treatment providers, including ongoing supervision for therapists, can provide the foundation that many trained professionals did not obtain during their original training. Going forward, professional training programs in neurology, psychiatry, and psychology should incorporate experience with functional neurological disorders such as PNES as a fundamental part of training. In particular, clear and sensitive communication with patients and other providers around these diagnoses should be a key learning objective for trainees.[44]

In geographic areas without sufficient trained behavioral health clinicians, distance-delivery treatment modalities or teletherapy should be considered. Remotely delivered therapy has been shown to be effective in a randomized trial for the treatment of depression in patients with epilepsy and might be particularly promising for patients with PNES given their poor treatment adherence and the driving restrictions often imposed on these patients.[45]

There are also interventions that individual providers or practices can undertake to improve systemic obstacles to nonadherence, such as the gaps in care between neurologists and behavioral health professionals as they attempt to transition patients from diagnosis to treatment. If possible, mental health professionals should be included in the workup prior to or during the diagnosis of PNES, as previously discussed. If this is not possible, neurologists should clearly communicate the basis of the diagnosis including an explanatory model, and discuss the plan for mental health treatment with the patient. The neurologist should also initiate open communication with the treating mental health provider and make clear to the patient that communication and cooperation is occurring on an ongoing basis. The neurologist should explain to the mental health provider the diagnosis, the evidence for and against the diagnosis, and the degree of confidence regarding the diagnosis. (For example: were all seizure types captured on vEEG? Is there any remaining concern for a dual diagnosis [PNES and epilepsy]? Is there any concern that these might be frontal lobe epileptic seizures or otherwise originate from a deep epileptic focus not appreciated on EEG?) It is also essential for the psychiatrist or mental health professional to have an opportunity to raise questions or concerns and to be able to contact the neurologist if new putatively neurological symptoms develop. Such open communication greatly improves the comfort of the behavioral health team, minimizes patients' feelings of abandonment, and significantly diminishes the chances that the patient will re-present to another neurologist or emergency department during mental health treatment.

Both the neurologist and psychiatrist (or mental health professional) should function as members of an integrated healthcare team with a single medical gatekeeper—ideally the PCP. Recall that the majority of patients with PNES suffer additional medically unexplained symptoms and that these can become *more* frequent during treatment of the nonepileptic seizures.[22] Those symptoms will need to be assessed by the PCP, with referrals back to the neurologist as necessary.

Published guidelines for the team-based treatment of somatizing patients exist and can offer excellent guidance in the treatment of patients with PNES.[46-48] Besides identifying a single PCP and gatekeeper, these guidelines entail frequent but limited appointments with the PCP, eliminating the presence of symptoms as a contingency to remain connected to the healthcare system, setting an agenda of caring for rather than curing the patient, and utilizing diagnostic and therapeutic conservatism.[46,47] If such guidelines are not followed, a long list of emergency department visits, consulting specialists, negative tests, and unnecessary treatments (e.g., antiepileptic medications, analgesics, narcotics, even surgeries) can quickly accumulate. This integrated team approach also serves as a containing environment for those patients who refuse to accept the diagnosis of PNES but who nonetheless continue to seek help for their various functional symptoms.

In order to minimize stigmatization experienced by patients, it is again recommended to involve mental health providers early and especially during the joint delivery of the diagnosis to the patient along with the neurologist. It is also important to openly raise the possibility of psychogenic seizures as a legitimate candidate on the differential diagnosis prior to the definite diagnosis. In discussing this possibility, it is important to describe it as a real and serious problem, requiring real treatment (albeit treatment that is very different from that indicated for epileptic seizures). PNES should not be dismissed as a "fake" or minor problem. A common response of neurologists when delivering the diagnosis of PNES is to congratulate patients that they do not have epilepsy and to tell them that PNES is a much "better" disorder to have. While it may be fortunate not to have epilepsy, PNES entails comparable disability and, as we have seen, often results in poor long-term outcomes.[9-12,48] It is therefore inaccurate as well as dismissive of patients' concerns to portray PNES as a "good news" disorder to have. Rather, neurologists should make it clear that PNES is a serious problem requiring intensive and sometimes extended treatment consisting of psychotherapy and that they will be available as needed to communicate with and support their behavioral health colleagues during this treatment.

Finally, interventions by the provider team can also minimize liability concerns. The open communication previously discussed allows behavioral health providers to achieve confidence in the diagnosis of PNES and to reassure themselves that if new symptoms develop they will be supported as needed by the PCP and neurologist in ruling out new medical or neurological illnesses. Careful planning for emergencies (e.g., what to do if an event occurs during a treatment session, using furniture pads, making sure an emergency contact is available should the patient have an event) can make psychotherapists more comfortable in treating patients with PNES and allow them to focus on the treatment program.[35]

5. SUMMARY

This chapter has reviewed the obstacles to initiating and completing successful treatment for PNES. We have examined the three stages at which patient dropout tends to occur in clinical practice and in studies. We have discussed patient-related, provider-related, and systemic causes of nonadherence. Finally, we have reviewed potential interventions to address obstacles to treatment.

- High rates of patient dropout occur following the diagnosis of PNES, at the point of referral to behavioral health specialists, and during psychotherapy.
- Patient-related factors contributing to nonadherence to treatment include a failure to accept or understand the diagnosis, psychiatric comorbidities, ambivalence about change, social isolation, and low socioeconomic status.

- Provider-related and systemic factors contributing to nonadherence include gaps in care between neurologists and mental health providers, a shortage of behavioral health specialists, a lack of familiarity with the disorder, and stigmatization of patients.
- Potential interventions to improve adherence to treatment include an integrated treatment team and joint presentation of the diagnosis, rapid and streamlined transition into psychotherapy, motivational interviewing, and engagement of patients' family members and support systems.

REFERENCES

1. LaFrance WC, Miller IW, Ryan CE, et al. Cognitive behavioral therapy for psychogenic nonepileptic seizures. *Epilepsy Behav*. 2009;14:591–596.
2. Goldstein L, Chalder T, Chigwedere C, et al. Cognitive-behavioral therapy for psychogenic nonepileptic seizures: a pilot RCT. *Neurology*. 2010;74:1986–1994.
3. Hopp JL, LaFrance WC. Cognitive behavioral therapy for psychogenic neurological disorders. *Neurologist*. 2012;18:364–372.
4. LaFrance WC, Baird GL, Barry JJ, et al. Multicenter pilot treatment trial for psychogenic nonepileptic seizures: a randomized clinical trial. *JAMA Psychiatry*. 2014;71:997–1005.
5. Barry J, Wittenberg D, Bullock K, Michaels J, Classen C, Fisher R. Group therapy for patietns with psychogenic nonepileptic seizures: a pilot study. *Epilepsy Behav*. 2008;13:624–629.
6. Lesser RP. Treatment and outcome of psychogenic nonepiletic seizures. *Epilepsy Curr*. 2003;3:198.
7. Santos N, Benute GR, Santiago A, Marchiori PE, Lucia MC. Psychogenic nonepileptic seizures and psychoanalytical treatment: results. *Rev Assoc Med Bras*. 2014;60-577-584.
8. Zaroff CM, Myers L, Barr WB, Luciano D, Devinisky O. Group psychoeducation as treatment for psychological nonepileptic seizures. *Epilepsy Behav*. 2004;5:587–592.
9. Reuber M, Pukrop R, Bauer J, Helmstaedter C, Tessendorf N, Elger CE. Outcome of psychogenic nonepileptic seizures: 1 to 10 year follow-up in 164 patients. *Ann Neurol*. 2003;53:305–311.
10. Lancman ME, Brotherton TA, Asconape JJ, Penry JK. Psychogenic seizures in adults: a longitudinal study. *Seizure*. 1993;2:281–286.
11. Walczak TS, Papacostas S, Williams DT, Scheuer ML, Liebowitz N, Notarfrancesco A. Outcome after diagnosis of psychogenic nonepileptic seizures. *Epilepsia*. 1995;36:1131–1137.
12. Duncan R, Graham CD, Oto M, Russell A, McKernan L, Copstick S. Primary and secondary care attendance, anticonvulsant and antidepressant use and psychiatric contact 5–10 years after diagnosis in 188 patients with psychogenic non-epileptic seizures. *J Neurol Neurosurg Psychiatry*. 2014;85:954–958.
13. Duncan R, Graham C, Oto M. Neurologist assessment of reactions to the diagnosis of psychogenic nonepileptic seizures: relationship to short- and long-term outcomes. *Epilepsy Behav*. 2014;41:79–82.
14. McKenzie P, Oto M, Russell A, Pelosi A, Duncan R. Early outcomes and predictors in 260 patients with psychogenic nonepileptic attacks. *Neurology*. 2010;74:64–69.

15. Kanner AM, Parra J, Frey M, Stebbins G, Pierre-Louis S, Iriarte J. Psychiatric and neurologic predictors of psychogenic pseudoseizure outcome. *Neurology*. 1999;53:933–938.
16. Baslet G, Prensky E. Initial treatment retention in psychogenic non-epileptic seizures. *J Neuropsychiatry Clin Neurosci*. 2013;25:63–67.
17. Garfield SL. Research on client variables in psychotherapy. In: Bergin AE, Garfield SL (Eds.), Handbook of Psychotherapy and Behavior Change, 4th ed. Chichester, UK: John Wiley & Sons; 1994.
18. Wierzbicki M, Pekarik G. A meta-analysis of psychotherapy dropout. *Prof Psychol Res Pr*. 1993;24:190–195.
19. Mayor R, Brown RJ, Cock H, et al. Short-term outcome of psychogenic non-epileptic seizures after communication of the diagnosis. *Epilepsy Behav*. 2012;25:676–681.
20. O'Brien FM, Fortune GM, Dicker P, et al. Psychiatric and neuropsychological profiles of people with psychogenic nonepileptic seizures. *Epilepsy Behav*. 2015;43:39–45.
21. Krishnamoorthy ES, Brown RJ, Trimble MR. Personality and psychopathology in nonepileptic attack disorder and epilepsy: a prospective study. *Epilepsy Behav*. 2001;2:418–422.
22. McKenzie PS, Oto M, Graham CD, Duncan R. Do patients whose psychogenic nonepileptic seizures resolve, 'replace' them with other medically unexplained symptoms? Medically unexplained symptoms arising after a diagnosis of psychogenic non-epileptic seizures. *J Neurol Neurosurg Psychiatry*. 2011;82:967–969.
23. Baslet G. Psychogenic non-epileptic seizures: a model of their pathogenic mechanism. *Seizure*. 2011;20:1–13.
24. Goldstein LH, Mellers JDC. Ictal symptoms of anxiety, avoidance behavior and dissociation in patients with dissociative seizures. *J Neurol Neurosurg Psychiatry*. 2006;77:616–621.
25. Cunningham PJ. Beyond parity: primary care physicians' perspectives on access to mental health care. *Health Aff (Millwood)*. 2009;28:490–501.
26. Kessler RC, Demler O, Frank RG, et al. Prevalence and treatment of mental disorders, 1990 to 2003. *N Engl J Med*. 2005;352:2515–2523.
27. Brown RJ, Syed TU, Benbadis S, LaFrance WC, Reuber M. Psychogenic nonepileptic seizures. *Epilepsy Behav*. 2011;22:85–93.
28. LaFrance WC. Psychogenic nonepileptic seizures. *Curr Opin Neurol*. 2008;21:195–201.
29. Harden CL, Burgut FT, Kanner AM. The diagnostic significance of video-EEG monitoring findings on pseudoseizure patients differ between neurologists and psychiatrists. *Epilepsia*. 2003;44:453–456.
30. Benbadis SR. The problem of psychogenic symptoms: is the psychiatric community in denial? *Epilepsy Behav*. 2005;6:9–14.
31. McMillan KK, Pugh MJ, Hamid H, et al. Providers' perspectives on treating psychogenic nonepileptic seizures: frustration and hope. *Epilepsy Behav*. 2014;37:276–281.
32. "Dr. Slicy." Doctor has pseudoseizure to avoid patient with pseudoseizures. Gomer Blog 2014. http://gomerblog.com/2014/06/pseudoseizure/. Retrieved October 5, 2015.
33. "Harvey Wallbanger." Pseudoseizure: please practice before coming to the ED. Gomer Blog 2014. http://gomerblog.com/2014/05/psuedoseizure-hilarious/. Retrieved October 5, 2015.
34. Whitehead K, Kandler R, Reuber M. Patients' and neurologists' perception of epilepsy and psychogenic nonepileptic seizures. *Epilepsia*. 2013;54:708–717.
35. Baslet G, Seshadri A, Bermeo-Ovalle A, Willment K, Myers L. Psychogenic non-epileptic seizures: an updated primer. *Psychosomatics*. 2016;57(1):1–17.

36. Baslet G, Qureshi N, Zinser J, et al. Attendance to first follow-up appointment after psychogenic non-epileptic seizures diagnosis. Presented at American Neuropsychiatric Association Meeting, Lake Buena Vista, FL, March, 2015.
37. Miller W, Rollnick S. *Motivational Interviewing: Helping People Change*, 3rd ed. New York: Guilford Press; 2013.
38. Miller W. Motivational interviewing with problem drinkers. *Behav Psychother*. 1983;11:147–172.
39. Armstrong M, Mottershead T, Ronsky P, Sigal R, Campbell T, Hemmelgarn B. Motivational interviewing to improve weight loss in overweight and/or obese patients: a systematic review and meta-analysis of randomized controlled trials. *Obes Rev*. 2011;12:709–723.
40. Golin C, Earp J, Tien H, Stewart P, Porter C, Howie L. A 2-arm, randomized, controlled trial of a motivational interviewing-based intervention to improve adherence to antiretroviral therapy (ART) among patients failing or initiating ART. *J Acq Immun Deficien Syndr*. 2006;42:42–51.
41. Lundahl B, Moleni T, Burke B, Butters R, Tollefson D, Butler C, Rollnick S. Motivational interviewing in the medical care settings: a systematic review and meta-analysis of randomized controlled trials. Patient education and counseling 2013;93:157–168.
42. Lundahl B, Burke B. The effectiveness and applicability of motivational interviewing: a practice-friendly review of four meta-analyses. *J Clin Psychol*. 2009;65:1232–1245.
43. Fagerlin A, Pignone MP, Abhyankar P, et al. Clarifying values: an updated review. *BMC Med Inform Decis Mak*. 2013;13(Suppl 2):S8.
44. Dworetzky, BA. What are we communicating when we present the diagnosis of PNES? *Epilepsy Curr*. 2015;15:1–5.
45. Thompson NJ, Walker ER, Obolensky N, Winning A, Barmon C, Diiorio C, Compton MT. Distance delivery of mindfulness-based cognitive therapy for depression: project UPLIFT. *Epilepsy Behav*. 2010;19:247–254.
46. Barsky AJ. Clinical practice: the patient with hypochondriasis. *N Engl J Med*. 2001;345:1395–1399.
47. Barsky AJ, Borus JF. Functional somatic syndromes. *Ann Intern Med*. 1999;130:910–921.
48. Krawetz P, Fleisher W, Pillay N, Staley D, Arnett J, Maher J. Family functioning in subjects with pseudoseizures and epilepsy. *J Nerv Ment Dis*. 2001;189:38–43.

Section V
Treatment Interventions

14

Evidence-Based Treatments

W. Curt LaFrance Jr., MD, MPH

and Laura H. Goldstein, PhD, MPhil

1. INTRODUCTION

In this chapter, we review treatments for psychogenic nonepileptic seizures (PNES) that are based on models associated with the development of disorders involving psychological factors or psychiatric mechanisms. The models include psychodynamic, cognitive-behavioral (CB), mindfulness/dialectical-behavioral (DB), hypnosis, and pharmacological models. Specifics for each approach are given in the next section, but as an introduction brief descriptions of the theoretical foundations for the models are provided here, as described by LaFrance and Bjornaes.[1]

The psychodynamic theory model is based in intrapsychic conflict between drives and desires, between appetites and morality. Past or present trauma generates unpleasant thoughts that are forbidden and repressed from conscious awareness. The unconscious conflict is expressed in symbolic form through somatic symptoms. CB models are based in learning theory, in which classical and operant conditioning pair stimuli with responses, and behaviors are progressively shaped and reinforced with subsequent exposures. Cognitive distortions and their influence on maladaptive coping strategies are addressed in relation to symptoms of a disorder. Mindfulness and DB models are offspring of CB theory and target affective instability,[2] where stress can be conceptualized as an unpleasant emotional response to some exterior-world threatening event that becomes internalized. Dysfunctional and self-injurious behaviors are addressed with safety behaviors and distress tolerance; a shift in perspective with present-moment intentional and nonjudgmental attention is followed by acceptance and "effective" behavioral choices. These are based on high-value roles (a conceptualization that has some overlap with acceptance and commitment therapy [ACT]). Hypnosis methods address syntactic and affective cognitions that coincide with past sensitizing event(s) and can be used to induce and suppress PNES.[3] Pharmacotherapy employs a biomedical approach in which disruption of neuronal/synaptic flow and neurotransmitter levels are hypothesized as neuropathophysiological dysfunction influencing somatoform symptoms.[4]

Historical approaches for PNES and other conversion disorders (then referred to as "hysteria," which are documented in a review of the medical literature[5]) included faradization (electric current applied to the skin), hydrotherapy (a jugful of water to an open mouth), and a vigorous tug at the pubic hair, used in England, or the ovarian compression belt, used in France. Hypnosis and psychoanalysis were commonly used in the early and mid-20th century to treat conversion disorder. Anecdotal references were followed by occasional publications of case reports, case series, and open-label trials.

Treatment advances in the past decade involve rigorous trials comparing pharmacotherapies and psychotherapies, providing an evidence-based medicine approach to somatic symptom disorders (SSDs). Examples of trials include those involving cognitive-behavioral therapy (CBT), CBT-informed psychotherapy (CBT-ip) using a manualized treatment workbook, and psychotropic medications for SSD and for PNES. These controlled trials are described in detail in this chapter.

2. REVIEW OF THE EVIDENCE BASE

Management of PNES approaches is reviewed extensively in the International League Against Epilepsy (ILAE) Nonepileptic Seizure Task Force's report.[6] The first step in appropriate treatment is proper diagnosis. Diagnostic accuracy has improved over the past 30 years with the use of video-EEG, and standards have been set by the ILAE for establishing the diagnosis.[7] A Cochrane Review published in February 2014 examined psychological and behavioral treatments for adults with PNES and identified two studies with low bias risk[8]; however, the publication predated the U.S. multicenter pilot randomized clinical trial (RCT)[9] and the current U.K. RCT for PNES,[10] which are described below.

2.1. Uncontrolled and Open-Label Data

Psychopharmacological interventions for conversion disorder have been used to attempt to treat the SSDs directly and to treat the common comorbidities (i.e., depression, anxiety, posttraumatic stress disorder and personality disorders). Historically, medication treatment approaches have been symptomatic. Fully powered phase III controlled studies of the benefit of psychotropics in patients with PNES, however, have not been conducted, and apart from largely anecdotal reports, their efficacy is unknown. The pharmacological references for PNES treatment using intravenous barbiturates, tricyclic antidepressants, selective serotonin reuptake inhibitors, mixed mechanism antidepressants, dopamine receptor antagonists, beta blockers, analgesics, or benzodiazepines are largely anecdotal references in case reports, journal review articles, and book chapters, with only three prospective open-label trials.[1,4]

Psychotherapy appears to have a stronger effect in SSDs than pharmacological approaches. Reviews of psychotherapies for patients with PNES report on the application of a variety of modalities, including psychodynamic, paradoxical intention, DB/mindfulness, CB, interpersonal, hypnosis, and eye movement desensitization and reprocessing (EMDR) therapies, delivered to children and adults in individual, group, and family therapies.[6,11] Other approaches to SSDs and PNES use patient education books and psychodynamic methods[12–14]; however, no data from controlled studies have been published using these approaches. The Cochrane Review notes the limitations of the studies based on small sample sizes, lack of blinded outcome measurement, and absence of control group.[8] It is beyond the scope of this chapter to review every open-label and uncontrolled study of PNES. The controlled trials are reviewed next.

2.2. Controlled Studies

2.2.1. Psychotherapeutic Treatments for PNES

In terms of randomized controlled studies, the evidence base remains very limited (see Table 14.1). For many years, the literature highlighted three randomized controlled studies,[15–17] the first two of which employed a hypnosis-based intervention and did not focus specifically on patients with PNES but treated patients with motor conversion disorder more widely; the studies also did not include seizure frequency as an outcome measure. While focusing on seizure frequency, Ataoglu et al.[17] did not adopt a typical psychotherapeutic approach, instead opting to deliver paradoxical intention therapy to hospitalized patients, at the rate of 2 paradoxical intention treatment sessions daily for 3 weeks. Patients were asked to imagine anxiety-provoking situations and/or experiences so that they might re-experience their traumas and experience PNES episodes. The study was small (Table 14.1), but the paradoxical intention group responded better than the control group both in terms of reduced PNES occurrence ($p = 0.034$) and anxiety symptoms ($p = 0.015$).

Although not included in Cochrane reviews, a behavior therapy intervention was documented by Aamir et al.[18] (Table 14.1). This is one of the few non-Western treatment studies to focus on PNES and tested 15 sessions of behavior therapy for patients with PNES administered over 2½ months, compared to treatment as usual (pharmacotherapy and outpatient review), in a predominantly rural Pakistani sample. The behavior therapy intervention consisted of positive reinforcement on a variable ratio and variable interval schedule to increase PNES-free behavior, along with punishment (the withdrawal of privileges) to reduce inappropriate (presumably seizure-related) behavior and also reduce opportunities for negative reinforcement. Both groups of patients were initially treated as inpatients for 1 week, discharged, and followed for 15 weeks. During the inpatient week, caregivers of the behavior therapy group received intensive training so that they could administer positive reinforcement and punishment and avoid negative reinforcement of the patients' behavior in the home environment. At the final follow-up session, there was a significant difference ($p < 0.001$) in PNES frequency, as well as anxiety and depression scores, between the two groups, in favor of those who had received behavior therapy. The small sample size and the very simple statistics applied to the data in this study render the findings interesting but requiring replication.

More conventionally, a CBT approach has been tested in a pilot RCT.[19] This approach is based on the two-process learning-theory derived, fear escape-avoidance model (see Goldstein et al.[20] for a description). The pilot RCT[19] compared specially tailored CBT (based on work by Goldstein et al.[21] and Chalder[22]) with standard medical care (SMC) in an outpatient neuropsychiatric clinic. Sixty-six patients with PNES were randomized to receive either SMC alone or 12 sessions of weekly/fortnightly CBT plus SMC, scheduled to occur over a 4-month period. The majority of patients (83%) had video-EEG

Table 14.1 Randomized Controlled Trials of Psychotherapeutic and Other Interventions for PNES

Reference	Treatments	N	Design	Comments
Moene et al. (2002)[15]	Inpatient group centered-activities (including group psychotherapy, social skills training), planning and evaluating goals, creative therapy and sports, individual physiotherapy, exercises, and bed rest either with an introductory session + 8 weekly 1-hour sessions with a therapist designed to optimize nonspecific or common therapy factors (control group) or with the addition of an introductory session + 8 weekly 1-hour sessions of manualized hypnosis (hypnosis group)	From an initial sample of 49 patients: Hypnosis group $N = 24$ Control group $N = 21$	RCT	Did not specifically focus on PNES patients but rather on motor conversion disorder patients. Eight patients had "seizures or convulsions" but no information was given about previous/comorbid epilepsy. Outcome measures did not include seizure frequency. Authors did not perform an ITT analysis.
Moene et al. (2003)[16]	Outpatient manualized hypnosis (introductory session + 10 hypnosis sessions over 3 months) or waiting list control	From an initial sample of 49 patients: Hypnosis $N = 20$ Waiting list controls $N = 25$	RCT	Did not specifically focus on PNES patients but rather on motor conversion disorder patients. Only two patients had "seizures or convulsions" but no information was given about previous/comorbid epilepsy. Outcome measures did not include seizure frequency. Authors did not perform an ITT analysis.
Ataoglu et al. (2003)[17]	Three weeks of inpatient paradoxical intention therapy (two sessions/day) vs. 6 weeks of diazepam (5–15 mg per day)	$N = 15$ per group	RCT	Participants with an abnormal EEG were excluded. Authors did not perform an ITT analysis but not clear that there was any notable data loss.

Study	Intervention	N	Design	Notes
Goldstein et al. (2010)[19]	12 sessions of CBT modified for PNES + standard medical care vs. standard medical care alone	$N = 33$ per group	RCT	Patients with past history of epilepsy or current comorbid epilepsy were excluded. An ITT analysis was conducted.
LaFrance et al. (2010)[24]	Flexible dose of sertraline (up to 200 mg) vs. placebo over 12 weeks. Seen in 6 biweekly 30-minute long sessions	Sertraline $N = 19$ Placebo $N = 19$	Double-blind placebo-controlled RCT	Two patients with both epilepsy and PNES were included as they were reportedly able to distinguish between seizure types. An ITT analysis was conducted.
Aamir et al. (2011)[18]	15 sessions of behavior therapy (positive reinforcement and withdrawal of privileges) on an in- and outpatient basis (administered by primary caregivers who received training) vs. routine treatment (pharmacotherapy)	$N = 9$ in each group	RCT	Patients with comorbid epilepsy were excluded. Authors did not perform an ITT analysis.
Sharpe et al. (2011)[34]	Four sessions of CBT-based guided self help + usual care vs. usual care	GSH+ usual care $N = 64$ Usual care $N = 63$	RCT	Did not specifically focus on PNES patients but rather on patients with a broad range of functional neurological symptoms. Only 12 patients were reported as having "blackouts."
LaFrance et al. (2014)[9]	12 sessions of CBT-ip vs. 12 sessions of CBT-ip plus flexible-dose sertraline vs. flexible-dose sertraline vs. TAU	CBT-ip $N = 9$ CBT-ip+sertraline $N = 10$ Sertraline $N = 9$ TAU $N = 10$	RCT	Study excluded patients with comorbid epilepsy. Main analyses of primary outcome were conducted within rather than between groups. An ITT analysis was conducted.

CBT, cognitive-behavioral therapy; CBT-ip, CBT-informed psychotherapy; GSH, guided self-help; ITT, intention to treat; PNES, psychogenic nonepileptic seizures; RCT, randomized controlled trials; TAU, treatment as usual.

telemetry-confirmed PNES. Patients with fewer than two PNES/month and an IQ below 70 were excluded.

Goldstein et al.'s[19,20] intervention was structured in five stages: engagement and rationale giving; seizure control techniques; reducing avoidance behavior; addressing seizure-related cognitions; and relapse prevention. In the initial stage, therapists delivered a treatment rationale that included the interaction between cognitions, physiological/emotional, and behavioral responses; patients were reassured that their PNES were viewed as real and distressing events for the person. Dissociation as a mechanism (namely "switching off") was explained as an extreme occurrence of normal changes in selective attention, in this context as a means of preventing experiencing extreme fear, distress, and anxiety. Factors including the role of risk avoidance and safety behaviors in maintaining PNES occurrence were outlined. Therapists would also deal with any persisting uncertainty by the person concerning the accuracy of their diagnosis and would consider contributions made by low mood, the role of significant others, and the potential for the sick role to be a maintaining factor. With the person's consent, the approach also involved, as part of the engagement process, his or her caregivers or significant others who would also be included later in treatment, where possible, to evaluate and also assist with generalization of treatment gains.

The second stage of treatment focused on development of techniques to help directly with PNES control. These techniques included distraction, attention refocusing, or relaxation with a view to improving the person's ability overall to better tolerate arousal-provoking stimuli and reduce seizure occurrence. Stage three focused on reducing emotional and behavioral avoidance, using standard exposure techniques but incorporating competing behaviors to prevent the person from dissociating.

In the fourth treatment stage, the therapists addressed seizure-related cognitions that might serve to maintain PNES occurrence. Therapy addressed negative automatic thoughts (NATs) that might relate to seizures, the person's self-esteem, and, where relevant, previously experienced trauma. Standard cognitive therapy techniques were employed to challenge NATs to improve mood more generally and increasing the person's beliefs in his or her ability to control the seizures. Where traumas had been identified during the treatment process, a range of techniques was used to facilitate appropriate emotional processing. In practice, the therapy approaches in stages 3 and 4 were incorporated flexibly as considered appropriate.

The final stage of treatment involved reviewing therapeutic progress and reformulating goals for any outstanding issues, planning a time frame for their achievement, and focusing on relapse prevention and the maintenance of achieved goals, often using a problem-solving approach. Table 14.2 indicates the structure of the treatment adopted in Goldstein et al.'s (2010)[19] study, based on information previously presented online.

Goldstein et al.'s pilot RCT indicated, in an intention-to-treat (ITT) analysis, that seizure reduction following CBT+SMC was superior to that in SMC alone (group × time interaction $p < 0.0001$). At the end of treatment, seizure reduction following CBT+SMC was greater than following SMC alone ($p = 0.002$), and there was a trend for lower seizure frequency at the 6-month follow-up following CBT+SMC versus SMC alone ($p = 0.082$). This reduction in between-group significance may in part have been attributable to the observation that the SMC group showed some improvement (i.e., reduction in PNES

Table 14.2 Approach to Sessional Content Used by Goldstein et al. (2010)[19]

Session Number	Content	Homework Tasks
1	This session includes the following: • Assessment and clarification of the person's main presenting problem, including its development, as well as the person's family history and background • Providing a description of CBT and rationale for treatment using a CBT model • Providing a formulation of the person's main/current problem and seeking the person's agreement to this	Completion of self-monitoring seizure diaries
2	This session includes the following: • Review of seizure diaries and homework as previously agreed; any difficulties experienced with these are discussed • Further discussion and clarification of treatment rationale and/or formulation • Agreement on long-term targets so that patient identifies something he or she would like to do in the future that the person cannot currently do • Agreement over two homework tasks to be completed by the next session; these should be based on the patient's avoidance behavior (e.g., avoiding going out in case of having a seizure); these have to be realistic and achievable and may take considerable discussion.	Completion of self-monitoring seizure diaries and two goals based on patient's avoidance behavior. This homework should be supplemented by asking patients to read a handout on Cognitive-Behavioral Therapy and Psychogenic Nonepileptic Seizures.
3	This session includes the following: • Review of seizure diaries and homework as previously agreed; any difficulties experienced with these are discussed • Involvement, where possible, of family members in the session to discuss ways in which factors in the person's life and role of significant others may be contributing to maintenance of the patient's problems (e.g., reinforcing PNES occurrence). • Introduction to seizure-directed techniques, such as attention refocusing and distraction techniques, in cases where the patient can identify warning signs for PNES	Completion of self-monitoring seizure diaries and practice of distraction and refocusing techniques to be implemented in response to seizure warnings. This homework should be supplemented by asking patients to read a handout on distraction and refocusing techniques and encouraging family members to read a handout providing an account of CBT and PNES for partners and family members.

(continued)

Table 14.2 Continued

Session Number	Content	Homework Tasks
4	This session includes the following: • Review of seizure diaries and homework as previously agreed; any difficulties experienced with these are discussed • Identification of past or present traumas or problems that may be contributing to PNES occurrence or making progress difficult • Introduction to breathing techniques and relaxation exercises to be used as seizure-interruption techniques or as stress- and anxiety-management techniques • Introduction to cognitive therapy techniques, i.e., recognizing negative thinking styles	Completion of self-monitoring seizure diaries. Practicing application of breathing techniques and relaxation exercises when seizure warnings occur. Patients should be encouraged to continue to apply distraction and attention refocusing techniques and to deal with avoided behaviors through exposure to avoided situations. This homework should be supplemented by asking patients to read a handout on progressive muscle relaxation exercises and cued relaxation.
5	This session includes the following: • Review of seizure diaries and homework as previously agreed; any difficulties experienced with these are discussed • Further cognitive therapy work involving clarification of patients' thinking errors, e.g., catastrophizing, all-or-nothing thinking, overgeneralizing • Further review of avoidant behavior and setting further goals • Consolidation of PNES interruption techniques (e.g., relaxation and breathing techniques, distraction, attention refocusing) • Introduction to problem-solving approaches	Completion of self-monitoring seizure diaries. Commencing identification of negative thoughts and recording these in thought diaries. This homework should be supplemented by asking patients to read a handout on identifying negative automatic thoughts and alternatives to negative thoughts.

Table 14.2 Continued

Session Number	Content	Homework Tasks
6	This mid-treatment review session includes the following: • Review of seizure diaries and homework as previously agreed; any difficulties experienced with these are discussed • Review of progress to date • Identification of remaining issues to be addressed in therapy • Meeting with family members to evaluate progress thus far	Completion of self-monitoring seizure diaries. Negotiate goals as considered suitable.
7–9	These sessions include the following: • Review of seizure diaries and homework as previously agreed; any difficulties experienced with these are discussed • Ongoing goal setting • Ongoing discussion of negative thoughts and how to address these • Ongoing consideration of past or present traumas or problems that may be contributing to PNES occurrence or making progress difficult • Ongoing consideration of both behavioral and cognitive avoidance in the person's difficulties • Continued use of breathing, relaxation distraction, and refocusing techniques • Encouraged use of problem-solving strategies for actual and potential problems	Completion of self-monitoring seizure diaries. Negotiate goals as considered suitable.
10	This session includes the following: • Review of seizure diaries and homework as previously agreed; any difficulties experienced with these are discussed • Identification of potential or ongoing problems and how they may be addressed using CBT techniques once the person has been discharged from CBT treatment	Completion of self-monitoring seizure diaries. Identification of potential difficulties; the person then has to address these using problem-solving techniques. This would be supplemented by reading a handout on preparing for the future.

(continued)

Table 14.2 Continued

Session Number	Content	Homework Tasks
11	This session includes the following: • Review of seizure diaries and homework as previously agreed; any difficulties experienced with these are discussed • Review of treatment to date • Allocation of time to reflect on the treatment process • Discussion of outstanding issues	Completion of self-monitoring seizure diaries. Negotiate homework as appropriate.
12	This session includes the following: • Review of seizure diaries and homework as previously agreed; any difficulties experienced with these are discussed • Review of progress made over the course of the treatment • Identification of goals to be reviewed at follow-up booster session • Positive reinforcement of gains made within treatment and how they were made • Meeting with family members to review progress that has been made	
Follow-up	In this session the agenda is structured to take into account the content of session 12 and may include negotiation of future homework tasks.	Plan for any further needed follow-up sessions.

Adapted from Goldstein et al. (2010).[19]

occurrence) over time; longer term, patients in the CBT arm may have benefitted from further CBT booster/maintenance sessions. At 6-month follow-up, the CBT+SMC group tended to be more likely to have experienced 3 months of seizure freedom ($p = 0.086$), but it was not possible to evaluate seizure freedom in 7/66 of the participants. Both groups demonstrated improvement on some of the health service use measures employed and on the Work and Social Adjustment Scale.[23] However, anxiety, depression, and employment status showed no change. A fully powered multicenter RCT is now underway in the United Kingdom to test the effectiveness of this CBT model in patients with PNES.[10] The care pathway for this study takes patients from their diagnosis by a neurologist or epilepsy specialist to a subsequent psychiatric assessment, prior to randomization to CBT+standard medical care versus standard medical care alone.

2.2.2. Pharmacological Treatments for PNES

Selective serotonin reuptake inhibitors (SSRIs) have, in addition to their demonstrated effectiveness in treating anxiety and depression, shown potential beneficial effects in patients with other comorbidities common to the PNES population, namely somatic symptom or conversion disorders, as well as some personality disorders. Based on this, a small double-blind pilot (not powered for efficacy) randomized placebo-controlled trial of pharmacological treatment for PNES[24] (Table 14.1) investigated the effects of flexible-dose sertraline versus placebo on PNES frequency. Following a 2-week baseline period, the flexible dosing regimen involved patients increasing their daily dose of sertraline or placebo from 25 mg to 50 mg in biweekly stages and then to a maximum of 200 mg/day, depending on the development of adverse effects. In this study, 26/38 people with telemetry-confirmed PNES produced end-of-study data.

Of the 38 enrolled patients, 19 received sertraline and of these, 16 tolerated at least 100 mg; 10 tolerated the maximum dose of 200 mg. Of these 38 patients, 33 were included in an ITT analysis.

The patients receiving sertraline experienced a 45% decrease in bi-weekly seizure frequency over the 12-week study. In contrast, the placebo group showed an 8% increase in seizure frequency over the corresponding period. Adjusting for different baseline seizure frequency, there was evidence for a reduced rate of seizure occurrence in the sertraline arm relative to placebo. In the ITT analysis, 47.1% of the sertraline and 18.8% of placebo patients demonstrated ≥50% reduction in seizures ($p = 0.18$). Within these "responders", there was a nonsignificant trend ($p = 0.08$) for the sertraline-treated patients to be more likely to demonstrate complete seizure cessation.

Interestingly, measures of anxiety, depression, quality of life, psychosocial functioning, somatic symptoms, and impulsivity did not show any between-group differences in terms of change across the study, adjusting for baseline differences. Thus, while this pilot study provided suggestive evidence that sertraline reduced seizure rates relative to that seen with placebo, the results suggested a direct effect of sertraline on PNES, rather than being mediated by change on measures of psychological/psychosocial status. The efficacy of sertraline as a psychopharmacological intervention for PNES has not yet been tested in a fully powered double-blinded pharmacological RCT. The findings from this pilot study remain intriguing in that the conversion/somatic symptom disorder symptoms appeared to exhibit a lower threshold for responding to SSRIs than the traditional targets of depression and anxiety. The findings suggested that while the SSRI did not lead to complete resolution of PNES, their reduction indicated the potential value of SSRIs as an adjunct to psychotherapeutic intervention for PNES.

2.2.3. Combined Pharmacological and Psychotherapeutic Treatments for PNES

LaFrance et al. have combined their previously tested psychopharmacological[24,25] and psychotherapeutic interventions for conversion disorders[26,27] in a four-arm pilot RCT[9] (Table 14.1).

LaFrance et al. refer to their psychotherapeutic approach for PNES as a Beckian-based, CBT-informed psychotherapy (CBT-ip). This intervention is structured, delivered over

12 one-hour-long sessions, and focused on present issues, addressing mood-cognition-environment associations, similar to Goldstein et al.'s[19] CBT approach, where it recognizes the importance of cognitive distortions in contributing to PNES occurrence and aims to facilitate behavioral change. It similarly also includes approaches to manage comorbidities (e.g., anxiety, depression) and targets the occurrence of seizures directly. The 2 approaches differ in that the Goldstein studies are based on conventional CBT, whereas the CBT-ip incorporates other psychotherapeutic modalities, including aspects of psychoeducation and transtheoretical, psychodynamic, interpersonal, and dialectical psychotherapies, described next.

The approach is modified from a program initially developed to treat epileptic seizures,[28,29] and the therapist guide has also been manualized to facilitate delivery by different counselors.[30] The workbook-based intervention fosters a self-management approach to dealing with seizures on the part of the patient.[31] The treatment approach takes account of the patient's environment, identifying moods, situations, and cognitions (e.g., automatic thoughts, catastrophic thinking, and somatic misinterpretations) that are relevant to PNES occurrence, and examines relevant external stressors and internal triggers. In addition, it emphasizes training adaptive communication styles and obtaining support in the person's environment for the necessary change to take place. Functional behavioral analysis (i.e., thought record) is used to understand more about factors maintaining PNES occurrence, including schemas (core beliefs). Other important components of this more eclectic intervention include a psychoeducational approach concerning central nervous system drugs (and their potential impact on PNES), learning relaxation techniques, and preparing for life after completing the 12-session intervention. The intervention incorporates techniques that address interpersonal communication and dialectical aspects, teaching mindfulness to help improve distress tolerance. Finally, dynamic therapy techniques are included to address relevant developmental aspects of patients' presentations.[32] Table 14.3 describes the sessions in the treatment workbook for seizures.

LaFrance et al.[9] randomized 38 patients across 3 different sites to four treatment arms (Table 14.1); of these, 34 patients provided outcome data in the mixed modelling analysis. As the study was not powered for between-group analyses, comparisons were undertaken within groups. At the end of treatment, the CBT-ip group reported a 51.4% reduction in PNES frequency ($p = 0.01$), in addition to improved anxiety, depression, quality of life, and global functioning scores. The CBT-ip+sertraline group showed a reduction in seizure frequency of a broadly similar magnitude (59.3%; $p = 0.008$), along with improvement in secondary outcomes, including depression, quality of life, and global functioning. A trend toward reduction in PNES frequency (26.5%, $p = 0.08$) was observed in the sertraline-only group, with a significant reduction in depression and no significant improvement on other secondary outcomes. No improvement in either PNES frequency ($p = 0.19$) or secondary outcomes was found in the treatment as usual (TAU) group. In all groups other than TAU, a majority of patients showed at least a 50% reduction in PNES frequency. Health service use (visits to emergency departments) was reduced in the CBT-ip group relative to baseline.

This pilot RCT demonstrated the potential value of LaFrance et al.'s therapeutic approach for PNES using a manualized workbook with or without adjunctive sertraline. The study also raised the possibility that the use of sertraline alone may not facilitate

Table 14.3 Taking Control of Your Seizures Workbook Sessions

Session	Title	Goal
Session Intro	Introduction for Patients: Understanding Seizures	Describes epileptic and nonepileptic seizures
Session 1	Making the Decision to Begin the Process of Taking Control	Patient makes the choice to engage in treatment
Session 2	Getting Support	Addresses communication styles and goals
Session 3	Deciding about Your Medication Therapy	Discusses central nervous system medications
Session 4	Learning to Observe Your Triggers	Examines physical, internal, and external triggers
Session 5	Channeling Negative Emotions into Productive Outlets	Explores emotions, cognitions, and relieving actions
Session 6	Relaxation Training	Teaches relaxation techniques
Session 7	Identifying Your Pre-seizure Aura	Identifies aura using self-awareness techniques
Session 8	Dealing with External Life Stresses	Addresses relational and psychosocial stresses
Session 9	Dealing with Internal Issues and Conflicts	Examines past trauma and unconscious processes
Session 10	Enhancing Personal Wellness	Sets healthy lifestyle priorities
Session 11	Other Seizure Symptoms	Describes comorbid symptoms
Final Reading	Taking Control: An On-going Process	Provides perspective on life after treatment

Modified permission from Reiter JM, Andrews DJ, Reiter C, LaFrance WC Jr. (2015). *Taking Control of Your Seizures: Workbook*. New York: Oxford University Press.

better secondary outcomes (e.g., mood, anxiety) in a somatically focused patient group. The longer-term outcome for the open-label trial revealed a maintained reduction in PNES at the 12-month follow-up, demonstrating durability of the therapy.[33]

2.2.4. Treatments for Conversion Disorders/Functional Neurological Disorders Including PNES

Of potential relevance more widely for the treatment of patients with PNES are brief, self-help treatments devised for patients with functional neurological symptoms/conversion disorder that might include PNES. While the approaches of Goldstein et al.[19]

and LaFrance et al.[9] involve the delivery of more traditional packages of therapy, not all patients want to attend formal psychotherapy,[34] and not all patients have access to intensive psychotherapy for their PNES.[35] Sharpe et al.[34] have suggested that a brief, self-help (bibliographic) intervention, combined with face-to-face guidance, could be delivered via neurology clinics to increase treatment uptake and address somatic symptoms.

Sharpe et al.[34] examined self-rated health in neurology outpatients with functional neurological symptoms 3 months after randomization. One hundred and twenty-seven patients were randomized to continue to receive either usual care alone or usual care plus guided self-help (GSH). A total of 12 of these patients had a diagnosis of "blackouts." In order to enhance usual clinical care, patients' comorbid psychiatric diagnoses were communicated to the patient's primary care doctor and their neurologist. GSH involved the provision of a CBT-based self-help workbook and face-to-face sessions to provide guidance in its use. Four half-hour guidance sessions were delivered in person (or if necessary by telephone) by a psychologist or nurse trained in CBT, both of whom received supervision from a psychiatrist. The self-help workbook that has subsequently been published[36] covers the following main areas: 1) what functional neurological symptoms are and understanding how people respond to symptoms, 2) how the brain and body link to symptoms, 3) a five-areas approach to improving symptoms (e.g., by learning about how thoughts and symptoms affect each other, the impact of activity on symptoms), 4) changing behaviors, including avoidance, and 5) noticing and changing unhelpful thinking. In Sharpe et al.'s study[34] 62/64 (97%) of the patients allocated to the GSH arm received at least one session of GSH in the use of the workbook; an average number of three sessions were received. After 3 months, the GSH group exhibited a significantly better self-rating of clinical improvement ($p = 0.016$) compared to the usual-care group. There was a difference of 13% between groups in the percentage characterized as "better." In terms of secondary outcomes, the GSH group reported a greater improvement in their presenting symptoms and health anxiety concerns but there were no between-group differences in depression, anxiety, or physical function. The GSH group also reported greater satisfaction with treatment. The difference between groups on the primary outcome of self-rated clinical improvement, taken together with the secondary outcomes, was considered to be clinically useful.

A 6-month follow-up found that while the GSH group's improvement in self-rated clinical improvement and reduced health anxiety had not persisted, the GSH group had maintained the reported improvement in their presenting symptoms and now reported improved physical functioning and stronger beliefs that their condition was not permanent. The GSH group also maintained their greater satisfaction with treatment.

The very small proportion of patients with likely PNES in this study makes immediate generalization of this approach, which contained a strong psychoeducation component, to the PNES population challenging. However, some preliminary psychoeducational approaches devised specifically for people with PNES have been described.

2.2.5. Psychoeducational Approaches to Reducing PNES Occurrence

Preliminary findings from a small RCT that randomized 64 patients with PNES who had received their PNES diagnosis in an epilepsy monitoring unit have been described by Chen et al.[37] The intervention included a standardized approach to diagnosis delivery, followed by a brief psychoeducation intervention conducted over three 1.5-hour-long group sessions which took place 1 month apart. Chen et al. reported a significant improvement in psychosocial functioning in the psychoeducation group, when evaluated at 3- and 6-month follow-up, compared to that seen in the participants who only had routine seizure follow-up clinic visits. Chen et al. did not find any between-groups differences in PNES frequency, but there was a trend for less hospital service use in the psychoeducation group.

In the United Kingdom, a brief, manualized psychoeducation approach for PNES patients has been reported,[38] although only within the limitations of a nonrandomized feasibility study. This prospective multicenter study incorporated a four-session psychoeducational intervention for PNES that used as its basis the initial communication of the patient's diagnosis. The intervention was delivered by healthcare professionals with very limited experience in the delivery of psychological therapies. Twenty-nine patients enrolled in the study; of these, 20 began and 13 completed the intervention. At follow-up, 4/13 of patients reported complete seizure cessation and a further 3/13 reported more than a 50% reduction in seizure frequency. The effectiveness of this psychoeducational approach requires further testing within an RCT.

3. CONCLUSIONS

Since 2010, the treatment of patients with PNES has evolved in an important manner to incorporate a small number of RCTs that begin to hold promise for the psychotherapeutic interventions for this challenging group of patients. In the context of this evolving literature:

- Future studies still need to improve on as-yet limited sample sizes and provide insights into predictors of treatment outcome so that rational decisions can be made about which treatments offer the best outcome and who is likely to best respond to which treatment.
- The high rates of psychiatric comorbidity (particularly for other somatic symptom and conversion disorders) are challenges not always specifically addressed in prior studies, where PNES is the primary focus of a complex neuropsychiatric disorder. The interventions in the RCT studies reviewed here are largely predicated on a CBT-based model of psychotherapeutic interventions, although with some additions of other psychotherapeutic techniques.[9]
- As yet, there are only open-label studies of more psychodynamically oriented psychotherapy approaches, such as brief augmented psychodynamic interpersonal therapy,[39] and these too require investigation in more robust trial designs.
- Similarly, psychoeducational approaches[38] may hold promise and require more rigorous investigation in this patient population.
- The option of psychoeducation or guided self-help, whether for PNES specifically or functional neurological symptoms/conversion disorder, requires demonstration of efficacy in adequately powered RCTs and could broaden the existing options of currently available treatments that empower patients with PNES.

REFERENCES

1. LaFrance WC Jr, Bjørnæs H. Chapter 28. Designing treatment plans based on etiology of psychogenic nonepileptic seizures. In: Schachter SC, LaFrance WCJr, eds. *Gates and Rowan's Nonepileptic Seizures*, 3rd ed. Cambridge; New York: Cambridge University Press; 2010:266–280.
2. Bullock KD, Mirza N, Forte C, Trockel M. Group dialectical-behavior therapy skills training for conversion disorder with seizures. *J Neuropsychiatry Clin Neurosci*. 2015;27(3):240–243.
3. Miller HR. Psychogenic seizures treated by hypnosis. *Am J Clin Hypn*. 1983;25(4):248–252.
4. LaFrance WC Jr, Blumer D. Chapter 32. Pharmacological treatments for psychogenic nonepileptic seizures. In: Schachter SC, LaFrance WCJr, eds. *Gates and Rowan's Nonepileptic Seizures*, 3rd ed. Cambridge; New York: Cambridge University Press; 2010:307–316.
5. LaFrance WC Jr. 'Hysteria' today and tomorrow. *Front Neurol Neurosci*. 2014;35:198–204.
6. LaFrance WC Jr, Reuber M, Goldstein LH. Management of psychogenic nonepileptic seizures. *Epilepsia*. 2013;54(Suppl 1):53–67.
7. LaFrance WC Jr, Baker GA, Duncan R, Goldstein LH, Reuber M. Minimum requirements for the diagnosis of psychogenic nonepileptic seizures: a staged approach: a report from the International League Against Epilepsy Nonepileptic Seizures Task Force. *Epilepsia*. 2013;54(11):2005–2018.
8. Martlew J, Pulman J, Marson AG. Psychological and behavioural treatments for adults with non-epileptic attack disorder. *Cochrane Database Syst Rev*. 2014;2:CD006370.
9. LaFrance WC Jr, Baird GL, Barry JJ, et al. Multicenter pilot treatment trial for psychogenic nonepileptic seizures: a randomized clinical trial. *JAMA Psychiatry*. 2014;71(9):997–1005.
10. Goldstein LH, Mellers JD, Landau S, et al. Cognitive behavioural therapy vs standardised medical care for adults with dissociative non-epileptic seizures (CODES): a multicentre randomised controlled trial protocol. *BMC Neurol*. 2015;15:98.
11. Baslet G, Dworetzky B, Perez DL, Oser M. Treatment of psychogenic nonepileptic seizures: updated review and findings from a mindfulness-based intervention case series. *Clin EEG Neurosci*. 2015;46(1):54–64.
12. Myers L. *Psychogenic Non-epileptic Seizures: A Guide*. CreateSpace Independent Publishing Platform; 2014.
13. Woolfolk RL, Allen LA. *Treating Somatization: A Cognitive-Behavioral Approach*. New York: Guilford Press; 2007.
14. Kalogjera-Sackellares D. *Psychodynamics and Psychotherapy of Pseudoseizures*. Carmarthen, UK: Crown House Publishing; 2004.
15. Moene FC, Spinhoven P, Hoogduin KA, van Dyck R. A randomised controlled clinical trial on the additional effect of hypnosis in a comprehensive treatment programme for in-patients with conversion disorder of the motor type. *Psychother Psychosom*. 2002;71(2):66–76.
16. Moene FC, Spinhoven P, Hoogduin KA, van Dyck R. A randomized controlled clinical trial of a hypnosis-based treatment for patients with conversion disorder, motor type. *Int J Clin Exp Hypn*. 2003;51(1):29–50.
17. Ataoglu A, Ozcetin A, Icmeli C, Ozbulut O. Paradoxical therapy in conversion reaction. *J Korean Med Sci*. 2003;18(4):581–584.
18. Aamir S, Haymayon S, Sultan S. Behavior therapy in dissociative convulsion disorder. *J Depress Anxiety*. 2011;1(1):1–4.

19. Goldstein LH, Chalder T, Chigwedere C, et al. Cognitive-behavioral therapy for psychogenic nonepileptic seizures: a pilot RCT. *Neurology*. 2010;74(24):1986–1994.
20. Goldstein LH, LaFrance WC Jr, Chigwedere C, Mellers JDC, Chalder T. Chapter 29. Cognitive behavioral treatments. In: Schachter SC, LaFrance WCJr, eds. *Gates and Rowan's Nonepileptic Seizures*, 3rd ed. Cambridge; New York: Cambridge University Press; 2010:281–288.
21. Goldstein LH, Deale AC, Mitchell-O'Malley SJ, Toone BK, Mellers JDC. An evaluation of cognitive behavioral therapy as a treatment for dissociative seizures: a pilot study. *Cogn Behav Neurol*. 2004;17(1):41–49.
22. Chalder T. Non-epileptic attacks: a cognitive behavioral approach in a single case with a four-year follow-up. *Clin Psychol Psychother*. 1996;3(4):291–297.
23. Mundt JC, Marks IM, Shear MK, Greist JH. The Work and Social Adjustment Scale: a simple measure of impairment in functioning. *Br J Psychiatry*. 2002;180:461–464.
24. LaFrance WC Jr, Keitner GI, Papandonatos GD, et al. Pilot pharmacologic randomized controlled trial for psychogenic nonepileptic seizures. *Neurology*. 2010;75(13):1166–1173.
25. LaFrance WC Jr, Blum AS, Miller IW, Ryan CE, Keitner GI. Methodological issues in conducting treatment trials for psychological nonepileptic seizures. *J Neuropsychiatry Clin Neurosci*. 2007;19(4):391–398.
26. LaFrance WC Jr, Friedman JH. Cognitive behavioral therapy for psychogenic movement disorder. *Mov Disord*. 2009;24(12):1856–1857.
27. LaFrance WC Jr, Miller IW, Ryan CE, et al. Cognitive behavioral therapy for psychogenic nonepileptic seizures. *Epilepsy Behav*. 2009;14(4):591–596.
28. Reiter JM, Andrews DJ. A neurobehavioral approach for treatment of complex partial epilepsy: efficacy. *Seizure*. 2000;9(3):198–203.
29. Andrews DJ, Reiter JM, Schonfeld W, Kastl A, Denning P. A neurobehavioral treatment for unilateral complex partial seizure disorders: a comparison of right- and left-hemisphere patients. *Seizure*. 2000;9(3):189–197.
30. LaFrance WC Jr, Wincze JP. *Treating Nonepileptic Seizures: Therapist Guide*. New York: Oxford University Press; 2015.
31. LaFrance Jr WC, Ranieri R, Baird GB, Blum A, Keitner G. One year follow up of cognitive behavioral therapy-informed psychotherapy treatment trial for psychogenic nonepileptic seizures. Abstract 3.237. 2015, American Epilepsy Society Annual Meeting. www.aesnet.org.
32. Chen DK, LaFrance WC Jr. Diagnosis and treatment of nonepileptic seizures. Continuum (Minneap Minn) 2016;22(1, Epilepsy):116–131.
33. Reiter JM, Andrews D, Reiter C, LaFrance WC Jr. *Taking Control of Your Seizures: Workbook*. New York: Oxford University Press; 2015.
34. Sharpe M, Walker J, Williams C, et al. Guided self-help for functional (psychogenic) symptoms: a randomized controlled efficacy trial. *Neurology*. 2011;77(6):564–572.
35. Mayor R, Smith PE, Reuber M. Management of patients with nonepileptic attack disorder in the United Kingdom: a survey of health care professionals. *Epilepsy Behav*. 2011;21(4):402–406.
36. Williams C, Kent C, Smith S, Carson A, Sharpe M, Cavanagh J. *Overcoming Functional Neurological Symptoms: A Five Areas Approach*. London: Hodder Arnold; 2011.
37. Chen DK, Maheshwari A, Franks R, Trolley GC, Robinson JS, Hrachovy RA. Brief group psychoeducation for psychogenic nonepileptic seizures: a neurologist-initiated program in an epilepsy center. *Epilepsia*. 2014;55(1):156–166.

38. Mayor R, Brown RJ, Cock H, et al. A feasibility study of a brief psycho-educational intervention for psychogenic nonepileptic seizures. *Seizure*. 2013;22(9):760–765.
39. Mayor R, Howlett S, Grunewald R, Reuber M. Long-term outcome of brief augmented psychodynamic interpersonal therapy for psychogenic nonepileptic seizures: seizure control and health care utilization. *Epilepsia*. 2010;51(7):1169–1176.

15

The Role of the Neurologist after Diagnosis

Adriana Bermeo-Ovalle, MD and Andres M. Kanner, MD, FANA

1. INTRODUCTION

The process of suspecting or diagnosing psychogenic nonepileptic seizures (PNES) often starts in the neurology office. Patients present with sudden, recurrent involuntary and often violent events that interfere with their daily activities and alter their quality of life. More often than not, PNES are diagnosed during the evaluation of paroxysmal events thought to be epileptic seizures, which have been refractory to multiple antiepileptic drug (AED) trials, frequently during many years, and often complicated with debilitating side effects and numerous neurological consultations. In fact, the diagnosis of PNES is usually delayed by 5 to 10 years after their initial presentation.[1]

General neurologists and epilepsy specialists are often able to suspect the diagnosis of PNES and to recommend a diagnostic evaluation. Unfortunately, they are not as effective at communicating the diagnosis and at explaining the pathogenic mechanisms operant in these events. Furthermore, they are often reluctant to follow the patients after the diagnosis is reached; as a matter of fact, in many epilepsy centers the role of the neurologist or epileptologist is considered to end when the diagnosis of PNES is established.

Yet the neurologist's continued involvement is vital in ensuring the patient's understanding and acceptance of the diagnosis, promoting continuity of care, preventing feelings of abandonment (that result from the neurologist's premature disengagement), allowing for management of other neurological symptoms, ensuring rationale pharmacological therapy with AEDs, promoting communication among healthcare providers, and preventing iatrogenic interventions. In short, and contrary to general practice, the neurologist's role only begins with the establishment of the diagnosis of PNES.

Neurologists and epileptologists need to recognize the clinical similarities and differences between PNES and epileptic seizures, the common neurological comorbidities associated with PNES, and, more important, the positive impact that the relationship between neurologists and these patients can have in the overall management of this condition. The objective of this chapter is to review the role of the neurologist in the comprehensive management of patients with PNES following establishment of the diagnosis.

2. EARLY INTERVENTION FOLLOWING A DIAGNOSTIC EVALUATION

The epilepsy monitoring unit (EMU) can be a very confusing environment for patients who are electively admitted to record their typical events. Medications are changed, mobility is restricted, and patients are expected to have their "seizures" or "events," which in turn often cause insecurity and fear in patients and family members. Yet a greater problem begins when the diagnosis of PNES is established. Indeed, for a significant number of these patients who had been diagnosed and treated as suffering from chronic, treatment-resistant epilepsy, the news that their paroxysmal events are not epileptic seizures may take some time to digest and understand the information communicated by the neurologist and an even longer time to accept the diagnosis. Therefore, it is helpful for patients to be seen in follow-up at the neurologist's office (with a supportive family member, if possible) within 2 weeks of hospital discharge, regardless of any therapeutic intervention started during the hospital stay.

The first task for the neurologist at the office visit is to carefully review again all aspects of the diagnostic evaluation. A good place to start is by asking patients about their understanding of the information presented in the hospital, keeping in mind that their level of education, cultural background, and belief systems may color their interpretation of the explanations provided at the time of diagnosis. The neurologist must next inquire how the patient feels about the diagnosis, what has changed in the way he or she perceives him- or herself or how others perceive the person since discharge from the EMU, and what is their understanding of the recommended therapeutic plan. While the participation of close family members and caregivers has proven to be very important in the management of all patients with PNES, it is crucial when dealing with children and adolescents.

Clinicians often assume that patients and family members can understand the difference between "epileptic" seizures and "psychogenic" seizures. Yet, the reality is that following their diagnostic evaluation, approximately two thirds of patients report being "confused" regarding the nature and meaning of the diagnosis of PNES,[2] which may persist for some time even after sessions dedicated to educate them about the diagnosis.[3] Often, the use of the term *seizures* when referring to their events contributes to the persistent confusion.

Several misconceptions about PNES are common among patients and family members and these may become obstacles to accepting the diagnosis. These include the assumption that since the events are nonepileptic, patients may have faked them or that they may be able to control them. This specific misconception should always be addressed openly. Stressing the involuntary nature of the events may free the patient from this burden.[4] The loss of economic benefits and difficulty adjusting to the "new" reality that they do not and probably never suffered from epilepsy pose additional barriers to the acceptance of the diagnosis. Clearly, each and every one of these potential concerns should be raised during that first office visit, as they are often the big elephant in the room.

Studies have highlighted the fact that the mere communication of the diagnosis (e.g., "You do not have epilepsy. Your events are caused by stress or psychiatric disorders.") has limited impact on the frequency of events and quality of life in the long term.[5]

Furthermore, not infrequently, patients refuse to accept a psychogenic cause of their events. Insisting on the psychogenic nature of the events may not be the best strategy in such cases, particularly when no evidence of a psychogenic cause is available at the time of the diagnosis. The neurologist must interpret the patient's rejection of a potential psychogenic cause as a clear message to the neurologist, "I am not ready to hear that my events are psychogenic." In such circumstances, helping patients and family members to understand and accept that the events are not epileptic seizures achieves one of the important therapeutic aims (discussed in the next section). Patients should be encouraged to start to use a journal that includes a description of the type and severity of each event and the identification of possible precipitants.

In the case of coexisting epileptic seizures, the clinical semiology of the two types of events should be reviewed in detail with patients and family members together, and the need for different types of management should be explained in detail.

The patient and caregiver's understanding of the condition and support of the recommended therapy have proven to be important for successful long-term outcomes, including reduced frequency of events and healthcare utilization.[6] A referral to psychiatry or psychotherapy should be made and encouraged as part of the management plan for the events and comorbid psychiatric disorder. It is the responsibility of the neurologist to ensure that the patient gets access to the appropriate providers, since in most cases the neurologist is the only health care professional with whom the patient and family have established a relationship and hence the only health care provider available to help and support the patient during this very crucial part of the treatment. Furthermore, engagement of the neurologist and his or her continued interest in the patient may dissipate the feelings of abandonment many PNES patients experience when facing this diagnosis and that are triggered by a premature discharge from their practice. In fact, the neurologist's failure to offer follow-up visits and care is very often associated with the patient's refusal to accept the diagnosis and follow treatment recommendations.

3. MANAGEMENT OF NEUROLOGICAL COMORBIDITIES

3.1. Coexisting Epileptic Seizures

Coexistence of epilepsy with PNES has been reported in 10% to 30% of patients with PNES, with higher prevalence rates reported among patients with cognitive impairement.[7] In around 10% of patients with PNES, videoEEG (vEEG) monitoring studies reveal interictal epileptiform discharges supportive of the diagnosis of comorbid epilepsy,[8] which may be active or in remission with AED therapy. Therefore, it is essential to identify clinical characteristics that can help the patient and family members to differentiate epileptic seizures from PNES. Careful review of the seizure description provided by the patient and caregivers independently can give the neurologist sufficient information to differentiate one type of event from the other. With the patients' permission, video of the epileptic and nonepileptic events can be reviewed during the clinic visit, the neurologist pointing out the semiological differences between the two types of events. Giving a different name to the events (e.g., *events* or *episodes* instead of *seizures*) may better enable the patient and caregivers to communicate among themselves and with their healthcare providers. It is important to emphasize that the two conditions can coexist but are different in nature, have a different cause, present with different signs and symptoms, and require a different treatment. Tracking and recording their occurrence in a seizure journal becomes even more important, as the response of each of the events to treatment can thus be ascertained. Family members can use a smartphone to videorecord events, which may differ from those recorded during the video-EEG monitoring study. A recent study showed better long-term outcome for event cessation in patients with coexisting epileptic seizures and PNES than for patients with lone PNES.[9] The authors of the study suggest that a more aggressive intervention plan in the double pathology group, such as closer follow-up with mental health consultations and avoidance of unnecessary treatment, may have contributed to this outcome.

3.2. Antiepileptic Medications

The decision to discontinue AEDs when facing the diagnosis of PNES is complex and needs to be individualized to each patient. Furthermore, keeping patients on these drugs while telling them that the recorded events are nonepileptic sends a conflicting message. Thus, the decision to discontinue AEDs has to be based on the following variables: 1) the presence of current comorbid epileptic seizures or suspicion of epileptic seizures that have been in remission on AEDs; 2) the presence of comorbid mood and anxiety disorders that may worsen with discontinuation of AEDs with mood stabilizing (e.g., carbamazepine, oxcarbazepine, valproic acid and lamotrigine) or anxiolytic properties (gabapentin, pregabalin, benzodiazepines); 3) the presence of comorbid headaches, which are common in patients with PNES and may have benefitted from treatment with AEDs with prophylactic analgesic properties (e.g., topiramate, valproic acid, gabapentin); and 4) the number and type of AEDs at the time of the video-EEG monitoring study. In fact, a majority of these patients who are admitted with a suspected diagnosis of treatment-resistant epilepsy are typically on polytherapy regimens.[10]

Lowering the dose of AEDs and discontinuing them often occurs during the vEEG monitoring study, with the expectation of increasing the occurrence of epileptic seizures. Yet, when patients are suspected to have PNES (but diagnosis not yet confirmed with videoEEG), often they may be left on their home AED regimen until events are recorded and characterized and only then are AEDs stopped or the dose lowered if a suspicion of comorbid epileptic seizures remains. While discontinuation of AEDs in the hospital is preferable, it requires a longer hospitalization. Thus, at the conclusion of the diagnostic evaluation, patients may still be taking one or more AEDs. If patients are discharged on AEDs, it is essential that a clear explanation be provided to the patient and family with reasons to continue taking these drugs, along with a concrete schedule of the tapering process until their discontinuation is achieved. If the patient has comorbid mood and anxiety disorders, the decision to maintain AEDs with positive psychotropic properties must be clearly explained as well.

Benzodiazepines and barbiturates are the only AEDs that can cause withdrawal seizures in nonepileptic patients when the drugs are abruptly discontinued. Furthermore, rapid tapering of benzodiazepines can result in worsening of a comorbid anxiety disorder, which can interfere with the diagnostic evaluation. Accordingly, these drugs should be tapered slowly over a period of time. Among the other AEDs, withdrawal seizures in nonepileptic patients are not expected; the only limiting factors are the trigger or exacerbation of underlying mood and anxiety disorders and of headaches with the abrupt discontinuation of AEDs with positive psychotropic and analgesic properties, respectively.

A review of the progressive tapering process of AEDs is essential with the patient and family members at each office visit until the drug is completely discontinued. The neurologist must inquire about the emergence of new psychiatric symptoms and new types of paroxysmal events that could suggest the possibility of recurrence of epileptic seizures that may have been in remission for a long time with the prior AED regimen. If there are doubts regarding the nature of the newly reported events and these cannot be resolved in the clinic, a repeat EEG evaluation may be in order. It is not unusual for the process of discontinuing AEDs to take several months in some patients. Clearly, if at any given time during the titration period the patient experiences spells or new symptoms, these should be discussed and analyzed in light of prior information available and shared with the mental health care clinician.

Occasionally, diagnostic evaluations may not rule in or out the possibility of a history of comorbid epileptic seizures. Accordingly, continuation of one AED that treats potential coexisting epileptic seizures and has positive psychotropic properties at doses that do not yield adverse events should be discussed with the patient. The AED should be continued until the issue is clarified in future vEEG monitoring studies, and this diagnostic uncertainty should be openly discussed with the patient and his/her family. As stated earlier, smartphone recording of the patient's paroxysmal events may yield invaluable information for establishing the nature of these events. All of these aspects clearly support the need for active involvement by the neurologist.

3.3. Headaches

Comorbid migraines and other types of headaches are relatively frequent comorbid neurological conditions in persons with epilepsy, with postictal headaches reported in up to 40% of patients.[11] Preictal headache, on the other hand, is rarely seen as an epileptic aura but is frequently described (in up to 87.3%) as a prodromal symptom in patients with PNES.[10] Furthermore, daily headaches are frequent in patients with PNES, which are worsened and facilitated by the excessive use of over-the-counter and prescription analgesic medications. Accordingly, mixed type of headache disorders occurs relatively frequently in these patients, which often meet criteria for treatment-resistant headaches. In fact, comorbid severe headaches are common complaints reported in the course of the vEEG monitoring study, which tend to cause friction between the patient and the treating team that refuses to accede to the patient's request for opiates or other strong analgesic medications. In such patients, the discharge plans must incorporate a therapeutic strategy to address the comorbid headaches. The treatment of headaches in this population should continue to be tailored in the outpatient clinic according to their clinical characteristics and severity, which may require additional consultations in subspecialty headache clinics.

In the case of migraine headaches, the use of AEDs with analgesic properties such as valproic acid and topiramate may be an attractive option. Their teratogenic effects limit their use in women of child-bearing age, especially valproic acid. Furthermore, topiramate is often associated with iatrogenic cognitive and psychiatric adverse events. Gabapentin has been used in the treatment of tension headaches, and its anxiolytic properties may yield an additional advantage in PNES patients. Just as described in relation to mood disorders, if there is an indication to continue an AED for headache prophylaxis, this indication should be specifically explained to the patient in order to avoid ambivalent messages with regard to the diagnosis of PNES.

A common error of neurologists is to minimize the headaches of these patients as "another conversion symptom." Failure to address these headaches can lead to repeated visits to the emergency department (ED), where patients may again be misdiagnosed with epilepsy and restarted on AEDs. Frequent and debilitating headaches may also be a reason that patients cite for their inability to engage in mental health treatment. Clearly, these are not conditions that can be expected to be handled solely by mental health professionals and require ongoing involvement of the neurologist.

4. RECOGNITION OF NEW FUNCTIONAL NEUROLOGICAL SYMPTOMS

Other functional symptoms and disorders have been identified in approximately 70% of patients with PNES, and their frequency has been reported to increase (e.g., up to 76.5%) after the diagnosis of PNES is established, regardless of the degree to which the paroxysmal events are controlled.[11] Some of these symptoms are neurological in nature, such as headaches, chronic pain, weakness, and numbness, and often include cognitive complaints as well, which may be associated with untreated mood disorders. While persons with epilepsy and other neurological disorders may experience several physical and neurological symptoms other than seizures for which an organic cause may not be readily identified,[12] the frequency of such symptoms is significantly higher in patients with PNES. The relatively frequent occurrence of such symptoms in these patients is another reason for continued involvement of the neurologist. Together with the patient's primary care physician and mental health professionals, the neurologist's input will minimize the need for repeated ED visits and unnecessary diagnostic and costly studies.

5. SEIZURE PRECAUTIONS AND RESTRICTIONS

Patients with PNES have been advised to follow seizure precautions during the time (often years) they were treated for a suspected seizure disorder. Once this diagnosis is disproven, most patients want to know if they can stop following these precautions and, in particular, if they can start driving again. Driving restrictions differ across different states and countries. The neurologist should know these regulations and discuss them with patients according to their place of residence.

In general terms, driving privileges are restricted in individuals who have sudden, unpredictable, and involuntary episodes of loss of awareness or decreased ability to respond to the surrounding environment; all of these events could certainly apply to most patients with PNES.

Studies in Europe and the United States have demonstrated that neurologists and epilepsy experts vary with respect to allowing their patients to drive. For example, in a survey of epileptologists conducted in the United States, 46% indicated that they wait for PNES patients to remain free of events for the same time period required for persons with epilepsy; 14% indicated that they wait for shorter time periods, 34% had no set rules, while only 5% allowed patients to drive.[13] Recommendations and driving restrictions have to be clearly documented in the medical record along with a statement of the understanding and acceptance of the restriction by the patient.

Other surveys have reported the occurrence of motor vehicle accidents related to PNES.[14,15] The Driver and Vehicle Licensing Agency in the United Kingdom provides guidelines that specifically address driving privileges for patients with PNES, as follows: "license will be issued after medical records confirm that behavioral disturbances have been satisfactorily controlled."[14] To our knowledge, there are no such specific regulations regarding PNES in the United States.

Driving restrictions result in limitations in mobility, socialization, and employment. The need and desire for resuming driving are often a great motivation for patients to engage in treatment, follow up with related appointments, and achieve better awareness and control of their events. Similar guidelines can be followed with respect to other restrictions, including work- and sport-related precautions. Work restrictions due to safety concerns need to be balanced against assurance that there is a functional recovery plan in place. The decision to lift all of these restrictions could very well be made by mental health professionals, but not infrequently they request the neurologist's opinion and often demand that the decision be made by the neurologist.

6. ADVOCACY FOR ACCESS TO MENTAL HEALTH CARE

Advocating access to mental health care is a daily task of providers who care for persons with epilepsy. Anxiety and depression are the most frequent psychiatric comorbidities in this population, with lifetime prevalence rates hovering around 30% for each condition.[16–18] Unfortunately, more often than not, the mental health needs of these patients go unmet. The main obstacles to care include limited access to psychiatry providers due to insurance and availability constraints, negative preconceptions about mental health that prevent patients from seeking or accepting psychiatric or psychological care, limited knowledge and understanding by mental health providers regarding the psychiatric comorbidities of epilepsy and specifically PNES, and lack of communication between epilepsy providers and mental health care providers.[18] In fact, a recent study showed that PNES patients feel unsure about the fact that psychological therapies may meet their needs or help them "return to normality."[19]

The role of the neurologist is pivotal in ensuring that PNES patients have access to psychiatric care and plan a comprehensive treatment strategy with a psychiatrist or other mental health providers. As stated earlier, mental health providers are often unfamiliar with the treatment of PNES and may be unwilling or unable to participate in the management of these patients. Often psychiatrists and other mental health professionals question the diagnosis and perpetuate the confusion about the nature of the events in the patient's (and their family members') mind. Clearly, this type of misinformation can have devastating consequences and can be prevented by active engagement of the treating neurologist with mental health providers. Ongoing active communication with the psychiatrist and psychotherapist provides neurologists with reassurance that their patients' neurological needs are met.

It is important to remember that there are other members of the healthcare team who may have even less information about PNES, their presentation, and their treatment. Primary care providers, subspecialists, social workers, and other clinicians should be made aware of the positive diagnosis, ongoing relationship with a neurologist, and treatment plan. When the neurologist takes the initiative to reach out to these providers, he or she may prevent the perpetuation of very well-intended but confusing information and, in some instances, prevent the relabeling of symptoms as epilepsy or the escalation of antiepileptic medication use and its consequences.

7. PREVENTION OF IATROGENIC INTERVENTIONS AND COMPLICATIONS

The first and most important goal in the management of patients with PNES is to ensure that patients and their families understand and accept that they do not suffer from epileptic seizures and that visits to the ED can frequently result in serious iatrogenic events, unnecessary reloading with intravenous AEDs, admission to ICUs, and intubation. In fact, patients with PNES taken to the ED often present with prolonged and recurrent events mimicking status epilepticus, referred to as "nonepileptic psychogenic status (NEPS)."[20] NEPS has been reported in 23% to 78%[21,22] of patients. When the condition is not recognized, patients may be aggressively treated as if they were in status epilepticus.[4,23] These treatments may include intravenous AED infusions, which may be associated with cardiac, respiratory, and neurological side effects; sedation; and the need for advanced airway management devices and even mechanical ventilation, with admission to an intensive care setting in 30% to 50% of patients. All of these procedures result in extended hospitalizations with their consequences, including infections, thrombotic complications, and deconditioning.

Providing patients and their families with guidance when they are experiencing their events at home can be the difference between a self-limited episode at home and a prolonged hospital admission. Providing families with an in-home action plan and a contact number for the neurologist may be a life-saving intervention.

Unfortunately, patients may experience their events away from home and may end up being taken to the ED by ambulance. The availability of a contact neurologist at those times is pivotal to clarify the nature of the events and prevent the iatrogenic complications just listed. Furthermore, families may at times feel compelled to bring their loved one to the ED when they are at a loss of what to do with recurrent and prolonged events associated with new signs and symptoms. While a treatment plan should never discourage patients or families to reach out to emergency services when they feel the safety of their loved one may be compromised, they should be encouraged to have the ED physician contact the treating neurologist to get an objective account of the patient's history and diagnostic data. Communication with the ED provider, once the patient reaches the hospital, is important. Such communication is typically welcome by ED providers, who are usually forced to make decisions with in adequate information and are often not equipped to make elaborate diagnostic considerations when they are presented with a patient in crisis who seems to be having a life-threatening neurologic emergency such as status epilepticus. Transferring patients to the EMU for reassurance and to de-escalate the situation out of the ED may be indicated in certain situations. In summary, continuous involvement of the neurologist in the patient's management prevents the reinstatement of unnecessary AED therapy when PNES recur, which unfortunately happens in 70% to 80% of patients at some point after the diagnosis.[24]

8. WHEN IS IT TIME TO LET THE PATIENT GO?

There are no guidelines regarding how long patients with PNES should be followed in the outpatient neurology clinic, just as there are no guidelines on how long patients with epilepsy, headaches, multiple sclerosis, or other medical conditions should be followed. The answer is simple: they should be followed until the patient and the neurologist decide together that the neurologist's involvement in the overall management of the PNES is not needed. That time is different for each patient.

Certain goals need to be reached, however (Table 15.1). The first goal is for the patient to achieve complete discontinuation of AEDs (unless they are needed for comorbid psychiatric conditions for which there is an identified and willing prescriber) and be off these drugs for a long enough period to be certain that there are no comorbid epileptic seizures. Likewise, the patient needs to have remission of comorbid headaches and other active neurologic conditions.

The frequency of outpatient visits should also be tailored according to the patient's clinical status. In general, patients are scheduled every 3 months or more frequently in case of persistent headaches and if undergoing medication changes. Visits can be scheduled every 6 months when the patient is stable and PNES have remitted and the patient is fully engaged in psychiatric or psychological treatment with satisfactory results. Finally, patients can be scheduled on a yearly basis when PNES are controlled, no therapy changes are foreseen, and the patient feels confident and in control with the treatment. Patients are always encouraged to request a resumption of follow-up visits if their condition worsens at any given time.

Some of our patients decide eventually not to continue follow-up as they remain seizure-free after adequate treatment or when they feel adequately engaged in psychiatric care.

Ultimately, it is the patient who determines when it is time to let go of a neurologist's involvement in their care.

Table 15.1 Indications to Continue Neurological Follow-up for Patients with PNES

Indication	Actions
Revise and explain diagnosis and treatment plan	• Review all available data. • Explain the diagnosis to patient and caregivers. • Try to understand PNES in the context of a social and cultural frame of the patient and family. • Review the treatment plan. • Encourage keeping of a seizure journal.
Management of coexisting epileptic seizures	• Try to establish the difference between the two types of spells. • Give them a different name. • Encourage patients to track them differentially in the seizure journal (using different colors or symbols). • Explain the different treatments for each type of spell.
De-escalation of AEDs	• AEDs do not treat PNES. • Start reducing AEDs in the EMU, if possible. • Make a plan for de-escalation of treatment. • Lower AED dosage slowly and one at a time. • Start with medications causing side effects or medication interactions. • Be available and have a plan in case new spells or epileptic seizures develop.
Management of other neurological symptoms	• Evaluate patients for headaches or other neurologic symptoms and treat as necessary.
Seizure precautions and restrictions	• Seizure precautions and driving restrictions are in order for PNES patients with active episodes of altered awareness and decreased responsiveness. • Restrictions should be explained and documented. • Follow local regulations for driving privileges.
Access to mental health care	• Identify and start management of psychiatric comorbidities, if indicated. • Assist in identifying psychiatry and psychotherapy providers. • Communicate with mental health providers regarding the diagnosis. • Educate mental health providers as needed regarding the diagnosis and management of PNES. • Be available and encourage open communication. • Be available to address new symptoms or concerns.
Prevention of iatrogenic complications	• Provide the patient and family with a seizure action plan and access to a provider (on-call number). • Encourage ED physician communication for information and support in case of emergency or NEPS.

Table 15.1 Continued

Indication	Actions

Clinic follow-up	• Be available.
	• Follow up patients according to their clinical needs:
	  • Every 3 months or more frequently when spells are active or during medication changes
	  • Every 6 months while undergoing active treatment for specific condition
	  • Every year when spells are controlled and no treatment changes are foreseen
	• Let the patient decide when it is time to let go of the neurologist's involvement.

AED, antiepileptic drug; ED, emergency department; EMU, epilepsy monitoring unit; NEPS, nonepileptic psychogenic status; PNES, psychogenic nonepileptic seizures.

9. SUMMARY

- In the management of patients with PNES, the role of the neurologist begins with establishment of the diagnosis and, as with any other neurological or medical condition, continues until the overall condition is considered to be stable or in remission.
- It falls to the neurologist to ensure that patients and families alike have understood and accepted the diagnosis of PNES. A premature abandonment of a case is likely to be followed by the patient's failure to accept the diagnosis and follow the recommendations for psychotherapy and may contribute to the persistence or worsening of PNES and comorbid neurologic conditions.
- Multiple specific tasks including 1) management of comorbid neurologic conditions, such as epileptic seizures and headaches; 2) management of AEDs; and 3) recommendations regarding work and driving restrictions require continued involvement of the neurologist.
- The neurologist is an integral member of a multidisciplinary team responsible for assisting in the establishment of appropriate mental health care and providing care for a period of time that will vary according to the individual patient's needs.

REFERENCES

1. Alessi R, Valente KD. Psychogenic nonepileptic seizures: should we use response to AEDS as a red flag for the diagnosis? *Seizure*. 2014;23(10):906–908.
2. Carton S, Thompson PJ, Duncan JS. Non-epileptic seizures: patients' understanding and reaction to the diagnosis and impact on outcome. *Seizure*. 2003;12(5):287–294.
3. Gordon PC, Valiengo Lda C, Proenca IC, et al. Comorbid epilepsy and psychogenic non-epileptic seizures: how well do patients and caregivers distinguish between the two. *Seizure*. 2014;23(7):537–541.
4. Kanner AM. Is the neurologist's role over once the diagnosis of psychogenic nonepileptic seizures is made? No! *Epilepsy Behav*. 2008;12(1):1–2.

5. Mayor R, Brown RJ, Cock H, et al. Short-term outcome of psychogenic non-epileptic seizures after communication of the diagnosis. *Epilepsy Behav*. 2012;25(4):676–681.
6. Duncan R, Graham CD, Oto M. Neurologist assessment of reactions to the diagnosis of psychogenic nonepileptic seizures: relationship to short- and long-term outcomes. *Epilepsy Behav*. 2014;41:79–82.
7. Baslet G, Roiko A, Prensky E. Heterogeneity in psychogenic nonepileptic seizures: understanding the role of psychiatric and neurological factors. *Epilepsy Behav*. 2010;17(2):236–241.
8. Benbadis SR, Agrawal V, Tatum WO 4th. How many patients with psychogenic nonepileptic seizures also have epilepsy? *Neurology*. 2001;57(5):915–917.
9. Sadan O, Neufeld MY, Parmet Y, Rozenberg A, Kipervasser S. Psychogenic seizures: long-term outcome in patients with and without epilepsy. *Acta Neurol Scand*. 2015; doi:10.1111/ane.12458
10. Patidar Y, Gupta M, Khwaja GA, Chowdhury D, Batra A, Dasgupta A. Clinical profile of psychogenic non-epileptic seizures in adults: a study of 63 cases. *Ann Indian Acad Neurol*. 2013;16(2):157–162.
11. McKenzie PS, Oto M, Graham CD, Duncan R. Do patients whose psychogenic non-epileptic seizures resolve, 'replace' them with other medically unexplained symptoms? Medically unexplained symptoms arising after a diagnosis of psychogenic non-epileptic seizures. *J Neurol Neurosurg Psychiatry*. 2011;82(9):967–969.
12. Stone J, Carson A, Duncan R, et al. Which neurological diseases are most likely to be associated with "symptoms unexplained by organic disease." *J Neurol*. 2012;259(1):33–38.
13. Mintzer S. Driven to tears: epilepsy specialists and the automobile. *Epilepsy Curr*. 2015;15(5):279–282.
14. Morrison I, Razvi SS. Driving regulations and psychogenic non-epileptic seizures: perspectives from the united kingdom. *Seizure*. 2011;20(2):177–180.
15. Jirsch J, Siddiqi M, Smyth P, Maximova K. Bias in counseling of seizure patients following a transient impairment of consciousness: differential adherence to driver fitness guidelines. *Seizure*. 2015;30:21–25.
16. Kanner AM. Epilepsy and mood disorders. *Epilepsia*. 2007;48(Suppl 9):20–22.
17. Tellez-Zenteno JF, Patten SB, Jette N, Williams J, Wiebe S. Psychiatric comorbidity in epilepsy: a population-based analysis. *Epilepsia*. 2007;48(12):2336–2344.
18. Kanner AM. Is it time to train neurologists in the management of mood and anxiety disorders? *Epilepsy Behav*. 2014;34:139–143.
19. Fairclough G, Fox J, Mercer G, Reuber M, Brown RJ. Understanding the perceived treatment needs of patients with psychogenic nonepileptic seizures. *Epilepsy Behav*. 2014;31:295–303.
20. Reuber M, Pukrop R, Bauer J, Helmstaedter C, Tessendorf N, Elger CE. Outcome in psychogenic nonepileptic seizures: 1- to 10-year follow-up in 164 patients. *Ann Neurol*. 2003;53(3):305–311.
21. Asadi-Pooya AA, Emami Y, Emami M, Sperling MR. Prolonged psychogenic nonepileptic seizures or pseudostatus. *Epilepsy Behav*. 2014;31:304–306.
22. Dworetzky BA, Bubrick EJ, Szaflarski JP, Nonepileptic Seizure Task Force. Nonepileptic psychogenic status: markedly prolonged psychogenic nonepileptic seizures. *Epilepsy Behav*. 2010;19(1):65–68.

23. Dworetzky BA, Weisholtz DS, Perez DL, Baslet G. A clinically oriented perspective on psychogenic nonepileptic seizure-related emergencies. *Clin EEG Neurosci.* 2015;46(1):26–33.
24. Kanner AM, Parra J, Frey M, Stebbins G, Pierre-Louis S, Iriarte J. Psychiatric and neurologic predictors of psychogenic pseudoseizure outcome. *Neurology.* 1999;53(5):933–938.

16

The Roles of the Patient and Family

Julia L. Doss, PsyD, LP and Jeffrey Mark Robbins, MSW

1. INTRODUCTION

Psychogenic nonepileptic seizures (PNES) often take years to diagnose, on average 3.5 years for youth and more than 7 years for adults. As such, when an accurate diagnosis is made, it is after years of evaluations, misdiagnoses in some cases, and often years of taking unnecessary antiepileptic drugs (AEDs).[1,2] The family and patient must understand this new diagnosis but also relinquish identification with another diagnosis the patient may have had for years, often epilepsy.[3] In order to successfully navigate this shift and ultimately get the patient and family members into appropriate treatment, providers must honor the patient's complicated history, aide the person in understanding this new diagnosis, and manage any defensiveness that the patient might experience about accepting a psychological diagnosis instead of a medical one. Without these key considerations during the diagnostic process, patients may not buy into their diagnosis, one of the most important factors in helping them get to appropriate treatment.[4]

Literature on family functioning and its impact on the development of PNES is sparse. Studies of youth with functional disorders have shown that there are higher rates of somatization, more frequent incidence of internalizing disorders, such as anxiety and depression, and higher degrees of family conflict.[5,6] Studies of adults with PNES have found high rates of psychopathology and histories of trauma.[3] Understanding, assessing, and then managing the factors that predispose individuals toward PNES is integral during both the diagnostic and treatment phases.

2. THEORIES OF SOMATIZATION AND FAMILY INFLUENCE

Theoretical models for PNES are currently in development. Several theories of somatization or functional syndromes and the influence of family in developing these exist. In youth, parental response to somatic complaints and pain, such as minimizing instead of focusing on the symptoms, leading to either distraction from symptoms in the former or solicitation of symptoms in the latter, may contribute to whether these symptoms are reinforced.[7] Perception of somatic symptoms as being dangerous can also contribute to their

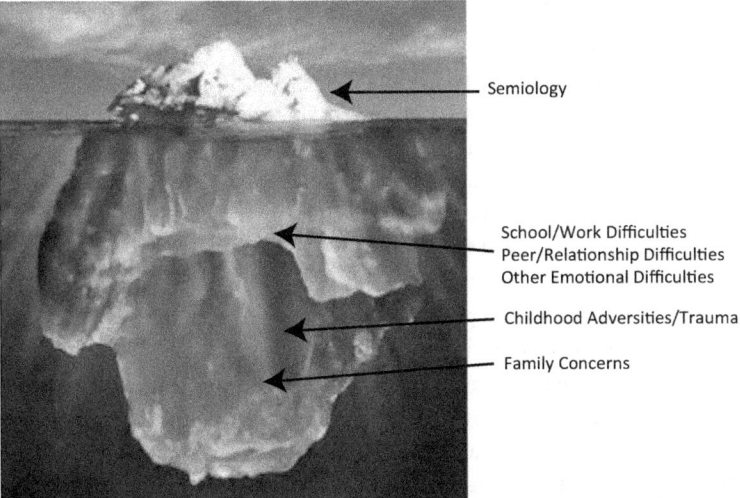

Figure 16.1 The iceberg illustrates the complexity of the presentation of functional, nonepileptic symptoms, with semiology being the most obvious challenge the person is facing, but the factors that lie below the surface contribute to the development of these physical symptoms.

exacerbation.[8] Still other theories postulate that struggles with communication of negative emotion play a role in the repression of these emotions within the family; the subsequent emergence of physical symptoms is how these negative emotions get channeled.[9]

All of these theories represent only parts of the overall picture of individuals with functional disorders. An illustration of the multiple factors that influence the development of somatic symptoms is the example of an iceberg. The somatic symptoms themselves are the tip of the iceberg, the part that we see and the part that the patient is most aware of. However, just below the surface are the factors that contribute to the development of those symptoms. It is often a combination of both individual and family factors that get combined to create the symptom. Figure 16.1 illustrates this concept with a picture of an iceberg, in which what we see is only a small part of the overall difficulty that the person has and the source of the struggle lies below the surface. This figure illustrates the common factors found in pediatric PNES. Adult patients' struggles also fit with this model, although the order and source of struggles might be slightly different.

3. DIAGNOSING PNES WITH THE PEDIATRIC PATIENT

"I don't understand why they can't find what's wrong with me."
Jenny, *16-year-old, with PNES for 2 years*

Given the lengthy time it takes to get an accurate diagnosis of PNES, it is important that the diagnostic environment enable appropriate time for the physician and mental health providers to build rapport with the patient. As such, an important aspect of the initial diagnosis is listening to the patient's story. This can be accomplished in several ways, but is often best accomplished with the patient and family members during the initial interview. The physician and mental health professional should inquire about past diagnoses, past treatments, and, perhaps most importantly, what patients have been told and believe about their physical symptoms.[10] This will allow the provider to develop a better understanding of how the patient feels about the diagnosis and will enable the provider to more successfully engage with the patient. If the patient or parents are upset or defensive about prior suggestions that the condition could be psychogenic, the provider can adjust the approach and respond to this defensiveness with more education. A common example that one may hear from patients is that they were told "this is all in your head," which often causes patients to feel that they are either "crazy" or "faking it." Should this concern be raised during the diagnostic process, the provider can respond to it directly by explaining the complicated interplay between the mind and the body and directly refuting that the symptoms are fake. A more in-depth discussion about the role of the mental health provider during the diagnostic phase can be found in Chapter 8.

If the patient and family have been able to explain their journey seeking treatment and have had a thorough evaluation, acceptance of the diagnosis starts during the feedback session when the PNES diagnosis is explained. Often, in the context of an admission for video-electroencephalogram (v-EEG) monitoring, patients can discuss with the physician and the mental health provider together both physical and emotional aspects of the illness. It also can send an important message to the patient and family that a thorough evaluation was completed and that the medical provider is handing off treatment to the mental health team. If this session is successful, the patient will understand his or her diagnosis, buy into the diagnosis and treatment, feel validated in the complexity of this emotional disorder, and have a sense of hope that treatment can begin soon to reduce symptoms and improve function.

The patient and family must then make the transition from seeking answers to treating the problem. While always true in the case of the pediatric patient, with adult patients the involvement of family may begin during treatment, rather than at diagnosis.

4. TREATMENT

After the diagnostic process is complete, it is important for the patient and family to begin treatment as soon as possible, as the shorter the duration from onset of symptoms to treatment, the better the outcome, according to some studies.[11] Literature on medically unexplained symptoms or functional symptom disorders supports the role of symptom management and maximizing functioning in the initial stages of treatment.[4] Treatment for children and adults differs in these initial stages.

4.1. Treatment with the Pediatric Patient

"We don't know where to go for help, all the people I've called say they have never worked with PNES."
Mark, father of Dylan, *a 14-year-old with PNES*

A significant challenge that families face in getting treatment for their child is the provider's lack of knowledge about this diagnosis. There have been few PNES treatment studies conducted with children.[6] The literature on somatization and pain disorders supports the use of cognitive-behavioral therapy (CBT)-informed and family treatments as useful in decreasing frequency and severity of symptoms and improving function.[4] Opinions differ somewhat in the approach to identifying stressors in these initial stages. Some models propose early identification of stressors coupled with anxiety reduction strategies,[12] while other models encourage first management of symptoms and then active identification of stressors.[12,13] There are no known studies to date examining these approaches in children with PNES. For the purpose of this chapter, description of the latter approach may be most beneficial, for several reasons. Primarily, aiding the patient in improving function, learning strategies for managing anxiety, and developing rapport with the therapist allows the patient to feel some success with even a small improvement in symptoms. This approach helps to reduce anxiety associated with symptoms, and it enables patients to develop the skills necessary to manage the emotions that will arise when they start addressing their stressors directly.

Return to normal functioning or promotion of function is an important part of the initial stage of treatment in any type of functional disorder.[14] At times, avoidance of function, such as school attendance or maintaining a job, serves as a primary means of reinforcing the symptoms. Thus, it is necessary to promote function even while symptoms continue, in order to reinforce that function is not contingent upon symptom resolution. This also serves to de-emphasize the focus of treatment on the "symptom" and starts shifting the focus to behavioral responses or thoughts about other life factors.

While much of the initial work of symptom management is the patient's responsibility, the parent or other family members must learn how to function around the symptoms and not inadvertently reinforce them. Techniques aimed at promoting independence with regard to symptom management, helping family members identify and cope with their own reaction to symptoms and developing strategies for family members to support the patient's struggle to gain control, are all important parts of this stage of treatment. An example of this can occur at the beginning of treatment: when teaching how to respond to episodes, encourage the patient to respond with relaxation strategies to sensations that signal an impending episode, and at the same time encourage caregivers to move to a place away from the patient and allow the patient to work on his or her own to manage the symptoms.

When the child has developed some control of his or her physical symptoms and has built rapport with the therapist, identifying and managing stressors will become a more prominent part of treatment. Some stressors may already be clear, particularly those that are easier for the child to discuss. It is important to allow the child to lead when exploring initial stressors. The child should be encouraged to discuss what is hard and how it impacts him or her. This will allow the child to feel that some of his or her concerns are going to be addressed and provides the therapist with a better sense of the child's current coping strategies (or lack thereof).

4.2. Treatment with the Adult Patient

"I've been to therapy before, how is this going to be different from what I have already done?"

Samantha, *25-year-old, with PNES for 5 years*

For adults, identification of stressors that contribute to PNES symptoms is a primary aspect of initial treatment.[15] Patients may be resistant to identifying precipitating stressors that contributed to symptom development. Moreover, it is often not true that there is a direct link between a precipitant and the onset of episodes. Often, it is the accumulation of stress over a long period of time that accounts for the development of PNES symptoms. Helping the patient to understand this phenomenon is necessary in order for treatment to be successful. If a patient is resistant to exploring stressors that may facilitate his or her symptoms (either historically or for each episode in particular), helping the person to instead explore current strategies for managing challenging life events in general may provide a gradual way to engage the patient in the treatment process. In addition, it allows the clinician to understand some current or past stressors and learn about the patient's coping strategies.

PNES symptom management is similar in adults and children. The patient should be provided with methods for reducing symptoms associated with physiological anxiety, such as relaxation strategies. As improvement in function is necessary in the management of PNES, it is important to use stress reduction strategies in daily life, not only in the face of distressing symptoms. Identification of stressors that interfere with daily life and direct management of these stressors will be necessary in the early stages of treatment.

4.3. Symptom Resolution (or Significantly Reduced)

Resolution of PNES symptoms is a first step in treating the underlying conversion or somatic symptom disorder. Literature has suggested that if treatment ceases after the functional symptoms cease, quite often a new form of functional symptom will appear within weeks or months.[16] This is likely because the symptoms themselves represent emotional difficulties usually related to maladaptive stress management, trauma, or difficult family interactions or communication that are often not the focus of the initial stages of treatment because the focus is on symptom resolution.[13] During the next stage of treatment, the patient must explore the underlying cause or causes of the symptoms, how he or she communicates and copes with stressors, and address any underlying comorbid emotional difficulties, such as anxiety or depression.

Family members are quite involved throughout treatment, from managing the symptoms in the initial stages to participating in managing ongoing stressors and family struggles later in treatment. After symptom resolution or improvement, in the pediatric population, the focus tends to be on managing family conflict and communication, providing support to the patient, and helping the parents and caregivers to cope with their own emotional struggles. In the adult population, the focus is on helping the individual symptomatic patient renegotiate relationships within the family and between adults outside the family in ways that are healthier and promote successful independence.

4.4. Challenges to Treatment

"The school won't allow my child to return until the episodes have resolved."
Jackie, *13-year-old, with PNES for 3 months*

It is not uncommon for school programs and employers to request that the individual with PNES remain home until symptom-free. This may be due to concerns about liability or fears about watching or managing the episodes. Education is key at this stage and is often best received through either the treating neurologist or the mental health provider. Working to improve and return to the patient's "normal" functioning even in the face of symptoms is a key part of treatment.[4] Avoiding or preventing return to normal function may exacerbate the symptoms and prolong their occurrence.

"Jack does not want to return to work until the symptoms have fully resolved."
Jack, *35-year-old, with PNES for 2 years*

At times employers request that patients stay home until symptoms have resolved, and at other times patients do not want to return. As in the prior example, this could be due to concerns about liability, anxiety on the part of the patient, or even the symptoms serving a purpose to enable the person to avoid function. Regardless of the reason, it is necessary to begin to transition the patient back to more normal function even while symptoms continue. Exploration of motivational factors and problem-solving barriers may help those patients who resist engagement in activities that promote functioning.

"Steven hasn't had any PNES for a month, we are so relieved, I don't think we need to continue therapy."
John, Steven's dad; *Steven is 12 and had PNES for 6 months*

As explained earlier in the chapter, managing the PNES symptoms is only part of the treatment. In both the pediatric and adult patient, addressing the underlying stressors that contributed to PNES onset is critically important to ensuring ongoing management and prevention of future functional symptoms. When this question is posed, it is important for the clinician to address the positive improvement but explain the importance of continuing to work toward a better understanding of the underlying mechanisms that allowed the symptoms to develop.

"Becky's PNES have improved significantly, but now I'm worried that she is really depressed; she's crying all the time and I'm worried that the therapy is making her worse, not better."
Joyce, Becky's mom; *Becky is 15 and had PNES for over a year*

While this is not always the case, occasionally, once the PNES symptoms are better, significant anxiety or depression may emerge. It is important for the treating clinician to recognize that the PNES symptoms represented a coping mechanism for stressors or underlying psychopathology, as in the iceberg figure illustrated in Figure 16.1. As such, providing the patient with coping strategies for managing these emotional difficulties will be important and should begin early in the treatment process.

Given the nature of the stressors the patient is experiencing, it may be necessary to address factors that impact treatment success very early in treatment, such as safety concerns (domestic violence for adults, abuse situations for children, or unmasking of severe depression and suicidal ideation). Should any of these situations become clear, the treatment must naturally shift to acute management of these safety issues.

A common concern for both late-adolescent and adult patients is driving. States vary in their laws about driving, and spells involving loss of consciousness; it is necessary to learn the law of the particular state and problem-solve with patients about how to maintain as much function as possible in the face of this significant restriction.

Please see Table 16.1 for other challenges to treatment and ways to manage them.

4.5. Case Vignette 1: Child Case

Annie, a 14-year-old female, had been to four treatment centers before being diagnosed with PNES and attending treatment. Her most significant concern with prior assessments was feeling as if they were being dismissed. She had been told she was "faking" the symptoms or that the episodes were for attention. During Annie's fifth hospitalization, she had a prolonged (7 days) video-EEG, which captured multiple episodes, and she also met with a clinical psychologist. The PNES diagnosis was explained, and the family was provided with an understanding of how some of the stressors identified in the evaluation contributed to the presentation.

Annie and her family agreed to start treatment with the psychologist involved in the diagnostic evaluation. She struggled initially with identifying physical signs of impending PNES because they tended to happen very quickly. Thus, early stages focused on "tuning in" and mindfully experiencing body sensations and using relaxation strategies to reduce any discomfort. Her parents struggled with not reinforcing her symptoms, as she often sought them to help her manage the episodes rather than working to manage them herself. Once Annie was able to identify her physiological triggers, experience some success in managing them on her own, and have her parent's support but not their intervention during episodes, her symptoms improved significantly. After Annie's symptoms were nearly gone, the treatment shifted to identifying and managing general life stressors.

Factors that influenced Annie's treatment include the following:

1) The family struggled to accept the diagnosis and buy into it because of previous misinformation about what the nature of the episodes was and not being provided with adequate education about PNES.
2) Annie's treatment began much like that described for other functional disorders, with a focus on symptom management.
3) Improving Annie's functioning was a key part of her initial treatment, as was helping her parents manage their own anxiety about her symptoms and encourage functioning.

Table 16.1. Treatment Challenges

Patient Concerns	Ideas for Response by Clinician
1. Misunderstanding the diagnosis	Provide explanation of mind–body connection; discuss physiological response to emotional stressors and highlight that the symptoms themselves are not physically harmful to the body.
2. Struggle with recognizing body cues of distress	Practice mindfulness with the patient and assist patient in identifying changes or responses in his or her body, both positive and negative, to emotional experiences and thoughts.
3. Resistance to becoming more functional	Assist patient in developing a list of attainable goals to increase function, and problem-solve through barriers, including ongoing PNES symptoms. Gain a better understanding of the patient's personal values about function and use this information in creating goals.
4. Family members who do not follow protocol for management of episodes	Meet with family members separately from the patient and explain the diagnosis and ways to help the person adhere to the plan, combating any fear they may have.
5. Patient is ready for change but family is not	Continue to meet with the patient and family separately. Coach patient in making changes and managing the family's resistance by using a "small steps" approach, where the patient recognizes what the family is sensitive to (example: in communication about emotion, have patient communicate more palatable emotion first and identify other "safe" people with whom to discuss more challenging emotions).
6. Patient's PNES have stopped, but now the patient is overwhelmed with symptoms of depression or anxiety	While continuing to encourage management of physical symptoms, shift the focus of sessions to more direct management of depression or anxiety and start to explore stressors that could be contributing.
7. Patient identifies significant family stressors but has little ability to make change with them	Assist patient in developing strategies for being aware of how the family stressors impact PNES and their emotional functioning. Encourage coping methods that allow for building additional positive relationships outside of the family, and identify ways of getting needs met that do not involve a change in that family member(s).
8. Patient struggles with identifying and working on concerns that are not associated with the physical symptoms	Work with the patient to understand how he or she has addressed other difficulties in life, and work on modifying this response style if it is a style that prevents change or growth.

4.6. Case Vignette 2: Adult Case

Maria is a 27-year-old Ecuadorian woman who was diagnosed with PNES 1 month before the birth of an unplanned pregnancy. She had been living with her parents and various members of her extended family of origin in a two-family home owned by her parents. Although Maria initially dismissed the idea that her PNES symptoms were a physiological expression of stress ("I don't believe in stress or depression"), following a video-EEG admission she came to understand that her symptoms were not a result of her having epilepsy, as she previously had been told. When she finally agreed to therapy, several stressors were identified, which included the following: 1) her ambivalence about becoming a parent at a young age with a man she barely knew; 2) the ongoing criticism leveled at her by her mother; 3) her father's alcoholism, in light of her paternal uncle's death related to alcoholism; 4) her worries about her brother, who was selling and using drugs; 4) her diminished sense of self-esteem for not having finished school and not being able to contribute to her nuclear family's finances; and 7) her general experience of feeling trapped by her living situation, which neither she nor her husband seemed able to change.

The identification of these stressors, coupled with the observation that Maria's way of being loyal to the culture of her family was by remaining silent about her worries, helped her to understand the evolution of her PNES symptoms. The therapy involved making the ongoing and continuous connection between symptoms and stressors. This, in turn, helped to establish the focus of treatment, which centered on helping Maria change how she related to members of her family with whom she had become enmeshed. Once she became able to establish independent relationships with family members and speak up and assert herself about the things that bothered or angered her, two important changes began to take place: 1) she became more able to be direct with her husband, which she had never been able to do, and 2) her symptoms began to diminish. In this case, the patient's family was a critical focus of treatment, even though they were not included in the therapy sessions.

5. SUMMARY

- Patients and families with PNES present challenges in diagnosis and treatment; pediatric and adult patients share some common characteristics but also have significant differences.
- Accurate diagnosis of PNES can take years, thus a component of a thorough evaluation involves hearing the patient's prior experience and better understanding of why acceptance of the diagnosis might be difficult for them.
- Pediatric patients with PNES must develop tools for improved management of their symptoms first and then proceed to working on underlying stressors.
- For adult patients, making the connection between symptoms and underlying stressors is an ongoing process that is woven throughout the course of treatment.
- For both children and adults, the "patient" refers to the symptomatic person and the family.

- There are many obstacles that can get in the way of treatment, from difficulty finding qualified providers to families or patients themselves wanting to terminate treatment prematurely. Managing these challenges requires the clinician to anticipate some of the questions that will arise and have an ongoing dialogue with the patient and family about the importance of adhering to treatment goals, which should be discussed early in treatment.

REFERENCES

1. Patel H, Scott E, Dunn D, et al. Non-epileptic seizures in children. *Epilepsia.* 2007;48:2086–2092.
2. LaFrance WC Jr, Benbadis SR. Avoiding the costs of unrecognized psychological nonepileptic seizures. *Neurology.* 2006;66:1620–1621.
3. LaFrance WC Jr, Kanner AM, Betts T. Psychogenic nonepileptic seizures and epilepsy. In: Engel J, Pedley TA, eds. *Epilepsy: A Comprehensive Textbook*, 2nd ed. Philadelphia: Wolters Kluwer Health/Lippincott Williams & Wilkins; 2007:2155–2161.
4. Ibeziako P, Bujoreanu S. Approach to psychosomatic illness in adolescents. *Curr Opin Pediatr.* 2011;23:384–389.
5. Kashikar-Zuck S, Lynch AM, Slater S, Graham TB, Swain NF, Noll RB. Family factors, emotional functioning, and functional impairment in juvenile fibromyalgia syndrome. *Arthitis Rheum.* 2008;59:1392–1398.
6. Plioplys S, Doss J, Siddarth P, et al. (2014). A multi-site controlled study of risk factors for pediatric psychogenic non-epileptic seizures. *Epilepsia.* 55(11):1739–1747.
7. Walker LS, Garber J, Greene JW. Somatization symptoms in pediatric abdominal pain patients: relation to chronicity of abdominal pain and parent somatization. *J Abnorm Child Psychol.* 1991;19:379–394.
8. Connelly M, Anthony KK, Schanberg LE. Parent perceptions of child vulnerability are associated with functioning and health care use in children with chronic pain. *J Pain Symptom Manage.* 2012;43:953–960.
9. Krawetz P, Fleisher W, Pillay N, Staley D, Arnett J, Maher J. Family functioning in subjects with pseudoseizures and epilepsy. *J Nerv Ment Dis.* 189: 38–43.
10. Gates J. Nonepileptic seizures: time for progress. *Epilepsy Behav.* 2000;1:2–6.
11. Caplan R, Plioplys S. Psychiatric features and management of children with psychogenic nonepileptic seizures. In: Schachter SC, LaFrance WC, eds. *Gates and Rowan's Nonepileptic Seizures.* Cambridge, UK: Cambridge University Press; 2010:163–178.
12. Kroenke K, Swindle R. Cognitive-behavioral therapy for somatization and symptom syndromes: a critical review of controlled trials. *Psychother Psychosom.* 2000;69:205–215.
13. Monsen K, Monsen J. Chronic pain and psychodynamic body therapy: a controlled outcome study. *Psychother Theory Res Pract Train.* 2000;37(3):257–269.
14. Palermo TM, Putnam J, Armstrong G, Daily S. Adolescent autonomy and family functioning are associated with headache-related disability. *Clin J Pain.* 2007;23:458–465.
15. LaFrance WC, Reuber M, Goldstein L. Management of psychogenic non-epileptic seizures. *Epilepsia,* 2013;54:53–67.
16. Walker LS, Greene JW. Negative life events and symptom resolution in pediatric abdominal pain patients. *J Pediatr Psychiatry.* 1991;16:341–360.

Section VI
Long-Term Outcomes and Prognosis

17

Long-Term Outcomes

Roderick Duncan, MD, PhD

1. INTRODUCTION

The scope of outcome studies in psychogenic nonepileptic seizures (PNES) has widened over the years, attention being increasingly focused on outcomes other than seizures, particularly social, economic, and psychiatric outcomes. While this has improved our understanding of the life trajectory of the PNES population, the quantity of available information remains modest.

The picture provided by this information has at least one straightforward aspect: it indicates that the population of patients with PNES does not, as a group, do well in the long term. However, the relationships between the various outcome measures that have been studied do not appear to be straightforward. Further, the obvious heterogeneity of the PNES population appears to extend to long-term outcome, and our understanding of why some patients remain free of seizures but unemployed, with or without obvious psychiatric morbidity, and why others do well on all three counts remains rudimentary.

Part of this relates to a more practical problem: obtaining long-term outcome data in patients with PNES is difficult. Patients with PNES are poor attenders at follow-up appointments, and it can be difficult to retain them in trials.[1,2] In the longer term, they may disengage with medical services entirely.[3] Truly prospective studies have not been possible, and in most of those studies that have been carried out, information has had to be obtained by telephone or postal survey rather than by face-to-face interview. This is compounded by the fact that in many medical systems, patients with PNES are diagnosed at specialist centers, then discharged back to their usual services, making it sometimes difficult to know how (if at all) they have been managed and how this may have impacted an outcome. These problems are reflected in the relative paucity of long-term outcome data in PNES and the limitations of those data. This chapter is focused on data on adults with PNES. There are some outcome data for children, which suggest that they may do better, in the medium term at least.[4] What happens to them as adults remains unknown.

The importance of measuring outcomes other than seizures has been stressed.[3,4] Employment, disability benefits, healthcare utilization, psychiatric morbidity, and quality of life have all been studied to some degree. One particular feature of outcome in PNES is that these variables tend to dissociate from each other—for example, many patients whose seizures appear to stop nonetheless remain economically dependent and have disabling psychiatric morbidity, with associated poor quality of life.[3,5-7] This suggests that, while it is important to recognize that outcomes other than seizure control are important in PNES, they may actually be, partially or wholly, the result (and therefore the outcome) of comorbid or underlying disorders other than PNES.

Two issues relating to current PNES outcome data are worth special mention: sampling problems and potential problems with seizure outcome measures.

2. SAMPLING PROBLEMS IN STUDIES OF PNES

There are no population-based long-term outcome data for PNES. All the long-term outcome data available are based on series from epilepsy centers. These series come from different territories with different medical systems,[3,7-12] so not only do referral patterns and follow-up practices likely induce bias, but this may well be different for different centers. It is difficult to gauge what role differences in management (management in the broad sense—for example, different follow-up practices, medication policies, and different psychological therapies) might play.

Even within center-based series, sampling is significantly limited. Two studies include information only on those patients whom investigators were able to follow up on or contact.[8,9] A telephone survey[10] obtained information from 67% of patients. One postal survey[7] obtained responses from 49.8% of patients, but others have obtained lower rates.[11,12] A study that obtained information from primary care medical records obtained information on 72.3% of patients.[3] While most studies[3,5,10,12] report no significant differences between responders and nonresponders in terms of demographic and other variables, it seems intuitively unlikely that in a disorder such as PNES, the fact that patients decide whether or not to be included in a study does not induce some kind of bias. In one study[11] females and older people were in fact overrepresented among responders.

While some variables (e.g., age, gender ratio) are relatively constant across follow-up studies, there are some obvious differences in population characteristics, possibly reflecting referral patterns, management, and follow-up practices. For example, the proportion of patients with comorbid epilepsy varies considerably, from 8.1% to 40.2%.[3,12] The proportion of patients with PNES that remains on antiepileptic drugs (AEDs) is similarly variable, ranging from 11% to 63.3%.[3,12] The degree to which these and other factors may have influenced measured outcome is discussed further later in the chapter.

3. PROBLEMS WITH SEIZURE MEASURES IN STUDIES OF PNES

Since seizures are by definition the main manifestation of PNES, most studies have recorded them as the main outcome measure. In patients with PNES and comorbid epilepsy, it is sometimes difficult even on the basis of a full face-to-face evaluation to know how many of a patient's seizures are PNES. It is doubly difficult to imagine an accurate estimation on the basis of a postal or telephone survey. The potential confounding effect of epileptic seizures (ES) will be least in series with low proportions of patients who have them. In one study with a large proportion of comorbid ES, there was no clear difference in seizure outcome between patients with and without comorbid ES,[7] though some data have suggested that patients with ES do worse, at least in terms of accessing healthcare for seizures.[3]

Seizure outcome has usually been expressed as the proportion of patients that are "seizure-free." In some studies, this has been recorded without any time period being specified.[6–8] Even when the time period is known, patient responses may be inconsistent. In one study of outcome 5–10 years after diagnosis,[12] responders to a postal survey were asked whether they were seizure-free and to give the date of their last seizure. Among patients who reported themselves "seizure-free," time from last seizure ranged from less than 1 month up to 8 years. Among patients who reported their last seizure a year or more previously, one quarter reported themselves as not seizure-free. In the same study, replies to the postal survey were compared with data from hospital and family doctors. Of 27 patients who reported themselves to be free of seizures, 6 had in fact presented to the family doctor or hospital complaining of seizures in the previous 6 months. Whether patients simply made mistakes, misunderstood the questions, or had some other motivation to return incorrect answers, this raises questions about the accuracy of data gathered by postal survey of patients. In one study, PNES patients' replies to questions about attacks during sleep appeared to have been influenced by considerations of losing Social Security payments,[13] and "self-protective" answers to research surveys have been encountered in other contexts.[14] This may account for some of the discrepancies seen. Whether this is relevant in jurisdictions with other social support systems is open to question.

4. THE RESULTS OF LONG-TERM OUTCOME STUDIES IN PNES

All that being said, several reasonably large outcome studies with reasonable diagnostic criteria are concordant in indicating that a majority of patients report that they continue to have seizures in the long term. The main studies are summarized in Table 17.1; in reading this table, it should be borne in mind that the studies are comparable only to a limited degree (see next discussion).

4.1. Seizure Outcomes

Meierkord et al.[8] studied 110 patients for a median of 5 years, finding that 40% had ceased to have seizures. Selwa at al.[10] obtained outcome information by telephone in 57 of 85 patients. They found that 23/57 patients (40.4%) reported that they had been free of seizures from 1 month after their monitoring until follow-up at 19 months to 4 years. An additional 9 patients (15.8%) had more than 90% reduction in seizure frequency. Lancman et al.[9] reported face-to-face outcomes in 93 patients for whom they had follow-up information, with a mean follow up of 5 years. They found that 25.4% were seizure-free. No duration was specified. Reuber et al.[7] studied obtained outcome information by postal survey in 148 of 329 patients with PNES and found that 71.2% reported continuing seizures. No duration was specified, but in a further study of 105 of these patients Reuber et al. found that 28.6% reported that they had been seizure-free for a year or

Table 17.1. Summary of Results of Long-Term Outcome Studies in PNES

Study	n	Follow-up Period	Seizures Continuing	On Antiepileptic Drugs	Unemployed/Disabled	Psychiatric Morbidity	Other Somatization
Meierkord et al. (1991)[8]	110	Mean 5 years	60%	n/a	20%	n/a	n/a
Selwa et al. (2000)[10]	57	19 months–4 years	59.6%	32%, PNES only	n/a	39%	n/a
Lancman et al. (1993)[9]	63	Mean 5 years	74.6%	n/a	n/a	n/a	n/a
Reuber et al. (2003)[7]	148	1–10 years	71.2%	40.7%, PNES only	53.8%	n/a	n/a
Jones et al. (2010)[11]	61	<10 years	83%	39%, all patients	n/a	52.6%	72.9%
Duncan et al. (2014)[12]	75	5–10 years	63.5%	n/a	29.3% in paid employment	n/a	n/a

more.[5] Jones et al.[11] obtained outcomes by postal survey in 61 out of 221 patients, finding that 83% had experienced seizures in the previous 12 months. Most had had more than one seizure per month, and 35.6% reported that they had been admitted to the hospital due to PNES. Duncan et al.[12] obtained seizure outcomes by postal survey in 75 out of 221 patients with PNES at 5–10 years from diagnosis, with 36.5% reporting that they were seizure-free.

4.2. Healthcare Utilization and Antiepileptic Drug Use

Patients with PNES consume large amounts of healthcare, heavily using both emergency and non-emergency services. Soon after diagnosis, there is considerable improvement in healthcare utilization among patients with PNES.[15,16] Longer term, there are relatively few data. Reuber et al.[7] found that 70% overall of patients with PNES continued to use emergency healthcare. This included 27 patients who said that their PNES had stopped. This series also included 42% of patients who had a diagnosis of comorbid epilepsy, so it was not clear for all patients what the healthcare use was for. The only other long-term study of healthcare utilization[3] found that 68.1% of 188 patients had no primary or secondary healthcare for seizures over a 6-month period, despite the fact that in many patients, the seizures had not stopped. In the same period, only 13.4% of patients went to the emergency department for seizures. This was similar to data gathered early after diagnosis. Thus, it appears that short-term gains in emergency healthcare utilization were maintained long term, independent of seizure outcome.

There is consensus that antiepileptic drugs (AEDs) should be withdrawn from patients with PNES who do not have comorbid epilepsy and that this should happen soon after diagnosis. In practice, the proportion of patients who remain on AEDs or are restarted on AEDs, short and long term, varies. Patients who are prescribed AEDs long term would appear to retain (or have regained) a diagnosis of epilepsy, either in their own minds or those of some of their medical caretakers. In either event, it is an aspect of healthcare utilization that has been included in some studies. In recent years, AEDs have been extensively prescribed for pain, migraine, and psychiatric indications. Thus, in more recent studies, unless specifically stated that the AED prescription is for seizures, this should be taken into account in interpreting this outcome.

In most studies, a substantial proportion of patients are prescribed AEDs at long-term follow-up, including some patients who are seizure-free. Reuber et al.[7] found that 78.6% of patients with PNES only who were still having seizures were taking AEDs 1–10 years after diagnosis, whereas 26.1% of those not having seizures were still taking AEDs (38.7% overall). Jones et al.[11] found that 39% of all their patients remained on AEDs up to 10 years after diagnosis, though only 8.1% had a diagnosis of epilepsy. A more recent study found that 11% of patients with a baseline diagnosis of PNES only were prescribed AEDs at 5–10 years from diagnosis,[3] and this figure did not exclude prescriptions for indications other than epilepsy. There may be multiple reasons for this difference. First, in more recent years there has been increased awareness that most patients with PNES do not have epilepsy, an increasing consensus that withdrawal should take place, and evidence that withdrawal is safe when appropriately monitored.[17] Second, this outcome is likely influenced by the nature of the system in which the study takes place. The last study mentioned took place in a system with unitary computerized medical records, access to specialists only through a single family doctor, and a single epilepsy service that maintained responsibility for the patient, making it relatively easy to "police" a diagnosis of PNES. There is also some evidence that reduced healthcare utilization may be linked to better caretaker acceptance of the diagnosis, medium and long term.[18]

4.3. Employment and Economic Dependence

As stated earlier, it is not clear in what sense employment and dependence can be regarded as outcomes of PNES (e.g., in the sense that the PNES simply cause the dependence). In one study,[9] 33.4% of patients were already unemployed at the time of PNES onset, and in another study,[19] 75.9% of patients were unemployed at PNES onset. In other studies, status of resolution of PNES appears to be independent to a degree from employment and dependence.[3,5,7,11,12] In one study, only 26.1% of patients who reported themselves seizure-free also reported that they were employed (unpublished data from Duncan et al.[12]). It is easy to see that seizures alone will make employment difficult; Lancman et al.[9] noted an additional group of patients who became unemployed after PNES onset and attributed their unemployment to the development of PNES. However, these data overall suggest that factors other than seizures are implicated in causing economic dependence in PNES patients, psychiatric morbidity and other medically unexplained symptoms (MUS) being among the more obvious possibilities.

Whatever the cause of the economic dependence, it appears to be highly prevalent among patients with PNES in the long term. In Reuber's study,[7] 41.4% of patients had "retired on health grounds," with an additional 12.4% being unemployed. Jones et al.[11] did not quote separate figures for unemployment, but their global outcome measure suggested low employment rates. Duncan et al.,[3] found that 22.8% of their patients were employed 5–10 years after diagnosis, a finding not significantly different from the proportion at the time of diagnosis.

4.4. Psychiatric Outcome and MUS Other Than PNES

As with employment, psychiatric morbidity may predate PNES onset: in one study[19] 38.9% of new-onset PNES patients had already had contact with secondary mental health services. Poor psychiatric health appears to persist long term. Duncan et al.[3] found that 26.5% of patients diagnosed with PNES 5–10 years earlier had recent contact with secondary mental health services and 39.5% were prescribed an antidepressant (both proportions were higher than at baseline, the antidepressant proportion significantly so). Selwa et al.[10] found that 39% of their patients were receiving ongoing mental health care at follow-up (25% of those patients were seizure-free, the same proportion as in patients who did not receive ongoing mental health care), and 35% were taking medication for psychiatric problems. Jones et al.[11] found that 52.6% of their patients had current mental health problems at the time of follow-up. The contribution of psychiatric morbidity to poor functional outcome in PNES has not yet been fully assessed, although Reuber et al.[5] did find an association between poor "productiveness" and psychiatric morbidity.

A substantial proportion of patients with PNES also have other MUS,[11,19-21] and in some, these predate the onset of PNES.[19] The contribution of such symptoms to other outcomes, such as dependency, and their long-term course are largely unknown. If our information on long-term outcome in PNES is limited, then information on long-term outcome of other somatic symptom disorders is even more so, as there are no good long-term studies to date.

4.5. Quality of Life Outcome

As in epilepsy, quality of life (QoL) appears to be related more to psychiatric status than to seizure frequency,[5,6] and it is probably significant that Reuber et al.[5] found QoL to be similar in patients who were economically dependent and having seizures, compared with those who were economically dependent and not having seizures. Jones et al.,[11] using a modified QOLIE-89 (Quality of Life in Epilepsy-89) inventory, found that their cohort of patients with PNES had QoL outcomes that were significantly poorer than those that might be expected for an epilepsy population, with poor physical function, physical symptoms, poor emotional well-being, and negative health perceptions being prominent themes.

5. PREDICTORS OF LONG-TERM OUTCOMES

In this context, what is meant by the term *predictor* is a variable that is collected at some time prior to the time of collection of the outcome variable and that is statistically associated with that outcome variable. The term *predictor* can also be used in a more statistical sense for a variable that predicts that the patient will be in a certain category: in this case the "predictive" variable may relate to a time frame that precludes causation, and so the relationship between it and the outcome variable might better be thought of as purely associative. While prediction can be tested in a number of ways, most studies have used bivariate techniques. These give a good indication of what one might experience clinically but do not take into account shared variance (e.g., comparing the proportion of patients with bad outcome between sexually abused and non–sexually abused subgroups might give a good indication of the relative outcome in both groups but does not indicate whether the association is primarily with sexual abuse or with an associated variable such as psychiatric status). Thus, the two techniques may well give somewhat different answers when applied to the same data set. In either case (and to state the obvious), only variables that have been recorded can be tested, and this varies from one study to the next. Potentially predictive and outcome variables may be measured in different ways (e.g., by face-to-face follow-up or by postal survey). For all these reasons, it is unsurprising that the results of analyses for predictors have varied and have in some cases seemed contradictory. The main predictors of outcome that have been found are summarized in Table 17.2.

Reuber et al.,[7] using bivariate analysis, found that seizure outcomes were poorer in patients who were younger at onset and at diagnosis, whose seizures had more dramatic features, who had a history of inpatient psychiatric care, and who remained on AEDs after diagnosis. Economic dependence long term was also associated with these

Table 17.2. Summary of Factors Found to Predict Long-Term Outcome in PNES

Study	Measure	Predictors of Good Outcome	Predictors of Poor Outcome	Nonpredictive Variables
Meierkord et al. (1991)[8]	Seizures	Female, independent, psychotherapy	Comorbid epilepsy	Duration of PNES Pre-existing psychiatric problems, type of seizure
Selwa et al. (2000)[10]	Seizures	Recent onset, swoon-type seizures		
Lancman et al. (1993)[9]	Seizures			Diagnostic delay, psychopathology
Reuber et al. (2003, 2005)[5,7]	"Global outcome measure"	Educational attainment, younger onset, less dramatic attacks	"Inhibitedness," emotional dysregulation, compulsivity	Diagnostic delay
Jones et al. (2010)[11]	"Global outcome measure"	None tested		
Duncan et al. (2014)[3,12]	Presentation to medical services with seizures, patient reported seizures	Disability benefit payments, comorbid epilepsy	Drawing state disability benefit	Delay to diagnosis, psychiatric morbidity

factors and with comorbid epilepsy. They also found that certain personality traits were associated with good outcome, in particular lower scores for inhibitedness, emotional dysregulation, and compulsivity, as was greater educational achievement. A later study of a subset of the same population[5] found that evidence of ongoing psychopathology (anxiety, depression, somatization index) was associated with poorer "productiveness" (employment) and seizure outcomes. Selwa et al.,[10] also using bivariate analysis, found that short delay to diagnosis was associated with good outcome and that patients with swoon-type seizures did better. It should be borne in mind that the subgroups they compared were quite small: they had only 19 patients who were seizure-free, for example. Duncan et al.[3] found that attendance at primary or secondary care for seizures at 5–10 years was predicted by comorbid epilepsy and was associated with Social Security payments at that time, but not predicted by earlier economic dependence. In a subgroup of 75 patients who had self-reported seizure outcomes, a report of being free of seizures was associated with being employed and by not being on Social Security benefits at 5–10 years, and was predicted by employment status at 12 months post-diagnosis.[12] Lancman et al.[9] found no associations with outcome. Jones et al.[11] did not analyze for predictors.

One potential predictor that is notable by its absence, with the exception of the study of Selwa et al.,[10] is delay to diagnosis. This has been analyzed in different ways in other large short- and long-term studies,[3,7,9,19] and was found not to be predictive of outcome. Whether the widely held belief that time reinforces somatization is incorrect (at group level in any event) or some other factor is in play is uncertain.

6. CONCLUSION

In the last two decades, we have come to understand that long-term outcome in PNES is poor at group level but that it is at the same time strikingly variable. Even if some data suggest that patients with poor psychiatric background and other factors may do badly, this is inconsistent across different studies, and we currently do not have reliable predictors of long-term outcome that might be useful to guide management. It has also become clearer that the seizures that define PNES are only part of the story. One important reason for studying the outcome of a disorder such as PNES is to be able to assess the effect of therapeutic interventions. In this respect, seizures provide a relatively uncomplicated measure. We can study other outcomes, but the limited follow-up information we have at present suggests that non-seizure outcomes may not necessarily respond to interventions that are directed specifically toward resolving the seizures. Some existing data help to pick apart relationships between seizures, other MUS, economic dependence, psychiatric morbidity, and other factors,[3,5,7,22] but this largely remains a challenge: understanding the disorder and its underpinnings will allow better understanding of what happens long term. A second challenge is to find ways of obtaining long-term outcome information that accurately reflects what happens to the patients so that we can measure the results of interventions with reasonable precision. This may turn out to be easier in some societies and healthcare systems than in others.

7. SUMMARY

- Practical and methodological issues have limited the quantity and quality of data on long- term outcome in PNES.
- Nonetheless, in the last two decades it has become clear that seizure outcome in PNES is poor, but highly variable.
- Social, employment, and psychiatric outcomes may also be poor, but are also highly variable.
- The relationships between different types of outcome and their implications for research into potential therapeutic interventions remain poorly understood.
- A major challenge for future research is to find better ways of obtaining long-term information on PNES patients.

REFERENCES

1. Oto M, Espie C, Duncan R. An exploratory randomised controlled trial of immediate versus delayed withdrawal of antiepileptic drugs in patients with psychogenic nonepileptic attacks (PNEA). *Epilepsia.* 2010;51:1994–1999.
2. LaFrance WC, Blum AS, Miller IW, Ryan CE, Keitner GI. Methodological issues in conducting treatment trials for psychological nonepileptic seizures. *J Neuropsychiatry Clin Neurosci.* 2007;19:391–398.
3. Duncan R, Graham CD, Oto M, Russell A, McKernan L, Copstick S. Primary and secondary care attendance, anticonvulsant and antidepressant use and psychiatric contact 5-10 years after diagnosis in 188 patients with psychogenic non-epileptic seizures. *J Neurol Neurosurg Psychiatry.* 2014;85:954–958.
4. Irwin K, Edwards M, Robinson R. Psychogenic non-epileptic seizures: management and prognosis. *Arch Dis Child.* 2000;82:474–478.
5. Reuber M, Mitchell AJ, Howlett S, Elger CE. Measuring outcome in psychogenic nonepileptic seizures: how relevant is seizure remission? *Epilepsia.* 2005;46:1788–1795.
6. LaFrance WC, Syc S. Depression and symptoms affect quality of life in psychogenic non-epileptic seizures. *Neurology.* 2009;73;366–371.
7. Reuber M, Pukrop R, Bauer J, et al. Outcome of psychogenic nondepileptic seizures: 1 to 10 year follow up in 164 patients. *Ann Neurol.* 2003;53:305–311.
8. Meierkord H, Will B, Fish D, Shorvon S. The clinical features and prognosis of pseudoseizures diagnosed following video-EEG telemetry. *Neurology.* 1991;41:1643–1646.
9. Lancman ME, Brotherton TA, Asconape JJ, Penry JK. Psychogenic seizures in adults: a longitudinal study. *Seizure.* 1993;2:281–286.
10. Selwa LM, Geyer J, Nikakhtar N, et al. Nonepileptic seizure outcome varies by type of spell and duration of illness. *Epilepsia.* 2000;41:1330–1334
11. Jones SG, O'Brien TJ, Adams SJ, et al. Clinical characteristics and outcome in patients with psychogenic non-epileptic seizures. *Psychosom Med.* 2010;72:487–497.
12. Duncan R, Graham C, Oto M. Outcome at 5-10 years in psychogenic nonepileptic seizures: what patients report vs. what family doctors report. *Epilepsy Behav.* 2014;37:71–74.
13. Duncan R, Oto M, Russell AJC, Conway P. Pseudosleep events in patients with psychogenic non epileptic seizures: prevalence and associations. *J Neurol Neurosurg Psychiatry.* 2004;75:1009–1012.

14. Van der Heijden PGM, Van Gils G, Bouts J, Hox J. A comparison of randomized response, computer-assisted self-interview and face-to-face direct questioning. *Sociol Methods Res.* 2002;32:384–410.
15. Martin RC, Gilliam FG, Kilgore M, et al. Improved health care resource utilization following video-EEG-confirmed diagnosis of nonepileptic psychogenic seizures. *Seizure.* 1998;7:385–390.
16. Razvi S, Mulhearn S, Duncan R, et al. New onset psychogenic nonepileptic seizures: healthcare resource utilization prior to and following diagnosis at a first seizure clinic. *Epilepsy Behav.* 2012;23:7–9.
17. Oto M, Espie C, Pelosi A, Selkirk M, Duncan R. The safety of antiepileptic medication withdrawal in patients with non-epileptic seizures. *J Neurol Neurosurg Psychiatry.* 2005;76:1682–1685.
18. Duncan R, Graham C, Oto M. Neurologist assessment of reactions to the diagnosis of psychogenic non epileptic seizures: relationship to short and long term outcomes. *Epilepsy Behav.* 2014;41:79–82.
19. Duncan R, Razvi S, Mulhearn S. Newly presenting psychogenic nonepileptic attacks: incidence, population characteristics and early outcome from a prospective audit of a first seizure clinic. *Epilepsy Behav.* 2011;20:308–311.
20. Bowman ES, Markand ON. Psychodynamics and psychiatric disagnoses of pseudoseizures subjects. *Am J Psychiatry.* 1996;153:57–63.
21. Lempert T, Schmidt D. Natural history and outcome of psychogenic seizures: a clinical study in 50 patients. *J Neurol.* 1990;237:35–38.
22. Lawton G, Mayor RJ, Howlett S, Reuber M. Psychogenic nonepileptic seizures and health related quality of life: the relationship with psychological distress and other physical symptoms. *Epilepsy Behav.* 2009:14:167–171.

18

An Integrated Approach to Other Functional Neurological Symptoms and Related Disorders

Jon Stone, MB ChB FRCP PhD and Alan Carson, MD

1. EPIDEMIOLOGY AND OVERLAP OF FUNCTIONAL SOMATIC DISORDERS AND DISSOCIATIVE SEIZURES

Functional symptoms and disorders are ubiquitous in clinical practice (see Table 18.1). Numerous studies of medical outpatient clinics in primary care[1] and secondary care[2] (including neurology services[3]) show that, depending how they are defined, around 15–50% of patients present with functional symptoms, either in combination with a more clearly defined disease or in isolation. More complex multisymptom functional disorder occurs with a prevalence of around 1–6% in the general population.[1]

In a study of 3,781 new neurology outpatients across Scotland, 16% had a primary diagnosis of a functional condition, making it the second most common reason to see a neurologist (after headache).[4] Analysis of these 587 patients presenting to the neurology service found that dissociative (nonepileptic) seizures (DS) were the most common diagnosis ($n = 85$). The list of the other most common diagnoses (functional sensory disorders [$n = 68$], functional motor disorders such as weakness, movement disorder, and gait disorder [$n = 56$], "nonspecific" functional disorder [$n = 97$], pain diagnoses [$n = 63$]) also gives some clues regarding common comorbidities experienced by patients with DS.

Patients with functional disorders in this study had similar levels of physical disability and disproportionate anxiety and depression compared to patients with recognized disease diagnoses.[3] This study also found that the level of unemployment was similar in cases and disease controls (50% vs. 50%), but patients with functional diagnoses were more likely not to be working for health reasons (54% vs. 37% of the 50% not working; odds ratio [OR] 2.0 [95% CI 1.6 to 2.4]) and also more likely to be receiving disability-related state financial benefits (27% vs. 22%; OR 1.3, 95%). Patients with these symptoms tend to be regarded as more "difficult to help"[5] but only exceptionally develop a neurological disease at follow-up that explains their original presentation.[6]

The associated healthcare costs are substantive. In the United States, a study of 1,914 patients in primary care found that those with high somatic symptom counts, adjusted for medical and psychiatric comorbidity, had more primary care visits, more specialty

Table 18.1 Functional Symptoms and Disorders in Clinical Practice

Gastroenterology	Irritable bowel syndrome (IBS), functional dyspepsia, chronic abdominal pain
Urology	Idiopathic overactive bladder
Rheumatology	Fibromyalgia
Infectious diseases	Post-viral chronic fatigue syndrome
Nephrology	Loin pain hematuria syndrome
Cardiology	Atypical chest pain, palpitations
Respiratory	Chronic cough, hyperventilation
ENT	Functional dysphonia, globus
Gynaecology	Chronic pelvic pain, dysmenorrhoea
Ophthalmology	Convergence spasm, functional visual loss
Neurology	Dissociative seizures, functional movement disorder

visits, more emergency department visits, and more hospital admissions than those with low symptom counts. The estimated annual direct medical costs extrapolated from these figures was $256 billion.[7]

It is clear across a range of functional disorders that these are problems with substantial and typically complex morbidity and costs[8] interfering with social and occupational functioning, typically in working-age adults.

1.1. Terminology

In this chapter, we will refer to dissociative seizures (DS) synonymously with psychogenic nonepileptic seizures (PNES) and nonepileptic attacks. This is the term used in ICD-10 and in our view is the best option. Our awkwardness on this point is not just pedantry. Later, when we discuss treatment, we emphasize the importance, in treatment of all functional disorders, of making a positive diagnosis based on assessment and sharing that with the patient. This cannot be easily done using a diagnosis which explicitly emphasizes the patient what they *don't* have. In addition, the term *dissociation* describes something about the mechanism of the symptom, without dualistic and potentially prematurely narrow conclusions about psychogenic etiology. Gastroenterologists do not use the term *psychogenic noncolitic bowel syndrome* because the terms *irritable bowel syndrome* and *functional gastrointestinal disorders*, among other advantages, provide a better framework for understanding and explaining the diagnosis, and we believe neurological and psychiatric practice has something to learn from this approach.

While the literature, including our own in the past, has conceived of these symptoms as "unexplained by disease," "medically unexplained," "somatoform" or "non-organic," our thinking, and that of others, has changed over the last 10 years. These are generally clinical presentations that are highly recognizable to physicians who are used to seeing them, often have positive diagnostic criteria, and can be usually diagnosed with a high degree of reliability, in the same way that we can recognize conditions such as epilepsy, migraines, or depression, some of which also have no identifiable "disease."

1.2. Comorbidity of Other Functional Somatic Disorders in Patients with Dissociative Seizures

Most clinicians seeing patients with DS would agree that comorbidity of other physical symptoms, typically functional symptoms, is the norm rather than the exception. It is surprising, therefore, that relatively little attention has been paid to this issue in research or treatment protocols. There is a particular lack of controlled studies examining the frequency of physical comorbidity in DS populations.

Studies reporting comorbidity of functional somatic disorders in DS are shown in Table 18.2. Most report high rates of both common functional disorders involving chronic pain and fatigue but also functional neurological symptoms, such as weakness and movement disorder, which are much less common and should not be occurring at these rates if the association was a generic effect of distress of having seizures.

Two studies have suggested that the presence of pain actually predicts a diagnosis of DS instead of epilepsy.[9,17] The presence of comorbid functional somatic disorders has unsuprisingly been demonstrated to predict worse outcome,[11] although a longitudinal study of 187 patients with DS did not find that DS was replaced with other functional symptoms if the DS improved.[18]

These studies are likely to overestimate the frequency of comorbidity to some extent, since they are mostly drawn from tertiary centers or patients attending for video telemetry. Our own experience is that the closer one sees the patient to initial diagnosis, the less likely these comorbidities are to be present. There is little doubt, however, that these comorbidities are often a major component of the distress and disability experienced by many patients with DS.

1.3. Classification of Dissociative Seizures in Relation to Other Functional Neurological Symptoms—the Problems of Lumping and Splitting

The data on comorbidity highlights a difficulty faced by those attempting to classify DS. Arguments for and against various categorizations can be summarized as follows:

1. Functional neurological symptoms (FNS) (as in *DSM-5*). FNS present most commonly to neurologists and commonly overlap with symptoms like functional movement disorder, which are rare in other settings. Patients with episodic functional tremor and other hyperkinetic movement disorders merge phenotypically into DS.[19] The hyperkinetic movements seen during the seizures themselves have all the features of a functional movement disorder (i.e., the quality of voluntary movement) if the patient was responsive. Patients with motionless unresponsive types of DS overlap patients who have episodic functional paralysis. Like functional movement disorders, DS is diagnosed on positive grounds and should not be a diagnosis of exclusion. Yet the experience of intermittent seizures compared to that of continuous leg paralysis

Table 18.2 Studies of Comorbid Functional Somatic Symptoms in Patients with Dissociative Seizures

Study	Population	Comorbidity Reported
Dixit et al.[9]	DS (n = 158) Epilepsy (n = 122)	66% had one or more of fibromyalgia, chronic fatigue syndrome, chronic pain, tension headache, or IBS vs. 27% epilepsy
Duncan et al.[10]*	DS (n = 54)	Single (57%) or multiple (19%) functional somatic disorder
Ettinger et al.[11]	DS (n = 56)	77% had moderate to severe pain in one or more areas of their body (e.g., headache, neck, back)
de Wet et al.[12]	DS (n = 102) Psychosis (n = 70)	26% vs. 9% had asthma. Authors suggest some asthma may have been hyperventilation
Lempert et al.[13]	DS (n = 50)	30% stance and gait; 22% sensory; 16% paresis; 16% pain; 10% visual symptoms; 6% bladder dysfunction; 4% contracture; 2% globus
Meierkord et al.[14]	DS (n = 110)	21% had another conversion symptom
Driver-Dunckley et al.[15]	DS (n = 116)	Pain (67%), fatigue (41%), sleep (21%), cognitive symptoms (60%), IBS (35%)
McKenzie et al.[16]*	DS (n = 120)	71% at baseline and 35% at 5–10 years follow-up had one or more of IBS, fibromyalgia, chronic fatigue, or tension headache

*Two study samples overlap. IBS, irritable bowel syndrome.

is arguably as intrinsically different as epilepsy is from multiple sclerosis, or panic disorder is from depression.

2. Functional somatic symptoms. Does it really make sense to separate out functional neurological symptoms from other somatic symptoms, which so commonly occur with them? Other functional disorders, such as functional gastrointestinal (GI) disorders, can also be diagnosed using positive diagnostic criteria.[20] On the other hand, DSM-5 no longer contains another category for somatic disorders diagnosed using features of the symptoms themselves (rather than their psychiatric presentation).
3. Dissociative disorder (as in ICD-10). The act of genuinely experienced loss of responsiveness and memory for episodic attacks can only be explained by dissociation. This is a strong argument for considering DS a dissociative disorder. On the other hand, many patients don't necessarily experience symptoms of dissociation other than the attack itself. It is worth remembering that dissociation can apply to two differing concepts: that of compartmentalization, which describes the phenomena above of a

disorder of voluntary motor system activity being perceived without consciousness or agency, and detachment, which may or may not be present.[21]

4. Anxiety disorder. Recent studies highlight how close in symptomatology, experience, and treatment DS is to panic disorder, another episodic condition in which the person loses control in a frightening and unpredictable way.[22]

Our view is that all of these arguments have some validity. Ideally, the ability to hold all these multiple perspectives provides an answer for clinicians and patients wishing to understand DS. The same arguments could all be made for other functional neurological symptoms.

Classification has other purposes in terms of research, coding, and reimbursement, but our natural desire, and those of our patients, to have an easy framework on which to hang our ideas about a condition can sometimes lead to oversimplified thinking in this area. It is useful in this context to consider what the literature tells us about the overlap between DS and functional movement disorders in particular, something that has been approached by several studies.

A review of 52 case series of DS and functional motor disorders found that, on average, 48% of the motor patients were female compared to 74% of the DS patients. Age of onset of functional motor symptoms was 34 years, whereas most studies of DS show an age of onset in the mid-20s.

A study of 20 patients with DS compared to 30 patients with functional limb weakness, all of recent onset and recruited in the same center, found that DS patients were younger by 12 years. DS patients also scored lower on several measures of perceived parental rearing.[23]

A study of 104 patients with DS compared to 35 patients with functional movement disorder found that the DS patients were a little younger (by 5 years, $p < 0.05$) and more likely to be female (86% vs. 67%, $p < 0.05$), but there were no differences in questionnaires assessing physical function, depression, "somatization," or measures of chronic disease management.[24]

A study of 116 patients with DS compared to 56 patients with functional movement disorder (FMD) also found that DS patients tended to be younger and had a lower age at symptom onset, although no difference in female proportion was found between the two groups.[15] In this study, there was fairly clear evidence that DS patients tended to present with a higher frequency of adverse childhood experience (41% DS vs. 21% FMD, $p = 0.003$). There were similarities in physical and psychological comorbidity.

Recently, we pooled data from the Illness Perception Questionnaire collected on two large cohorts of patients with DS ($n = 40$) and functional limb weakness ($n = 107$).[25] Although both groups tended to reject psychological factors as being relevant to their symptoms, patients with DS tended to do so less strongly than patients with functional limb weakness. This is perhaps understandable given the different nature of the symptoms, but provides some support for previous anecdotal observations that patients with DS tend to be a little more receptive to psychological explanations, where relevant, than patients with motor symptoms. This suggests that the approach to these symptoms required some differences in the treating clinician.

Table 18.3 Epidemiological Similarities and Differences between Dissociative Seizures (DS) and Functional Movement Disorder

	Dissociative Seizures	*Functional Movement Disorder*
Mean age of onset	Mid-20s	Mid to late 30s
Female:male	3:1	1.5–3:1
Physical symptoms	Episodic	Continuous
Scores on physical disability, depression/somatization scores	Higher than population	Higher than population—not clearly different from DS
Adverse childhood experience	2–3 times higher than the population	More common than population but often less than DS rates
Illness perceptions	Not keen on idea of "stress" being involved in symptoms	Even less keen on idea of "stress" than DS

The main findings are summarized in Table 18.3. Apart from age and sex, we have avoided extrapolating from individual studies, restricting our observations to those studies in which patients with both symptoms were studied using the same measure.

Our conclusion from these studies is that, leaving aside the obvious difference between an episodic attack disorder and one with persistent symptoms, there are some notable epidemiological differences, especially in age, gender, and adverse childhood experience, between patients who have DS and those with functional movement disorders which are worth highlighting. In many ways, it makes sense that if DS begins earlier, it will have a greater connection with events occurring in childhood rather than adulthood. Clearly, however, they must share some overlapping etiologies for the reasons already outlined, perhaps most persuasively because of the phenomenological overlap in the symptoms themselves.

2. ASSESSING FUNCTIONAL SOMATIC AND FUNCTIONAL NEUROLOGICAL DISORDERS IN THE PATIENT WITH DISSOCIATIVE SEIZURES

We now move on to more practical issues regarding the assessment of comorbid functional somatic disorders in the patient with DS.

2.1. History Taking and General Approach

We have described elsewhere a general approach to the assessment of the patient with functional neurological disorders which starts with obtaining a list of all physical symptoms, and not just those initially volunteered.[26] We would suggest asking everyone about pain (including headache), fatigue, limb symptoms, sleep, memory, dizziness,

GI symptoms, and bladder symptoms as a minimum. This is useful for the clinician in understanding the scope of the problem, especially in treatment, but also potentially therapeutic for the patient, for whom it may be the first time a health professional has bothered to ask the person, for example, about fatigue or dizziness. Contrary to stereotype, many patients are not forthcoming on this issue and are only too aware of how doctors usually respond to a long list of complaints.

Dissociative symptoms often occur immediately prior to dissociative seizures, usually briefly and in combination with symptoms of autonomic arousal and intense discomfort, which patients are typically reluctant to describe or may become unaware of as part of the seizure.[22,27,28] Similarly, patients with functional movement disorders, especially those with episodes that are of sudden onset or paroxysmal, may report dissociative symptoms of depersonalization ("my body didn't feel like mine") or derealization ("I felt disconnected from my surroundings") around the time symptoms first occur, which may be helpful later in the explanation of the disorder or treatment.[29,30]

The patient's view on the nature of their symptoms and their view on what treatment they are looking for is of paramount importance when tailoring initial explanation and treatment. We would suggest exploring this in relation to any functional somatic symptom as well as the dissociative seizures, as patients may have quite different views regarding etiology depending on the symptom.

2.2. Assessment of Other Functional Neurological Symptoms

The diagnosis of functional neurological symptoms should be made positively, usually on the basis of the examination. This should also be the case for DS, although we are aware that there is still a widespread tendency by many in the field to regard the diagnosis negatively (i.e., an attack with a normal EEG) rather than positively (e.g., an episode of sudden motionless unresponsiveness with eyes closed lasting 5 minutes, which can't be anything but DS).

Table 18.4 indicates a range of diagnostic maneuvers appropriate to various symptoms. What they mostly have in common is that the symptom can be demonstrated to be related to a state of abnormally focused attention. The more the patient focuses on the problem, the worse it gets. Conversely, these maneuvers generally use distraction techniques to demonstrate transiently normal function. This is what is meant by "internal inconsistency." In recent years, these physical signs, which neurologists have long used to make these diagnoses, have been shown in controlled studies to perform well in experienced hands. The interested reader is directed to a systematic review of motor and sensory signs,[31] a study of interobserver agreement,[32] and a study demonstrating the way in which the clinical diagnosis of functional tremor can be enhanced with laboratory investigations.[33]

Some of the signs rely on a difference between the examination findings in the patient and what we know should occur through scientific laws. For example, patients with functional visual symptoms commonly have a tubular visual field defect, which is incompatible with the laws of optics, which demand that the field should be conical. Even here, though, the findings can be interpreted as a sign of abnormally focused attention.

Table 18.4 Examples of Positive Signs in Functional Motor and Sensory Disorders That Can Be Shared with a Patient to Explain the Diagnosis*

	Positive Finding
Weakness	
Hoover's sign[31] (Figure 18.1)	Hip extension weakness that returns to normal with contralateral hip flexion against resistance
Hip abductor sign[31]	Hip abduction weakness that returns to normal with contralateral hip abduction against resistance
Other clear evidence of inconsistency	E.g., weakness of ankle plantar flexion on the bed but patient able to walk on tiptoes
Global pattern of weakness	Weakness which is global affecting extensors and flexors equally
Dragging gait	A gait in which the forefoot remains in contact with the ground, typically with hip externally or internally rotated
Movement Disorder/Gait	
Tremor entrainment test[35]	Patient with a unilateral tremor is asked to copy a rhythmic movement with the unaffected limb. The tremor in the affected hand either "entrains" to the rhythm of the unaffected hand, stops completely, or the patient is unable to copy the simple rhythmic movement.
Other tremor signs	Heel bouncing tremor (although can indicate clonus) Transient pauses during ballistic movements Tremor worsens with loading or immobilization
Fixed dystonic posture[36] (Figure 18.2)	A typically fixed dystonic posture, characteristically of the hand (with flexion of fingers, wrist, and/or elbow) or ankle (with plantar and dorsiflexion)
Typical "functional" hemifacial overactivity[37]	Orbicularis oculis or oris overcontraction, especially when accompanied by jaw deviation and/or ipsilateral functional hemiparesis
Truncal jerking	Axial myoclonus can relate to neurological disease but most cases are variable, functional, and preceded by a Bereitschafts potential on neurophysiological testing.
Distraction during standing[38]	Patients with an apparently positive Romberg's test are asked to guess numbers written on their back or carry out a complex motor task (e.g., with a phone). With a functional gait problem, balance will improve significantly.

(continued)

Table 18.4 Continued

	Positive Finding
Visual Symptoms[39]	
Fogging test	Vision in the unaffected eye is progressively "fogged" using lenses of increasing diopters while reading an acuity chart. A patient who still has good acuity at the end of the test must be seeing out of the affected eye.
Tubular visual field	A patient is found to have a field defect that has the same width at 1 meter as it does at 2 meters.

*Adapted with permission from Stone (2014)[34] and Stone and Carson (2015).[26]

Patients' a priori view that they have tunnel vision shapes their response even in the face of sensory input that must be contradictory to their beliefs.

Some signs, such as the presence of a new-onset clenched fist or inverted ankle in an adult found in functional dystonia, do not conform to these rules. In this case, however, the clinical presentation is so clearly associated with the features of a functional movement disorder that there is widespread agreement that they are clinically reliable.

Crucially, these signs and logical process of diagnosis can also be helpfully shared with the patient to ensure that transparency runs right through assessment, examination, explanation of the diagnosis, and treatment.

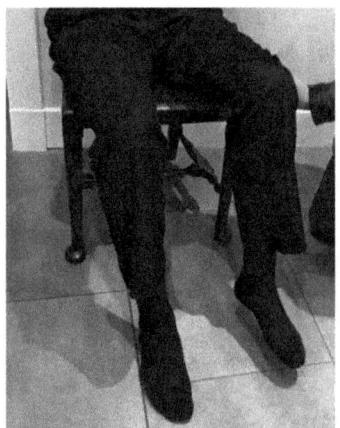
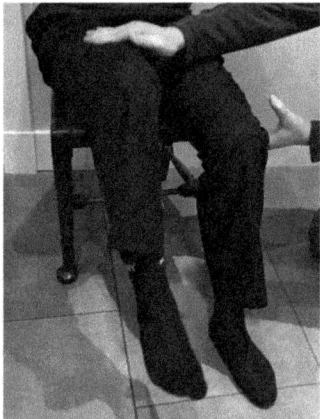

'Keep your left heel on the ground–don't let me lift it up'

LEFT hip extension is weak

'Lift up your right leg. Don't let me push it down'

LEFT hip extension returns to NORMAL

Figure 18.1 Hoover's sign of functional limb weakness. Test hip extension and demonstrate weakness. Test contralateral hip flexion against resistance and demonstrate that hip extension returns to normal.

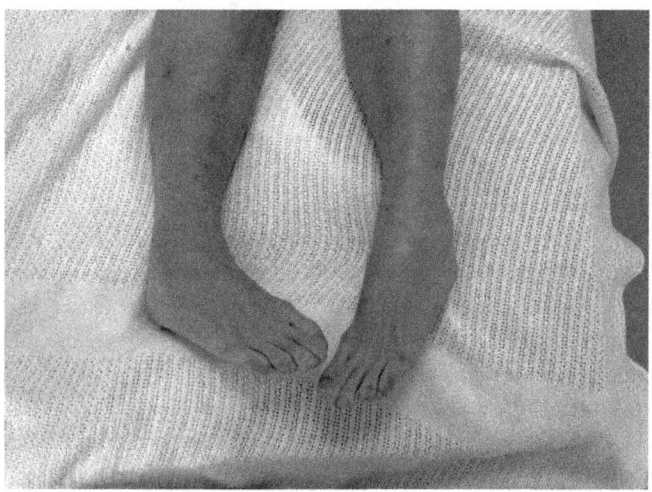

Figure 18.2 Functional dystonia with characteristic ankle inversion and plantar flexion (reproduced by permission from Stone and Carson [2015][26]).

2.3. Assessment of Pain, Memory, Sleep, Dizziness, Bowel and Bladder Symptoms

Ideally, any health professional seeing a patient with DS will also have some knowledge regarding the diagnosis of other common functional somatic symptoms that the patient may have and be able to incorporate these into an integrated formulation and treatment, especially with the help of relevant specialists. These are not diagnoses of exclusion in our view either, and in all patients, even when present, there needs to be consideration of whether there is another disease process explaining these symptoms as well.

2.3.1. Pain and Fatigue

The complaint of chronic widespread pain and tenderness affecting muscles and joints and associated with unrefreshing sleep and fatigue (fibromyalgia) is characteristic and arguably just as positively identifiable as a dissociative seizure. Complex regional pain syndrome (CRPS) is also highly recognizable as disproportionate pain in a limb associated with motor and sensory dysfunction, the clinical features of which have all the hallmarks of functional motor and sensory disturbance.[40] There is typically allodynia and hyperalgesia, and there may be swelling, color, and temperature change often relating to immobility. As models of functional motor and sensory disorders emerge from a constricted "conversion/psychogenic" model, then they can more logically align with existing models of chronic pain/CRPS and fatigue that already integrate biological, cognitive, and emotional factors without trying to pigeonhole the problem into one or the other.

2.3.2. Cognition

Cognitive symptoms are common in DS patients, an issue that has been highlighted in several studies.[41,42] These symptoms typically involve alterations of attention, memory, and executive function. Once again, with careful assessment, cognitive symptoms can often be demonstrated to be functional on the basis of the assessment.[43,44] Functional cognitive symptoms are recognizable by 1) patient's self-report of symptoms (rather than an accompanying caregiver); 2) ability to recall details of times when they did forget something; 3) dissociative symptoms (e.g., "I couldn't remember the whole car journey home"); 4) marked variability and inconsistencies of performance (e.g., complaint of terrible memory but no concerns from work colleagues). Patients with functional cognitive symptoms often develop a distorted and negative view of both their own memory function and an overly positive evaluation of how good their memory used to be (and how good everyone else's memory is). Anxiety about dementia is common and understandable and sometimes extends to a health anxiety disorder. Symptom validity testing (effort testing) may assist in diagnosis, although is not a black and white way of assessing wilful exaggeration. Chapters 5 and 9 cover this topic in detail.

2.3.3. Dizziness

In recent years, the phenotype of functional dizziness has been better described. Various terms, including phobic postural vertigo, chronic subjective dizziness, and, most recently, PPPD (persistent postural-perceptual dizziness), describe a type of dizziness that can be readily recognized in clinical practice.[45,46] The patient typically has an initial vestibular trigger such as a migraine or labyrinthitis which then persists as a sense of disequilibrium with movement and visual sensitivity, typically with fear of falling or going outside, and the same abnormal but involuntary attentional focus seen in motor disorders.

2.3.4. Gastrointestinal tract

Gastroenterologists have refined and researched diagnostic criteria for functional disorders over many years with the Rome Criteria.[47] These include disorders of bowel transit and pain but also disorders more closely aligned with functional neurological symptoms, such as globus pharyngitis (the feeling of a ball stuck in the throat)[48] and anismus (failure of the normal relaxation of the pelvic floor during defecation). These are an excellent starting point for dealing with patients' GI complaints.

2.3.5. Bladder

Primary disorders of bladder function are common in patients with multiple symptoms. Overactive bladder syndrome (colloquially, irritable bladder syndrome) describes a disorder of storage in which the patient has urgency and frequency. Conversely, the patient may have voiding dysfunction or sometimes even complete retention. This latter scenario commonly appears to occur in combination with acute back pain and opiate use.[49] Fowler's syndrome of chronic urinary retention is regarded as an "organic" disorder but appears to commonly co-occur with functional neurological symptoms, including 11% of patients having DS in one study.[50]

3. INTEGRATED APPROACH TO TREATMENT OF FUNCTIONAL DISORDERS IN THE PATIENT WITH DISSOCIATIVE SEIZURES

3.1. Explanation

As with DS, treatment begins with an explanation of the diagnosis. In a recent article (accompanied by a photo story!), we outlined some of the key components of a successful explanation, which are applicable to the whole range of functional disorders.[51]

1. Take the problem seriously.
2. Make it clear that there IS a diagnosis.
3. Demonstrate the rationale for the diagnosis.
4. Discuss the mechanism initially rather than etiology.
5. Convey the potential for reversibility.
6. Provide written information.
7. Triage for further treatment.

Our suggestions are, in large part, really just a recapitulation of what most health professionals would do anyway to explain most conditions—for example, stroke: take the patient seriously; tell the patient what he or she has; tell the patient something about what that condition is, how you know the diagnosis is correct, and explain how treatment may help, with written information. Discussions about etiology usually wait until later in most clinical situations.

What typically goes wrong for patients with functional disorders is that the normal sequence is disrupted or has omissions. Often patients are made to feel they are not being taken seriously; they are told what they don't have or are given no diagnosis at all; and instead of explaining what the problem is (a disorder of function), the clinician may jump immediately to speculative discussion about etiology, all of which tend to reinforce the patient's concern that he or she is being accused of "making it up."

In order to restore the normal sequence of explanation, it becomes crucial for patients to hear that they have a positive diagnosis. This is where terms such as *nonepileptic* or *medically unexplained* can be particularly antitherapeutic. The precise term may not matter that much as long as it's clear that it *is* a diagnosis.

For other functional neurological symptoms, there is particular value in demonstrating, sensitively, the physical signs to the patient.[52] For example, patients may be shown how their weakness of hip extension returns to normal with contralateral hip extension against resistance. Or they may be able to appreciate how their tremor improves with the entrainment test. Our experience is that this component is the one most valued by patients because it shows them that 1) the diagnosis is not one of exclusion and 2) there is the potential for improvement. This approach also helps patients make sense of variability that they themselves have usually already appreciated and sometimes felt bewildered about.

Explanation may have some therapeutic value in itself, but the evidence suggests that its true value lies in increasing the likelihood of benefit from subsequent therapy. Patients and doctors often get into unhelpful discussions about whether the symptoms are in the mind or the brain, when we know that such dualistic thinking is not appropriate. Instead, an emphasis on the potential for reversibility and a disorder of function (rather than structure) will map better onto a rehabilitation strategy. Jumping straight to a presumed etiological factor—(e.g., "I think this is stress related or related to your abuse") is akin to insisting to a stroke patient in the emergency department that the person has a "smoking-related left-sided weakness" without explaining properly how one can sometimes contribute to the other, among other risk factors. Such discussions are usually best left for later consultations, in our experience.

For patients with multiple types of functional symptoms, it is often helpful to explain to the patient how these problems are commonly linked together, and all have in common a disorder of nervous system functioning. Patients in this situation often feel as if they are "falling to bits" with so many different problems. Understanding that they have one vulnerability, to functional disorder, which comes out in different symptoms at different times can be empowering if handled carefully.

These are complex disorders which patients usually have never heard of. We think it is essential to provide patients with written information (e.g., available at http://www.neurosymptoms.org or http://www.nonepilepticattacks.info). This enables patients to discuss their condition with family and employers if necessary.

3.2. Physical Therapy

For patients with functional motor symptoms, emerging evidence and experience suggest that physical therapy, specific to functional disorders, can be highly effective.

Studies from the Mayo Clinic,[53] London,[54,55] and Glasgow,[56] as well as a randomized controlled trial (RCT) from Norway,[57] have all demonstrated remarkable improvements in patients with functional motor symptoms, even in patients with fairly long-standing symptoms lasting over 5 years.[54] It has been recognized in recent years that physical therapy in this patient group has some fundamental differences from that given for stroke or multiple sclerosis. For example, a recent RCT from London showed a 72% improvement in 30 patients, 6 months after a 5-day intervention compared to 18% in patients receiving usual physiotherapy.[58]

Ideally, physical therapy builds on a successful explanation by expanding on the idea that abnormally focused attention is at the root of many of the motor symptoms.[59] Practicing techniques that divert attention or use different motor "programs" can be framed as an intervention that is designed to "retrain the brain" or alter "bad habits." As physical therapy helps, the patients' diagnostic confidence and motivation can improve. Physiotherapy like this therefore has a significant cognitive-behavioral component even if it is not explicitly labelled as this.

Detailed recommendations for this type of intervention are now available in open access form.[60] The published evidence suggests that closely spaced sessions over 2 or 3 weeks are often more effective at effecting change than weekly sessions.

There is good evidence for graded exercise and physiotherapy especially in the context of a behavioral therapy for fibromyalgia,[61] chronic back pain,[62] and fatigue.[63] Studies of mediating factors suggest that improvement may relate primarily to overcoming fear avoidance, something that may be achieved by talking about it and practicing it (cognitive-behavioral therapy [CBT]) or just doing it (graded exercise).[64]

3.3. Psychological Therapy

Evidence for psychological therapy for functional motor symptoms is rather lacking, with the exception of an RCT that had 15 participants.[65] Many randomized trials have shown that psychotherapy of various forms can be effective to various degrees in aiding patients with functional disorders.[66] In functional neurological symptoms, there is some evidence for a guided self-help CBT-based brief intervention.[67] In chronic fatigue there is evidence for CBT being more effective than adaptive pacing but equally effective as graded exercise.[61] It is likely that other types of psychotherapy are effective on an individual basis but require careful patient selection.

3.4. Other Treatments

For functional motor symptoms, including speech symptoms, more unusual therapies may be worth considering, especially when ordinary approaches fail. Hypnosis has been used since the 19th century for these disorders, and some trial evidence suggests it may have a useful role.[68] There has been interest in the use of transcranial magnetic stimulation (TMS) in recent years. Some groups have reported dramatic benefit, although this has been in combination with other treatment modalities, including explanation and rehabilitation.[69] It is unclear whether any effect comes from the same combination of suggestion and possibly biofeedback, which has played such an important part of electrical therapy in functional disorders for over 200 years, or whether there may be a neuromodulatory role.[70] Finally sedation, not as a way of abreacting the patient but to promote movement or speech that otherwise cannot be induced on examination, may have a role for some more severely affected patients, especially those with functional dystonia.[71]

4. CONCLUSIONS

The assessment and treatment of comorbid functional somatic disorder (including functional neurological symptoms) in patients with dissociative seizures represents one of the most important aspects of an integrated approach to management. Enabling the patient to make links between the dissociative seizures and other physical symptoms allows a more comprehensive formulation and treatment plan. Ideally, services for patients with dissociative seizures should be multidisciplinary and include physical rehabilitation, where appropriate, for functional motor symptoms, pain, and fatigue.

5. SUMMARY

- Functional symptoms and disorders are common throughout medical practice. Patients with dissociative (nonepileptic) seizures often have other functional disorders.

- The diagnosis of functional neurological symptoms such as movement disorder, paralysis, and visual symptoms should be made on the basis of positive clinical signs of inconsistency and incongruity with neurological disease, such as Hoover's sign—this is not a diagnosis of exclusion and can be made in the presence of neurological disease.
- Functional disorders should not be diagnosed on the basis of psychosocial variables as these may or may not be present and are common in all neurological disorders.
- Treatment begins with a transparent explanation of the problem, preferably sharing positive evidence of the diagnosis with the patient and providing information about his or her condition.
- Treatment of functional disorders other than dissociative (nonepileptic) seizures should be multidisciplinary and focused on rehabilitation.

REFERENCES

1. Haller H, Cramer H, Lauche R, Dobos G. Somatoform disorders and medically unexplained symptoms in primary care. *Dtsch Arztebl Int.* 2015;112:279–287.
2. Nimnuan C, Hotopf M, Wessely S. Medically unexplained symptoms: an epidemiological study in seven specialities. *J Psychosom Res.* 2001;51:361–367.
3. Carson A, Stone J, Hibberd C, et al. Disability, distress and unemployment in neurology outpatients with symptoms "unexplained by organic disease." *J Neurol Neurosurg Psychiatry.* 2011;82:810–813.
4. Stone J, Carson A, Duncan R, et al. Who is referred to neurology clinics?—The diagnoses made in 3781 new patients. *Clin Neurol Neurosurg.* 2010;112:747–751.
5. Carson AJ, Stone J, Warlow C, Sharpe M. Patients whom neurologists find difficult to help. *J Neurol Neurosurg Psychiatry.* 2004;75:1776–1778.
6. Stone J, Carson A, Duncan R, et al. Symptoms "unexplained by organic disease" in 1144 new neurology out-patients: how often does the diagnosis change at follow-up? *Brain.* 2009;132:2878–2888.
7. Barsky AJ, Orav EJ, Bates DW. Somatization increases medical utilization and costs independent of psychiatric and medical comorbidity. *Arch Gen Psychiatry.* 2005;62:903–910.
8. Konnopka A, Schaefert R, Heinrich S, et al. Economics of medically unexplained symptoms: a systematic review of the literature. *Psychother Psychosom.* 2012;81:265–275.
9. Dixit R, Popescu A, Bagić A, Ghearing G, Hendrickson R. Medical comorbidities in patients with psychogenic nonepileptic spells (PNES) referred for video-EEG monitoring. *Epilepsy Behav.* 2013;28:137–140.
10. Duncan R, Razvi S, Mulhern S. Newly presenting psychogenic nonepileptic seizures: incidence, population characteristics, and early outcome from a prospective audit of a first seizure clinic. *Epilepsy Behav.* 2011;20:308–311.
11. Ettinger AB, Devinsky O, Weisbrot DM, Goyal A, Shashikumar S. Headaches and other pain symptoms among patients with psychogenic non-epileptic seizures. *Seizure.* 1999;8:424–426.
12. De Wet CJ, Mellers JDC, Gardner WN, Toone BK. Pseudoseizures and asthma. *J Neurol Neurosurg Psychiatry.* 2003;74:639–641.
13. Lempert T, Schmidt D. Natural history and outcome of psychogenic seizures: a clinical study in 50 patients. *J Neurol.* 1990;237:35–38.

14. Meierkord H, Will B, Fish D, Shorvon S. The clinical features and prognosis of pseudoseizures diagnosed using video-EEG telemetry. *Neurology*. 1991;41:1643–1646.
15. Driver-Dunckley E, Stonnington CM, Locke DEC, Noe K. Comparison of psychogenic movement disorders and psychogenic nonepileptic seizures: is phenotype clinically important? *Psychosomatics*. 2011;52:337–345.
16. McKenzie PS, Oto M, Graham CD, Duncan R. Medically unexplained symptoms in patients with PNES: do they explain poor employment outcome in patients with good seizure outcomes? *Epilepsy Behav*. 2016;59:9–12.
17. Benbadis SR. A spell in the epilepsy clinic and a history of "chronic pain" or "fibromyalgia" independently predict a diagnosis of psychogenic seizures. *Epilepsy Behav*. 2005;6:264–265.
18. McKenzie PS, Oto M, Graham CD, Duncan R. Do patients whose psychogenic non-epileptic seizures resolve, "replace" them with other medically unexplained symptoms? Medically unexplained symptoms arising after a diagnosis of psychogenic non-epileptic seizures. *J Neurol Neurosurg Psychiatry*. 2011;82:967–969.
19. Ganos C, Aguirregomozcorta M, Batla A, et al. Psychogenic paroxysmal movement disorders—clinical features and diagnostic clues. *Parkinsonism Relat Disord*. 2013;20:41–46.
20. Wessely S, Nimnuan C, Sharpe M. Functional somatic syndromes: one or many? *Lancet (London)*. 1999;354:936–939.
21. Holmes EA, Brown RJ, Mansell W, et al. Are there two qualitatively distinct forms of dissociation? A review and some clinical implications. *Clin Psychol Rev*. 2005;25:1–23.
22. Hendrickson R, Popescu A, Dixit R, Ghearing G, Bagic A. Panic attack symptoms differentiate patients with epilepsy from those with psychogenic nonepileptic spells (PNES). *Epilepsy Behav*. 2014;37:210–214.
23. Stone J, Sharpe M, Binzer M. Motor conversion symptoms and pseudoseizures: a comparison of clinical characteristics. *Psychosomatics*. 2004;45:492–499.
24. Hopp JL, Anderson KE, Krumholz A, Gruber-Baldini L, Shulman LM. Psychogenic seizures and psychogenic movement disorders: are they the same patients? *Epilepsy Behav*. 2012;25:666–669.
25. Ludwig L, Whitehead K, Sharpe M, Reuber M, Stone J. Differences in illness perceptions between patients with non-epileptic seizures and functional limb weakness. *J Psychosom Res* 2015; 79:246–9.
26. Stone J, Carson A. Functional neurologic disorders. *Behav Neurol. Neuropsychiatry*. 2015;21:818–837.
27. Reuber M, Jamnadas-Khoda J, Broadhurst M, et al. Psychogenic nonepileptic seizure manifestations reported by patients and witnesses. *Epilepsia*. 2011;52:2028–2035.
28. Stone J, Carson AJ. The unbearable lightheadedness of seizing: wilful submission to dissociative (non-epileptic) seizures. *J Neurol Neurosurg Psychiatry*. 2013;84:822–824.
29. Stone J, Warlow C, Sharpe M. Functional weakness: clues to mechanism from the nature of onset. *J Neurol Neurosurg Psychiatry*. 2012;83:67–69.
30. Pareés I, Kojovic M, Pires C, et al. Physical precipitating factors in functional movement disorders. *J Neurol Sci*. 2014;338:174–177.
31. Daum C, Hubschmid M, Aybek S. The value of "positive" clinical signs for weakness, sensory and gait disorders in conversion disorder: a systematic and narrative review. *J Neurol Neurosurg Psychiatry*. 2014;85:180–190.
32. Daum C, Gheorghita F, Spatola M, et al. Interobserver agreement and validity of bedside "positive signs" for functional weakness, sensory and gait disorders in conversion disorder: a pilot study. *J Neurol Neurosurg Psychiatry*. 2014;86:425–430.

33. Schwingenschuh P, Saifee TA, Katschnig-Winter P, et al. Validation of "laboratory-supported" criteria for functional (psychogenic) tremor. *Mov Disord.* 2016;31(4):555–562.
34. Stone J. Functional neurological disorders: the neurological assessment as treatment. *Neurophysiol Clin Neurophysiol.* 2014;44:363–373.
35. Zeuner K, Shoge R, Goldstein S, Dambrosia J, Hallett M. Accelerometry to distinguish psychogenic from essential or parkinsonian tremor. *Neurology.* 2003;61:548–550.
36. Schrag A, Trimble M, Quinn N, Bhatia K. The syndrome of fixed dystonia: an evaluation of 103 patients. *Brain A J Neurol.* 2004;127:2360–2372.
37. Fasano A, Valadas A, Bhatia KP, et al. Psychogenic facial movement disorders: clinical features and associated conditions. *Mov Disord.* 2012;27:1544–1551.
38. Wolfsegger T, Pischinger B, Topakian R. Objectification of psychogenic postural instability by trunk sway analysis. *J Neurol Sci.* 2013;334:14–17.
39. Chen CS, Lee AW, Karagiannis A, Crompton JL, Selva D. Practical clinical approaches to functional visual loss. *J Clin Neurosci.* 2007;14:1–7.
40. Marinus J, Moseley GL, Birklein F, et al. Clinical features and pathophysiology of complex regional pain syndrome. *Lancet Neurol.* 2011;10:637–648.
41. Strutt AM, Hill SW, Scott BM, Uber-Zak L, Fogel TG. A comprehensive neuropsychological profile of women with psychogenic nonepileptic seizures. *Epilepsy Behav.* 2011;20:24–28.
42. Demir S, Cam Çelikel F, Erdoğan Taycan S, Etikan I. [Neuropsychological assessment in conversion disorder]. *Turk Psikiyatri Derg.* 2013;24:75–83.
43. Stone J, Pal S, Blackburn D, Reuber M, Thekkumpurath P, Carson A. Functional (psychogenic) cognitive disorders: a perspective from the neurology clinic. *J Alzheimer's Dis.* 2015;48:S5–S17.
44. Jones D, Drew P, Elsey C, et al. Conversational assessment in memory clinic encounters: interactional profiling for differentiating dementia from functional memory disorders. *Aging Ment Health.* 2016;20:500–509.
45. Staab JP. Chronic subjective dizziness. *Continuum (Minneap Minn).* 2012;18:1118–1141.
46. Thompson KJ, Goetting JC, Staab JP, Shepard NT. Retrospective review and telephone follow-up to evaluate a physical therapy protocol for treating persistent postural-perceptual dizziness: a pilot study. *J Vestib Res.* 2015;25:97–104.
47. Drossman DA. The functional gastrointestinal disorders and the Rome III process. *Gastroenterology.* 2006;130:1377–1390.
48. Selleslagh M, van Oudenhove L, Pauwels A, Tack J, Rommel N. The complexity of globus: a multidisciplinary perspective. *Nat Rev Gastroenterol Hepatol.* 2014;11:220–233.
49. Hoeritzauer I, Doherty CM, Thomson S, et al. "Scan-negative" cauda equina syndrome: evidence of functional disorder from a prospective case series. *Br J Neurosurg.* 2015;29(2):178–180.
50. De Bock F, Dirckx J, Wyndaele J-J. Evaluating the use of different waveforms for intravesical electrical stimulation: a study in the rat. *Neurourol Urodyn.* 2011;30:169–173.
51. Carson A, Lehn A, Ludwig L, Stone J. Explaining functional disorders in the neurology clinic: a photo story. *Pract Neurol.* 2016;16:56–61.
52. Stone J, Edwards M. Trick or treat? Showing patients with functional (psychogenic) motor symptoms their physical signs. *Neurology.* 2012;79:282–284.
53. Czarnecki K, Thompson JM, Seime R, Geda YE, Duffy JR, Ahlskog JE. Functional movement disorders: successful treatment with a physical therapy rehabilitation protocol. *Parkinsonism Relat Disord.* 2012;18:247–251.

54. Nielsen G, Ricciardi L, Demartini B, Hunter R, Joyce E, Edwards MJ. Outcomes of a 5-day physiotherapy programme for functional (psychogenic) motor disorders. *J Neurol.* 2015;262:674–681.
55. Demartini B, Batla A, Petrochilos P, Fisher L, Edwards MJ, Joyce E. Multidisciplinary treatment for functional neurological symptoms: a prospective study. *J Neurol.* 2014;261:2370–2377.
56. Matthews A, Brown M, Stone J. Inpatient physiotherapy for functional (psychogenic) gait disorder: a case series of 35 patients. *Mov Disord Clin Pract.* 2016; doi:10.1002/mdc3.12325.
57. Jordbru AA, Smedstad LM, Klungsøyr O, Martinsen EW. Psychogenic gait disorder: a randomized controlled trial of physical rehabilitation with one-year follow-up. *J Rehabil Med.* 2014;46:181–187.
58. Nielsen G, Buszewicz M, Stevenson F, et al. Randomised feasibility study of physiotherapy for patients with functional motor symptoms. *J Neurol Neurosurg Psychiatry.* 2016; jnnp – 2016-314408.
59. Edwards MJ, Adams RA, Brown H, Pareés I, Friston KJ. A Bayesian account of "hysteria." *Brain.* 2012;135:3495–512.
60. Nielsen G, Stone J, Matthews A, et al. Physiotherapy for functional motor disorders: a consensus recommendation. *J Neurol Neurosurg Psychiatry.* 2015;86:1113–1119.
61. Bidonde J, Busch AJ, Bath B, Milosavljevic S. Exercise for adults with fibromyalgia: an umbrella systematic review with synthesis of best evidence. *Curr Rheumatol Rev.* 2014;10:45–79.
62. Kamper SJ, Apeldoorn AT, Chiarotto A, et al. Multidisciplinary biopsychosocial rehabilitation for chronic low back pain: Cochrane systematic review and meta-analysis. *BMJ.* 2015;350:h444–h444.
63. White PD, Goldsmith KA, Johnson AL, et al. Comparison of adaptive pacing therapy, cognitive behaviour therapy, graded exercise therapy, and specialist medical care for chronic fatigue syndrome (PACE): a randomised trial. *Lancet.* 2011;377:823–836.
64. Chalder T, Goldsmith KA, White PD, Sharpe M, Pickles AR. Rehabilitative therapies for chronic fatigue syndrome: a secondary mediation analysis of the PACE trial. *Lancet Psychiatry.* 2015;2:141–152.
65. Kompoliti K, Wilson B, Stebbins G, Bernard B, Hinson V. Immediate vs. delayed treatment of psychogenic movement disorders with short term psychodynamic psychotherapy: randomized clinical trial. *Parkinsonism Relat Disord.* 2014;20(1):60–63.
66. Koelen JA, Houtveen JH, Abbass A, et al. Effectiveness of psychotherapy for severe somatoform disorder: meta-analysis. *Br J Psychiatry.* 2014;204:12–19.
67. Sharpe M, Walker J, Williams C, et al. Guided self-help for functional (psychogenic) symptoms: a randomized controlled efficacy trial. *Neurology.* 2011;77:564–572.
68. Moene FC, Spinhoven P, Hoogduin CA, Van Dyck R. A randomized controlled clinical trial of a hypnosis-based treatment for patients with conversion disorder, motor type. *Int J Clin Exp Hypn.* 2003;51:29–50.
69. Pollak T, Nicholson T. A systematic review of transcranial magnetic stimulation in the treatment of functional (conversion) neurological symptoms. *J Neurol Neurosurg Psychiatry.* 2014;85(2):191–197.
70. McWhirter L, Carson A, Stone J. The body electric*: a long view of electrical therapy for functional neurological disorders. *Brain.* 2015;138:1113–1120.
71. Stone J, Hoeritzauer I, Brown K, Carson A. Therapeutic sedation for functional (psychogenic) neurological symptoms. *J Psychosom Res.* 2014;76:165–168.

19

Toward the Integration of Care

Gaston Baslet, MD and Barbara A. Dworetzky, MD

1. INTRODUCTION

Functional neurological symptom disorder (FNSD) is common in neurology practice, with nearly one third of patients seen in neurology clinics having symptoms that cannot be fully explained by a medical or neurological disease.[1] Functional neurological symptoms (FNS), the symptoms that are the hallmark of FNSD, have a negative impact on patients' quality of life and social functioning; many patients use medical resources ineffectively and become chronically disabled. Psychogenic nonepileptic seizures (PNES) represent one symptomatic expression of FNSD and ought to be considered within the larger context of other FNS and somatic complaints that have a limited physiological explanation.

Despite its relatively high prevalence, FNSD is poorly understood and underdiagnosed and receives little attention in the medical literature and research. In clinical practice, patients with FNS tend to receive suboptimal care owing to a number of factors: the nature of the disorder itself, the limited availability of evidence-based treatments, limited attention in training programs and, therefore, very limited or even lack of expertise, and factors related to the healthcare system.

This volume has discussed the practical challenges that PNES (and other FNSDs) pose to patients, families, and clinicians during the different stages of care: at the time of diagnosis, presentation of the diagnosis, engagement in treatment, treatment itself, and long term. Our hope is to not only show the frustration associated with the clinical management of PNES and related disorders but also shed light on potential and already existing solutions. An integrated care approach addresses these components in a seamless and coordinated fashion and helps patients achieve their maximum level of functioning.

2. A CHALLENGING DISORDER

Functional neurological symptoms, including PNES, are presumed to be an involuntary, automatic or reflexive expression of distress, usually not recognized by or not conscious to the patient, and are attributed to psychological defense mechanisms such as conversion, dissociation, or both. This quality distinguishes this disorder from other typical symptoms in medicine where the main complaint usually ends up fitting some pathophysiological explanation once the diagnosis is discovered. Patients with PNES will initially present to clinicians fearing that they suffer from epileptic seizures (or some other paroxysmal syndrome), only to be told their symptoms have a psychological origin, often without much further explanation. This psychological explanation sounds foreign to most patients who, at face value, are puzzled by their scary symptoms and see no clear association with emotional distress. Psychologically, the symptom represents the patient's unconscious effort of distancing him- or herself from painful affect (the traditional definition of conversion). Therefore, an explanation of the symptom as psychological in origin can only alienate most patients who have tried very hard, for the most part unconsciously, to distance themselves from their painful and uncomfortable emotional experiences or memories.

As discussed in detail in Chapter 3, the complexity of this disorder relies on not only its physical symptomatic expression but also its underlying psychopathological mechanisms. Individuals with PNES can have heterogeneous psychiatric backgrounds.[2,3] Nonspecific psychopathological factors associated with PNES have been identified in many studies. These include, but are not limited to, avoidance tendencies, alexithymia, external locus of control, insecure attachment, and under- or overmodulation of emotions.[4] None of these factors are likely to explain the etiology of PNES in all patients, and they may only offer one aspect of what needs to be addressed therapeutically. Therefore, from a psychiatric standpoint, it is difficult to offer a one-size-fits-all model to conceptualize this disorder and to clearly identify treatment targets that will fit all patients.

Despite FNS being described for centuries in the medical literature, there have been miniscule advances in terms of effective therapies, especially when compared to other neuropsychiatric disorders that have well-established treatment algorithms based on evidence-based studies. The last 10 years have seen a resurgence of interest in FNSD, generating a handful of randomized controlled trials and a few uncontrolled studies that support the use of effective therapies. Evidence-based treatments for PNES are summarized in Chapter 14. Still, the contrast with other neuropsychiatric disorders that have their own associations, foundations, journals and research funds is striking.

Why is it that healthcare professionals have not found a better understanding of this disorder, translating to a dearth of widespread effective treatments, as compared to other neuropsychiatric conditions? Why is it that we have not been able to agree on a term for the disorder that is both descriptive and acceptable to patients and clinicians? We can only hypothesize reasons for this neglected status that FNSD, and PNES in particular, have attained. As noted, FNSD is a truly complex disorder from both the neurologic and psychiatric perspectives. Additionally, our division of efforts in neurology and psychiatry as two separate fields does not fit this disorder that loudly conveys that there is no room for dualistic thinking in medicine. Chapter 11 discusses in detail why the functional or conversion nature of PNES can lead to attitudes among many clinicians that subtly send the message that FNSD (or PNES) is not important or only quasi-legitimate. Such an attitude is also already implicit in the limited research efforts, funding, and educational initiatives.

The response we have created as a profession recapitulates the individual story of many patients with PNES or other FNSDs. The reaction by many professionals generates a negative experience in these patients who carry histories in which abuse and neglect are common. The relationship with the healthcare system thus becomes toxic, making many patients feel retraumatized. It ultimately becomes clear that these patients are claiming, "Look, I am sick. . . . I just don't know how to verbally explain what this is about." As the diagnosis of FNSD or PNES is uncovered, patients and professionals can soon find each other speaking a very different language, with professionals forcing a psychological explanation that patients are not ready to embrace, and with patients feeling the need to speak their somatic language even louder. A recent survey among epilepsy experts showed that communicating to patients that the events are "not explained by epilepsy" and due to a "psychological cause" is the most commonly used explanation that patients receive.[5] As healthcare professionals, we should at least enlist an effort to validate our patients' complaints, even while we try to better understand this puzzling condition, without losing sight of the ultimate goal of getting them the care they need. Chapter 10 presents a communication strategy that integrates the physical experience of the patient with an underlying psychological cause.

3. THE LIGHT AT THE END OF THE TUNNEL: A WINDOW INTO THE NEUROBIOLOGY OF THIS DISORDER

Our affective experiences are important determinants of our decision making, as Damasio postulates in his "somatic marker" hypothesis.[6] While we are consciously aware of some aspects of our emotional lives, a significant portion of our emotional experiences plays its role outside of our awareness. This concept is not well understood by the general public, and therefore, explanations of affective processes directing other biological functions seem rather elusive when we try to explain to patients the link between emotion processing and FNS. Chapter 6 discusses a number of studies that provide scientific evidence of our long-held belief that emotion processes do influence motor control in PNES now explainable by changes in the brain.[7,8]

The fact that functional symptoms are experienced as "involuntary" often leads patients to believe that their symptoms cannot be explained by an underlying affective process. Again, in Chapter 6, the authors present evidence from psychogenic movement disorder, another FNSD, that parts of the brain that signal a certain behavior as "our own" have a lower degree of activation and connectivity with areas involved in generating the ultimate movement. This altered activation and connectivity is thought to underlie the perception of involuntariness in functional symptoms.[9] The overlap in "unawareness" between functional motor and somatosensory symptoms and lesional neglect has been noted and "functional unawareness syndrome" has been proposed as a conceptual framework to understand FNSD.[10]

As more and more evidence becomes available, our hope is that most clinicians will start to understand that FNS are not under the patient's volitional control. This is a concept already well accepted in primary psychiatric disorders such as major depression or panic disorder. Clinicians would not consider demanding patients to "stop being depressed" or "stop having panic attacks," as if symptoms in those disorders were volitionally produced.

Yet, it is not uncommon in PNES and other FNSD to hear such equivalent statements from clinicians and sometimes from angry and frustrated family members.

What is most therapeutically relevant is that while symptoms are involuntary, they can still have a transactional value. This means that detailed functional analysis in behavioral treatment can often identify a function to the symptom. This does not make the symptom more or less voluntary, but rather allows a point of intervention as the patient embarks on treatment.

Finally, while symptoms are involuntary, improvement can only occur with the active and very conscious participation of the patient in treatment for change to take place. This important message needs to be conveyed to patients before they initiate a therapeutic intervention. The expectation that "the treatment will take the symptoms away," as if treatment were an external force that the patient has no influence on, can negatively interfere with successful outcomes. Active treatment participation that promotes change and clearly understanding that there is "no magic pill" are essential to facilitate recovery, if explained in a supportive and validating manner.

4. A TEAM SPORT: IT TAKES A VILLAGE

FNSD, including PNES, has now scientific evidence of altered brain function. Patients and clinicians have questioned the functional nature of the diagnosis based on various factors such as the unclear unconscious influence of emotional factors and the involuntary versus voluntary nature of symptoms. Our evidence now supports FNS as being involuntary and heavily influenced by emotional processes with a neurologically mediated mechanism. These advances should be exploited therapeutically and should help further legitimize this disorder and dissipate any skepticism that may still remain. FNSD should be considered a true neuropsychiatric disorder: a neurobiologically based disorder at the intersection of mind and brain, neurology and psychiatry. Interestingly, dualistic thinking gets reflected in the suboptimal and fragmented care that many of our patients receive: diagnosed in one clinical setting, but treated in a different one.

It is only through the integration of care that patients with PNES and other FNSD will receive the comprehensive and multidisciplinary treatment they deserve. Integrated care involves not just gathering different disciplines that collaborate within a closed or connected system. It also involves enhancing the patient's functioning in the community and home by providing services that help monitor adherence, avert unnecessary crises or inappropriate treatment, and provide logistical and emotional support.

Integrated care serves a variety of purposes. At the most superficial level, it helps patients to not fall through the cracks as they are cared for by different disciplines. It ensures that patients do not get diverted toward new functional symptoms, by carefully examining new complaints and helping them get the appropriate medical care they need, while ensuring that they do not feel that care is denied. The support provided by an integrated system also helps family members become part of the care team by empowering them to become facilitators of change. School- and work-related supports are also enlisted, when appropriate, to ensure that appropriate measures are taken to maximize recovery. Treatment providers outside of the connected system become part of the team, at least virtually, so that a consistent and supportive message is received by the patient and his or her immediate support network. In short, integrated care is much more than a neurologist and a mental health provider talking to each other about PNES or another FNSD; it is making sure that all the components in the patient's life will reinforce therapeutic recovery.

At a psychological level, the function of the integrated treatment team is to re-create a containing and validating environment that facilitates change. The multiplicity of symptoms in PNES patients (within each episode, or when combined with other psychiatric and medical comorbidities) recapitulates the complex medical system necessary to help them. Providing care to PNES patients becomes an opportunity to model harmony and collaboration between providers and community supports. This process of collaboration and integration parallels the harmony between mind and body that, through treatment, we try to re-create for patients.

Chapter 12 outlines innovative models of care that are being and could be offered to PNES patients (and could probably be extended to other FNSDs, with minor adaptations). Our proposed integrated care model relies on this kind of organized and stepped care and oversees the therapeutic process to ensure that all components of treatment are properly deployed at the right time to optimize outcomes. Our integrated care approach ensures that the components outlined in the subsequent chapters are chained accordingly: patients are retained in treatment (Chapter 13); when possible, evidence-based interventions are implemented (Chapter 14); the neurologist and other medical providers remain available through the recovery process and actively collaborate with the mental health team (Chapter 15); and families and community supports take an active role (Chapter 16).

Even after all these interventions are properly delivered and monitored, some patients may remain disabled either by ongoing symptoms or by other psychiatric or medical comorbidities, as discussed in Chapter 17. Our integrated care approach proposes that, in such patients, a rehabilitative program maximizes any chances of vocational reintegration and minimizes any possibility of symptomatic decline or multiplication.

At a practical level, integrated care relies on more than different disciplines doing their job. Rather than thinking, "the neurologist diagnoses and the psychiatrist or mental health professional treats," our proposed model emphasizes a team approach in which each professional highlights his or her expertise but remains actively involved and available throughout the course of treatment for this chronic and recurring disorder. An essential care management professional oversees the recovery process and ensures that all providers and community resources (anyone involved in the patient's care—both within and outside of the same health system) are actively participating and in line with the same plan.

PNES is one symptomatic expression of a larger disorder. Chapter 18 illustrates many other functional disorders that can present in the context of PNES. Our goal for the future is to provide evidence-based data that will inform integrated care. As this approach targets the larger picture rather than one isolated symptom (PNES), new complaints, whether thought to be functional in nature or not, become the responsibility of the team to address (either directly or through facilitating the appropriate care) and are mapped onto the patient's recovery path. Ultimately, going through this process for a predefined period of time will lead patients to be in a position where symptoms are properly managed and functional outcomes improved.

5. THE ROLE OF EDUCATION AND TRAINING

PNES and other FNSD have existed for centuries. Despite our hopes for improved primary prevention, such as minimizing childhood adversities, unfortunately, these conditions will probably continue to exist. Therefore, our view goes beyond providing adequate care to existing patients: the next generations of professionals needs to be prepared to suspect, diagnose, and manage patients with PNES in a timely and effective fashion. There are many challenges involved with this process, for instance, the challenges in the diagnostic process that are outlined in Chapters 7, 8, and 9 for different disciplines. Only well-educated and informed clinicians will be prepared to confront these challenges.

Mark Hallett refers to psychogenic movement disorder, a subtype of FNSD, as a "crisis in neurology," alluding to the recognized prevalence but limited attention and resource allocation to address it.[11] Unfortunately, psychiatrists and other mental health professionals are not widely prepared either to manage these disorders or to champion multidisciplinary programs to do so.

Education and training programs in neurology and psychiatry could provide insight for trainees into PNES and other FNSD.[5] However, time and effort committed to training on this disorder tends to be limited and not proportional to the percentage of patients that general practitioners in neurology and primary care will evaluate throughout their careers.[1] Such numbers are more difficult to determine in psychiatry or psychology, since many PNES patients will not follow through with the recommended referral, as illustrated in Chapter 13. Even when they do, some mental health professionals either have no training on how to manage the disorder or are skeptical about the accuracy of the diagnosis.[12]

As our integrated care model borrows from all different aspects of a patient's life to facilitate change, so should our approach to improve education. Training in PNES and other FNSDs should address not only formal didactic learning but also attitude training. Many neurologists may feel that they did not pursue a career in neurology to manage a neuropsychiatric disorder; therefore, it should not be in the realm of their responsibility to treat these patients. This is where dualistic thinking showcases its limitations again. While most neurologists choose to specialize in other neurologic disorders, the commitment to provide the best care possible and ensure availability of adequate treatment should not be different for FNSD than for any other neurological disease. This is akin to having a patient with chest pain in the psychiatrist's office and the doctor ignoring the symptom because he or she is not a cardiologist or an emergency doctor: such a response would be considered negligent care. However, in the case of PNES, the disorder is, in fact, a disorder of the brain, and the symptom is, in fact, affecting motor or sensory or cognitive function. Therefore, the neurologist should be involved in the recovery process as the mental health team manages the underlying factors that cause the FNS.

Another strength of integrated care is that it models training to be free of division of responsibility. The argument that "this is the neurologist's or the psychiatrist's duty" has no place in the proposed approach. It is a team's responsibility to help patients receive the most appropriate treatment and navigate a complex healthcare system safely and effectively. This is a model for trainees to learn from. Medicine has already accepted such integrated models of care for complex disorders, such as in substance use disorder and other disorders with multiorgan involvement, such as diabetes mellitus.

In summary, training in PNES and related conditions must help trainees learn to conceptualize the disorder from a neurobiological and psychological perspective. Training must also include special attention to a compassionate, responsible approach to care. While these are words that can and should apply to training in any disorder, it is our impression that as a profession, we have failed to do so in PNES and other FNSDs. We now have an opportunity to change how we integrate this condition into the realm of modern medicine, where the distinction between mind and brain is a theoretical and archaic concept. We also have an opportunity to improve how we communicate about this condition, including finding a label acceptable to patients and clinicians, so we can all move on to focus on recovery. It is our hope that this new approach will help the next generation of neurologists and psychiatrists carry and further improve this message.

REFERENCES

1. Carson AJ, Brown R, David AS, et al.; UK-FNS. Functional (conversion) neurological symptoms: research since the millennium. *J Neurol Neurosurg Psychiatry*. 2012;83(8):842–850.
2. Baslet G, Roiko A, Prensky E. Heterogeneity in psychogenic nonepileptic seizures: understanding the role of psychiatric and neurological factors. *Epilepsy Behav*. 2010;17:236–241.
3. Rusch MD, Morris GL, Allen L, Lathrop L. Psychological treatment of nonepileptic events. *Epilepsy Behav*. 2001;2(3):277–283.
4. Baslet G, Seshadri A, Bermeo-Ovalle A, Willment K, Myers L. Psychogenic non-epileptic seizures: an updated primer. *Psychosomatics*. 2016;57(1):1–17.
5. Dworetzky BA. What are we communicating when we present the diagnosis of PNES? *Epilepsy Curr*. 2015;15(6):353–357.
6. Damasio A. *The Feeling of what Happens: Body and Emotion in the Making of Consciousness*. New York: Harcourt; 1999.
7. van der Kruijs SJ, Jagannathan SR, Bodde NM, et al. Resting-state networks and dissociation in psychogenic non-epileptic seizures. *J Psychiatr Res*. 2014;54:126–133.
8. Li R, Liu K, Ma X, et al. Altered functional connectivity patterns of the insular subregions in psychogenic nonepileptic seizures. *Brain Topogr*. 2015;28(4):636–645.
9. Voon V, Gallea C, Hattori N, Bruno M, Ekanayake V, Hallett M. The involuntary nature of conversion disorder. *Neurology*. 2010;74(3):223–228.
10. Perez DL, Barsky AJ, Daffner K, Silbersweig DA. Motor and somatosensory conversion disorder: a functional unawareness syndrome? *J Neuropsychiatry Clin Neurosci*. 2012;24(2):141–151.
11. Hallett M. Psychogenic movement disorders: a crisis for neurology. *Curr Neurol Neurosci Rep*. 2006;6(4):269–271.
12. Harden CL, Burgut F, Kanner AM. The diagnostic significance of video-EEG monitoring findings on pseudo-seizure patients differs between neurologists and psychiatrists. *Epilepsia*. 2003;44:453–456.

Index

accidents, 22. *See also* falls; traumatic brain injury
Alberta Children's Hospital (ACH) care model, 210, 211*f*
alexithymia, 47, 94–95, 147, 180, 222–23, 226
   definition and nature of, 47, 94, 222
   self-report measures to characterize, 165*t*
   and treatment adherence, 221*t*, 222
anterior cingulate cortex (ACC), 107, 108
antidepressants, 92–93
antiepileptic drugs (AEDs), 15–16, 69, 256–57, 262*t*. *See also* pharmacological treatment(s); PNES treatment
   adverse reactions, 92–93
      associated with specific AEDs, 16, 17*t*
      cognitive sequalae, 76, 158–59
      patients attributing cognitive difficulties to side effects, 158–59
   outcomes studies, 283–84
anxiety disorder, 294
attention regulation difficulties, 163–64
autonomic function, abnormalities of, 110–11
avoidance tendencies, 50, 51, 147, 165*t*, 168, 180, 221*f*, 222, 237. *See also* overmodulating patient(s)/overmodulator(s)

behavior therapy, 237. *See also* cognitive-behavioral therapy
below chance performance, 156
benzodiazepines, 256–57
biopsychosocial (BPS) model, 37, 38, 38*f*, 39–41*t*
bladder symptoms, assessment of, 300–301
borderline personality disorder (BPD), 23, 25

bowel symptoms. *See also* gastrointestinal (GI) tract; irritable bowel syndrome
   assessment of, 299
brain injury. *See* traumatic brain injury
brain regions, 100, 107–8. *See also* neuroimaging
brain surgery, prior, 72–73

car accidents, 250
care coordination, 209
care coordination activities, examples of, 209
care manager, 209, 214
case manager, role in emergency and urgent care, 27*t*
CBT. *See* cognitive-behavioral therapy
central sensitization, paradigm of, 77
Charcot, Jean-Martin, 106
children. *See* pediatric patients
children, PNES in, 15–16
chronic care model (CCM), 207, 212
chronic fatigue syndrome, 77
clinician characteristics, 139–43, 140*t*
clinician knowledge, barriers to care related to, 203–4
   case vignettes, 198
clinician-patient relationship. *See* patient-physician relationship
clinicians. *See also under* PNES treatment adherence
   attitudes toward PNES diagnosis, 194–95, 199–200
      case vignettes, 195
   response to the PNES diagnosis, 193–94, 199–200
      potential solutions and recommendations regarding, 198–99

cognitive-behavioral theory and cognitive-behavioral models, 235
cognitive-behavioral therapy (CBT), 55, 56, 168, 218, 237, 240, 244. *See also* psychotherapeutic treatment(s)
   CBT-informed psychotherapy (CBT-ip), 245–46
cognitive complaints, 75–76, 146, 300
cognitive function, 86, 100–101
   assessment of
      current, 87–88, 89f, 90, 300
      initial era of, 87
   cognitive dysfunction resulting from non-disease variables, 87–88, 89f, 90
   future research on, 96–97
      controlling for confounding variables, 97–100
      medications with known cognitive sequelae, 158–59
      potential factors affecting, 96f
      studies on, 90–91t
cognitive profiles, nonspecific, 163–64, 169
cognitive symptoms, 300. *See also* cognitive complaints; cognitive function
   improving insight into, 166
cognitive therapy, 240
complex regional pain syndrome (CRPS), 299
conversion disorder, 74, 183, 235–36. *See also* functional neurological symptom disorder
   treatments for, 247–48

depression, comorbid, 43, 46, 48
detailing block, 46
developmental disorders with PNES, treatment planning in, 167–68
diagnosis of PNES
   barriers to care related to, 204–5
   clinicians' attitudes toward, 194–95, 199–200
      case vignettes, 195
   clinicians' response to the, 193–94, 199–200
      potential solutions and recommendations regarding, 198–99
      communicating the, 188–89
      challenges involved in, 179–80
      choosing the best setting for, 180–82
      do's and don'ts in, 189t
      published strategies for, 183, 184–85t
      what to say about PNES, 183, 184–85t, 186–87
   elements to assess when screening a patient with suspected PNES, 144t
   explanation of the
      how to explain the diagnosis, 182–83
      outcome after, 187–88
   with the pediatric patient, 3, 7, 267–68
Diagnostic and Statistical Manual of Mental Disorders (*DSM*), 74
diagnostic challenges for the mental health team and psychiatrist, 139, 151
   clinician characteristics, 139–43, 140t
   patient characteristics, 143–47
   special patient groups, 147–50
diagnostic challenges for the neurologist, 123, 135–36
   data from outside providers, 133–34
   delivering the diagnosis, 134–35
   establishing the diagnosis, 125
      diagnostic challenges, 125–26
      electroencephalography (EEG), 128–29, 130f. *See also* EEG
      navigating diagnostic options, 132–33
      semiology, 127–28
      what to do if event is not captured or diagnosis remains unclear, 131–32
   suspecting the diagnosis
      history, 123–24
      observations, 124–25
diagnostic challenges for the neuropsychologist, 153, 162–65, 169
diagnostic levels of certainty, 126, 126t
diagnostic testing
   algorithm for navigating, 132f
   inpatient testing
      cons, 158
      pros, 157–58
diagnostic tests, 77–79
diaries. *See* seizure diaries
difficult patients, 149
diffusion tensor imaging (DTI), 107, 108
dissociation, 47, 95, 112, 240, 291

dissociative disorder, 293–94
dissociative seizures (DS), 303–4. See also PNES
  assessing functional somatic and functional neurological disorders in patients with, 295
    history taking and general approach, 295–96
  classification of
    in relation to other functional neurological symptoms, 292–95
  comorbidity of other functional somatic disorders in patients with, 292
  epidemiological similarities and differences between functional movement disorder and, 294–95, 295t
  epidemiology and overlap of functional somatic disorders and, 290–91
  integrated approach to treatment of functional disorders in patients with
    explanation, 301–2
    physical therapy, 302–3
    psychological therapy, 303
  terminology, 183, 186, 291–92
dizziness, assessment of, 300
Dodrill Discrimination Index (DDI), 89f
driving restrictions, 250
dystonia, functional, 299f
dystonic posture, fixed, 297t

economic dependence, 284. See also socioeconomic status
EEG (electroencephalography), 79, 110, 128–29. See also video-EEG (vEEG/v-EEG) monitoring; specific topics
  ambulatory, 72, 133
  data from outside providers, 133–34
  establishing the diagnosis, 125–29, 126t, 130f, 131–33
  interictal EEG patterns, 67, 68t, 69, 77–78, 126t
  as a neurobiological marker for PNES, 78
  reasons for misinterpreted, 134
  suspecting the diagnosis, 123–25
EEG dysrhythmias, 77

EEG research techniques, quantitative, 110
EEG sleep, 73
electroencephalography. See EEG
electrophysiology studies, 107–10
emergencies, PNES, 28–29
  handling, 24–25
    acute management, 24
    recommendations for, 26t
  preventing, 25–27
  understanding them from the perspective of borderline cases, 24–25
emergency department (ED), 14–15, 28–29
emergency department (ED) physicians, educating, 19–21
emergency presentation(s), 28–29. See also emergency treatments
  factors raising suspicion for PNES on, 19–20, 20f
  for non-seizure complaints, 21
    accidents and injuries, 22
    medically unexplained symptoms (MUS) other than seizure, 23–24
    suicide and self-injurious behavior, 22–23
  settings, 14–16
emergency treatments
  individualized treatment plans, 27–28
  morbidity associated with, 16–19
  roles for members of treatment team, 26–27, 27t
emotion regulation subgroups, 144–47, 165f, 168
employment and economic dependence, 284
epilepsy, 43
  PNES and, 67, 69, 70, 71t, 254
  evidence for coexistent epilepsy in PNES patients, 67, 68t, 69
epilepsy monitoring unit (EMU), 69, 72, 75
  diagnosis and, 18, 69–71, 75, 125, 126, 131, 132, 219, 220, 225, 226
  mental health care in, 207
  pregnant women in, 18–19
  problems related to, 18–19, 22, 131, 132, 220, 254
  transferring patients from emergency department (ED) to, 261
  traumatic brain injury (TBI) and, 70, 71
  videoEEG (vEEG) monitoring in, 125, 126, 225

epilepsy patients, PNES cognitive deficits initially appeared equivalent to those of, 87
epilepsy surgery, PNES events following, 98–99
epileptic seizures (ES), 124, 255–56, 262t, 280–81
  comorbid rates of, 43
  comparison of findings in PNES and, 127, 128t
escape-avoidance. *See* avoidance tendencies
evidence-based treatments, 235–36, 249. *See also* PNES outcomes; PNES treatment
  review of the evidence base, 236
  controlled studies, 236–39t, 240, 244–49
  uncontrolled and open-label data, 236–37
executive function impairment, 164

factitious disorder, 148
falls, 10
  case of pediatric PNES associated with, 11–12
  case of PNES associated with, 10–11
  spells associated with, 6t
family influence
  and predisposing factors, 47–48
  theories of somatization and, 266–67
family members and patients
  family and patient characteristics to evaluate in those with suspected PNES, 145t
  misconceptions about PNES among, 254
  roles of, 266, 274–75
    diagnosing PNES and, 267–68
    pediatric patients and, 267–69, 272
    treatment and, 268–72
      case vignettes, 272, 274
fatigue, assessment of, 299
fibromyalgia, 77
focusing resistance, 46
4P-BPS model, 37, 38, 38f, 39–41t
Freud, Sigmund, 106
frontal lobe seizures and PNES, comparison between, 128, 129t

functional connectivity (FC) findings, 108, 109f
functional imaging, 78–79
functional motor and sensory disorders, positive signs in. *See also* shaking/motor spells
  that can be shared with a patient to explain the diagnosis, 296, 297–98t, 298
functional movement disorder (FMD), 112, 294, 295, 295t. *See also* functional neurological disorders; functional neurological symptom disorder
functional neurological disorders, 77. *See also* functional movement disorder; functional neurological symptom disorder; medically unexplained symptoms
  treatment for, 247–48
functional neurological symptom disorder (FNSD), 43, 46, 47, 74, 224, 308. *See also* conversion disorder; functional movement disorder; functional neurological disorders; medically unexplained symptoms
  toward the integration of care, 308–14
functional neurological symptoms (FNS), 74–75, 106, 292–93, 303–4. *See also specific topics*
  assessment, 296, 297–98t, 298
  history of the concept of, 106
  terminology, 106
functional somatic symptoms, 293
functional symptoms and disorders in clinical practice, 290, 291t

gastrointestinal (GI) disorders, functional, 76–77, 291
  assessment of, 300
gender differences, 42
guided self-help (GSH), 248

headaches, 75, 77, 257–58
Hoover's sign (leg paresis), 297t, 298f
hyperventilation (HV), 125
hypo-/hypervigilant states secondary to anxiety and trauma, 95

hypothalamic-pituitary-adrenal (HPA) axis, abnormalities of, 111
hysteria, 106, 183. *See also* conversion disorder

ictal evaluation, 127
incapacitating events, patients with, 149–50
injuries, 22. *See also* traumatic brain injury
intellectual disability (ID), 43, 72, 147
   interview with ID patient, 148
intellectual disorders with PNES, treatment planning in, 167–68
intelligence quotient (IQ), 167–68
interictal epileptiform activity (IIEA), 67, 68t, 69, 77–78, 126t
irritable bowel syndrome (IBS), 76–77, 291

learning disabilities (LD), 72
lesion analysis studies, 98–100
loss of consciousness (LOC)
   case of adolescent PNES characterized by, 8
   case of adult PNES characterized by, 7–8
   causes in adults and children, 4t
   common presentations of, 7–8

magnetic resonance imaging (MRI), 78, 107, 108
malingering, 95–96, 148
medically unexplained symptoms (MUS), 23–24, 76–77, 79, 193, 284–85. *See also specific symptoms*
   and performance validity test (PVT) failures, 93
   terminology, 291, 301
memory, assessment of, 300
mental health care. *See also* diagnostic challenges for the mental health team and psychiatrist; psychotherapeutic treatment(s)
   access to, 262t
mild traumatic brain injury (mTBI), 43, 49, 70t, 71–72, 195. *See also* traumatic brain injury
Minnesota Multiphasic Personality Inventory-2 (MMPI-2), 94f
motivational interviewing (MI), 226

motivation and performance on PVT measures, 76, 95–96
motor disorders. *See* functional motor and sensory disorders; shaking/motor spells
motor vehicle accidents, 250
movement disorder, 297t
multidisciplinary approach. *See* treatment team
multiple sclerosis (MS), 73

negative automatic thoughts (NATs), 240
neurocognitive dysfunction. *See* cognitive function
neuroimaging, 78–79, 98–100, 107–10
neurological comorbidities, 43, 67–74, 124. *See also specific conditions*
neurological symptoms, 111–14. *See also specific symptoms*
neurologist, 204. *See also* diagnostic challenges for the neurologist
   most common reasons for seeing a, 290
   role after diagnosis, 253, 263
      advocacy for access to mental health care, 259–60
      early intervention following a diagnostic evaluation, 254–55
      indications to continue neurological follow-up, 261–62t
      management of neurological comorbidities, 255–58
      prevention of iatrogenic interventions and complications, 260–61
      recognition of new functional neurological symptoms, 258
      seizure precautions and restrictions, 258–59
      when it is time to let the patient go, 261
   role in emergency and urgent care, 27t
neuropsychological battery, comprehensive, 160, 161–62t
neuropsychological evaluation
   comprehensive evaluations vs. brief screens, 160, 161–62t, 162, 163f
   defined, 153
   defining objectives of, 154, 154t
   therapeutic goals of, 165, 169

neuropsychological evaluation (*Cont.*)
improving insight into cognitive symptoms, 166
informing treatment plans and directing patients to specific treatments, 167–69
promoting cognitive self-efficacy, 166–67
neuropsychological screens, brief, 160, 162, 163*f*
neuropsychologist, practical challenges for the, 155, 169
acute psychological distress, 159–60
clinical environment, 157–58
comprehensive evaluations vs. brief screens, 160, 161–62*t*, 162, 163*f*
medications with known cognitive sequalae, 158–59
performance validity test failures, 155–57
nonepileptic attack disorder, 183. *See also* dissociative seizures; functional movement disorder; functional neurological disorders; functional neurological symptom disorder; medically unexplained symptoms; PNES
nonepileptic psychogenic status (NEPS), the problem of, 16–18, 260
"nonepileptic," use of the term, 301

oppositional patients. *See* resistant and oppositional patient who does not want to engage with clinician
overmodulating patient(s)/overmodulator(s), 146, 168
psychiatric interview with an, 146–47

pain, assessment of, 299
pain complaints, 75
paradoxical intention therapy, 237
patient-centered care, 209
patient characteristics, 143–47
patient groups, special, 147–50
patient-physician connection
clinician factors that can affect, 139–41, 140*t*
resistant and oppositional patient who does not want to engage with clinician, 149
patient-physician relationship, 135, 199
4P-BPS model, 37, 38, 38*f*, 39–41*t*
pediatric patients
cases, 9–12
diagnosis of PNES with, 3, 7, 267–68
PNES care models and, 210, 211*f*, 212
role of family members, 267–69, 272
treatment, 268–69, 272
performance validity test (PVT) failures, 87–88, 89*f*, 90, 155. *See also* symptom validity testing
below chance performance, 156
below failure cutoff but well above chance performance, 155–56
clinical decision-making around, 156–57
clinical decision-making model, 156, 157*f*
reasons for
comorbid psychiatric conditions and medically unexplained symptoms, 93
general psychological variables, 93–96
medication effects, 92–93
periprocedure PNES, 15
perpetuating factors, 37, 40–41*t*, 50–52. *See also* 4P-BPS model
defined, 50
key points for treatment, 52
personality assessment and personality tests, 94*f*, 164–65, 165*f*
personality disorders. *See* avoidance tendencies; borderline personality disorder
pharmacological treatment(s), 245. *See also* antiepileptic drugs; PNES treatment
combined psychotherapeutic treatment and, 245–47
medication discontinuation and change in patient status, 159
physician-patient relationship. *See* patient-physician relationship
PNES (psychogenic nonepileptic seizures), vii. *See also* functional movement disorder; functional neurological

disorders; functional neurological symptom disorder; medically unexplained symptoms; *specific topics*
common presentations of, 7–12
comorbidities, 43, 67–74, 124. *See also specific conditions*
dualist perspective on, 224
neurobiology, 106–15, 310–11
patient and family characteristics to evaluate in those with suspected, 145*t*
prevalence, 3, 7
proposed disease mechanisms suggested by RCTs, 53, 54–55*t*, 55–56
stages during the evaluation and treatment of patients with, 219*f*, 219–20
terminology, 183, 186, 255–56, 291–92, 301
PNES care. *See also* PNES treatment
barriers to care, 206*t*
lack of empirical argument, 204
lack of integrated care models, 206
toward the integration of care, 308–14
role of education and training, 313–14
PNES care models, 202–3, 214
examples
adult PNES model considerations, 212, 213*f*, 214
pediatrics, 210, 211*f*, 212
future directions, 214
practical considerations, 208–9
recommended components of, 209, 210*t*
theoretical considerations, 206–8
PNES outcomes, long-term, 279–80, 287–88. *See also* prognostic factors
predictors of, 285, 286*t*, 287
sampling problems in PNES studies, 280
PNES outcome studies, long-term. *See also* PNES treatment studies
problems with seizure measures, 280–81
results of, 281, 282*t*
employment and economic dependence, 284
healthcare utilization and antiepileptic drug use, 283–84

psychiatric outcome and MUS other than PNES, 284–85
quality of life outcome, 285
seizure outcomes, 281, 283
PNES subgroups
emotion regulation subgroups, 144–47, 165*f*, 168
examination of, in relation to cognition, 97–98
psychopathological heterogeneity and, 164–65, 169
self-report measures to characterize pathophysiological and emotion regulation subgroups, 165*t*
treatment planning for, 168–69
PNES treatment, 235–36. *See also* emergency treatments; evidence-based treatments; PNES care; PNES outcomes; treatment team
with the adult patient, 270, 274
challenges to, 271–72, 273*t*
clinicians' attitudes toward, 196–98, 197*t*
informing treatment plans and directing patients to specific treatments, 167–69
key points for, 48, 50, 52, 53, 56–57
with the pediatric patient, 268–69, 272
and roles of the patient and family, 268–74
stages during, 219*f*, 219–20
what to do if episodes reoccur, 134
PNES treatment adherence, 139, 229–30
potential solutions to promote, 225–29
the problem of poor adherence, 218–20
time points at which poor adherence is known to arise, 219, 219*f*
underlying causes of the adherence problem, 220
patient-related factors, 220, 221*t*, 222–23, 225–27
provider-related and systemic factors, 221*t*, 223–25, 227–29
PNES treatment studies, 56–57. *See also* PNES outcome studies
and mechanistic clues, 53, 55–56
postictal evaluation, 128
post-long-term monitoring (LTM) clinic, 226

post-traumatic stress disorder (PTSD), 22, 50, 72, 98, 112, 124
precipitating factors, 37, 40t, 49. See also 4P-BPS model
    defined, 49
    immediate triggers, 49–50
    key points for treatment, 50
    symptom onset, 49
predictor, defined, 285
predisposing, precipitating, perpetuating, and prognostic (4 P's) system. See 4P-BPS model
predisposing factors, 37, 38, 39t, 42. See also 4P-BPS model
    biological, 42–44
    culture/family, 47–48
    demographics, 42
    key points for treatment related to, 48
    psychiatric illness, 44, 46
    psychological characteristics, 46–47
    traumatic experiences, 44, 45t
pregnancy, PNES in, 18–19
preictal evaluation, 127
preictal pseudosleep, 73
primary care physician(s), 203–4, 228
    role in emergency and urgent care, 27t
prognostic factors, 37–38, 41t, 52–53, 187–88. See also 4P-BPS model; PNES outcomes
    key points for treatment, 53
pseudostatus. See nonepileptic psychogenic status
psychiatrist. See also diagnostic challenges for the mental health team and psychiatrist
    role in emergency and urgent care, 27t
psychodynamic theory model of treatment, 235, 236
psychoeducational approaches to reducing PNES occurrence, 248–49
psychogenic nonepileptic seizures. See PNES
psychological risk factors for PNES, 46–47
psychological variables, general effect of, 93–96
psychotherapeutic treatment(s), 235–37, 240, 244. See also diagnostic challenges for the mental health team and psychiatrist
    combined pharmacological treatment and, 245–47
psychotherapist, role in emergency and urgent care, 27t

quality of life (QoL) outcome, 285

randomized controlled trials (RCTs), 53, 54–55t, 237, 238–39t
resistant and oppositional patient, 149
risk markers, 42

seizure diaries, self-monitoring, 241–44t. See also seizure journal
seizure journal, 255, 256, 262t. See also seizure diaries, self-monitoring
seizure measures, problems with, 280–81
seizures. See also specific topics
    proposed primary cause of, 70, 71f
    terminology, 183, 186, 255–56, 291–92, 301
self-injurious behavior, 22–23
self-monitoring seizure diaries. See seizure diaries
sensory disorders. See functional motor and sensory disorders
shaking/motor spells, 9
    in adults and children, 5t
    case of adult PNES associated with shaking, 9
    case of pediatric PNES associated with shaking, 9–10
single-photon emission computed tomography (SPECT), 78, 79
sleep problems and sleep disorders, 73, 299
social isolation, 223, 227
socioeconomic status, low, 223, 227. See also economic dependence
somatic marker hypothesis, 310
somatization, 45–46, 48, 77
    theories of, 266–67
somatoform/conversion personality style, 93–94
SPECT (single-photon emission computed tomography), 78, 79
status pseudoepilepticus. See nonepileptic psychogenic status

stepped-care model, 208–9
suicide, 22–23
supplementary motor area (SMA), 107–9, 112, 113f
surgery, epilepsy, 98–99
symptom onset, 49
symptom resolution and symptom reduction, 270
symptom validity testing (SVT), 76. *See also* performance validity test (PVT) failures

temporoparietal junction, 113–14, 114f
therapy. *See* diagnostic challenges for the mental health team and psychiatrist; psychotherapeutic treatment(s)
therapy refusal, 139. *See also* PNES treatment adherence
trauma, psychological, 111–12, 113f
traumatic brain injury (TBI), 22, 43, 49, 70–72, 195
  studies of prior TBI and subsequent development of PNES, 70t, 70–71
traumatic experiences, 44, 45t
  studies of childhood trauma comparing PNES and epileptic seizures (ES) populations, 44, 45t
treatment team, 311–12. *See also* diagnostic challenges for the mental health team and psychiatrist

setting up a, 150
suggested roles for members of, 26–27, 27t
triggers
immediate, 49–50

undermodulating patient(s)/undermodulator(s), 144–46, 168
psychiatric interview with an, 145–46
United States Veterans Affairs (VA) healthcare system, 202–3
urgent care. *See* emergencies; emergency presentations

values clarification therapy, 226
Veterans Affairs (VA) healthcare system, U.S., 202–3
video-EEG (vEEG/v-EEG) monitoring, 24, 69, 125, 132, 157, 195, 225, 255–57, 268
  and diagnosis, 19, 21, 22, 67, 78–79, 125–26, 128, 131, 132f, 132–35, 154, 160, 181, 186, 187, 194, 195, 224, 225, 236, 255
voxel-based morphometry (VBM), 107

Word Memory Test (WMT), 89f, 94f